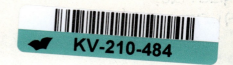

ORGAN AND TISSUE TRANSPLANTATION
Nursing Care from Procurement through Rehabilitation

M. K. Gaedeke Norris, RN, MSN

Clinical Nurse Specialist, Cardiology
Children's Hospital of Buffalo
Buffalo, New York
Former Director, Transplant Education
Ohio Valley Organ Procurement Center
Cincinnati, Ohio

and

Mary Anne House, RN, MSN

Administrator, Organ Procurement Program
Medical College of Georgia
Augusta, Georgia

 F. A. DAVIS COMPANY • Philadelphia

Printed in the United States of America

Last digit indicates print number: 10 9 8 7 6 5 4 3 2 1

NOTE: As new scientific information becomes available through basic and clinical research, recommended treatments and drug therapies undergo changes. The author(s) and publisher have done everything possible to make this book accurate, up-to-date, and in accord with accepted standards at the time of publication. The authors, editors, and publisher are not responsible for errors or omissions, or for consequences from application of the book, and make no warranty, expressed or implied, in regard to the contents of the book. Any practice described in this book should be applied by the reader in accordance with professional standards of care used in regard to the unique circumstances that may apply in each situation. The reader is advised always to check product information (package inserts) for changes and new information regarding dose and contraindications before administering any drug. Caution is especially urged when using new or infrequently ordered drugs.

Library of Congress Cataloging-in-Publication Data

Norris, M. K. Gaedeke, 1955–
    Organ and tissue transplantation: nursing care from procurement through rehabilitation/M. K. Gaedeke Norris and Mary Anne House.
        p. cm.
    Includes bibliographical references and index.
    ISBN 0-8036-6587-3 (hardbound: alk. paper)
        1. Transplantation of organs, tissues, etc.—Nursing. 2. Transplantation of organs, tissues, etc.—Patients—Rehabilitation. 3. Organ donors—Rehabilitation. I. House, Mary Anne, 1958–   . II. Title.
        (DNLM: 1. Organ Procurement—nurses' instruction. 2. Tissue Donors—nurses' instruction. 3. Tissue Preservation—nurses' instruction. 4. Transplantation—nurses' instruction. WO 660 N857o)
RD129.8.N67   1991
610.73'677—dc20
DNLM/DLC
for Library of Congress   90-14141
                                                                  CIP

Dedication

To my husband, Allyn, for his support and patience with the time this project has taken; to my sons, Jeff and Adam, who are all my inspiration; to my parents and sister, whose unconditional love has always made me believe anything is possible.

And to my best friend, who has always supported me, encouraged me, and believed in me.

M. K. Gaedeke Norris

To the many donor families whose courage at their time of tragedy has provided hope for others.

And to my staff and colleagues at the Medical College of Georgia and my peers in the organ procurement and transplantation profession, who have believed in me and continuously provided me support and encouragement.

Mary Anne House

To Remember Me

The day will come when my body will lie upon a white sheet neatly tucked under four corners of a mattress located in a hospital busily occupied with the living and the dying. At a certain moment a doctor will determine that my brain has ceased to function and that, for all intents and purposes, my life has stopped.

When that happens, do not attempt to instill artificial life into my body by the use of a machine. And don't call this my deathbed. Let it be called the bed of life, and let my body be taken from it to help others lead fuller lives.

Give my sight to the man who has never seen a sunrise, a baby's face or love in the eyes of a woman.

Give my heart to a person whose own heart has caused nothing but endless days of pain.

Give my blood to the teenager who was pulled from the wreckage of his car, so that he might live to see his grandchildren play.

Give my kidneys to one who depends on a machine to exist from week to week.

Take my bones, every muscle, every fiber and nerve in my body and find a way to make a crippled child walk.

Explore every corner of my brain. Take my cells, if necessary, and let them grow so that someday a speechless boy will shout at the crack of a bat and a deaf girl will hear the sound of rain against her window.

Burn what is left of me and scatter the ashes to the winds to help the flowers grow.

If you must bury something, let it be my faults, my weaknesses and all prejudice against my fellow man.

Give my sins to the devil.

Give my soul to God.

If, by chance, you wish to remember me, do it with a kind deed or word to someone who needs you.

If you do all I have asked, I will live forever.

Robert N. Test

Preface

Nurses have long expressed the need for a book that crosses the continuum of transplantation. While it is true that not all nurses work in medical centers where transplantation of lifesaving organs is an everyday occurrence, every nurse comes in contact with potential donors. No single segment of this transplant continuum is as important as identifying potential donors and beginning the process that will result in the procurement of organs and tissues. A reference that addresses organs as well as tissues and procurement as well as transplantation written expressly for the nursing discipline was needed.

Until now, the literature has been dominated by an orientation that addresses organ function but not human function. This is the unique focus of nursing that only *nurses* can address. Transplantation of organs and tissues is only part of the recovery. Restoration of activities of daily living such as regaining previous role functions through work, school, and play must be a focus to assist patients in a full and meaningful recovery.

The main reason transplantation is not saving even more lives is the lack of available organs and tissues. By addressing procurement in addition to transplantation, this book hopes to close a critical gap in the literature. Every nurse, from community to outpatient settings, and from medical-surgical to critical care units, is potentially part of the transplant team. Through simple contact with people inquiring about organ and tissue donation or intimate contact with grieving families, nurses can help close this disparity between our patients who are in need of transplants and our patients who may wish to give the gift of life.

This book has attempted to address procurement, transplantation, organs, tissues, adults, pediatrics, and special ethical and legal issues of transplantation important to all nurses. The care plans and nursing diagnoses will help translate organismic and physiologic information to the art and science of nursing. We believe this book will serve to guide the medical-surgical, critical care, and community health nurse as well as those working directly in transplantation. Transplantation touches all our practices, and we have now advanced our body of transplant knowledge as nurses.

M. K. Gaedeke Norris, RN, MSN
Mary Anne House, RN, MSN

Acknowledgments

We'd like to thank our contributors from around the country, who have so willingly taken their time to write for this volume. We are forever grateful to the F. A. Davis Company, who believed in the importance of this project and has given its constant support. Elaine Ewing, our editor, has carefully guided the manuscript to its completion.

Finally, we are most grateful to our consultants who have assisted in enriching this manuscript through their shared expertise.

M.K.G.N.
M.A.H.

Acknowledgements

Contributors

Sharon M. Augustine, RN, MS, CANP
Coordinator, Heart and Heart/
Lung Transplant Program
The Johns Hopkins Hospital
Baltimore, Maryland

Marguerite E. Brown, RN, BS
Donor Coordinator for the Heart
and Heart/Lung Transplant
 Program
Stanford University Medical
 Center
Stanford, California

Robert M. Duckworth, BS, CPTC (ARTC)
Director of Procurement
Nebraska Organ Retrieval
 System, Inc.
Omaha, Nebraska

Marilyn A. Groshek, RN, BSN
Transplant Coordinator
University of Wisconsin – Madison
Madison, Wisconsin

Tina C. Haberer-Weiss
Kidney Transplant Recipient
Patient Communications Advisor
Chicago, Illinois
Former Manager Patient Out-
 Reach Program
Sandoz Pharmaceuticals, Inc.
East Hanover, New Jersey

Carol Hill, RN, MSN(c)
Clinical Nurse II
Children's Hospital Medical
 Center
Cincinnati, Ohio

Jo Ann I. Lamb, MSN, RN-C
Cardiac Transplant Nurse
 Practitioner
Department of Surgery
Columbia Presbyterian Medical
 Center
New York, New York

Joan Miller, RNC, MSN
Clinical Coordinator
Department of Cardiovascular
 Surgery
Stanford University Medical
 Center
Stanford, California

Peggy Schreck Patella, BSN, RN

Senior Nurse Specialist
Kidney Disease Program
University of Louisville
Louisville, Kentucky

Rachel I. Rhude, MSN, RN, CCRN

Critical Care Clinical Nurse
   Specialist
Franciscan Health System of
   Cincinnati, Inc.
Cincinnati, Ohio

Joyce A. Slusher, RN

Clinical Nurse II
Children's Hospital Medical
   Center
Cincinnati, Ohio

Victoria L. Smith, RN, MSN

Extra-renal Transplant
   Coordinator
University of Cincinnati Hospital
   Medical Center
Department of Surgery/
   Transplant Division
Cincinnati, Ohio

Mary L. Stoeckle, RN, MSN, CCRN

Critical Care Instructor
Mercy Hospital Anderson
Cincinnati, Ohio

Patricia A. Weiskittel, RN, MSN, CNN

Renal Clinical Nurse Specialist
University Hospital
Cincinnati, Ohio

Laurel Williams, RN, MSN, CCTC

Clinical Nurse
   Specialist/Coordinator
University of Nebraska Medical
   Center
Omaha, Nebraska

Consultants

William A. Baumgartner, MD
Associate Professor of Surgery
Director Heart and Heart-Lung
Transplant Program
The Johns Hopkins Hospital
Baltimore, Maryland

Jeremiah P. Donovan, MD
Assistant Professor, Department
of Internal Medicine
University of Nebraska Medical
Center
Omaha, Nebraska

Ronald L. Dreffer, BS, CPTC
Executive Director
Ohio Valley Organ Procurement
Center
Cincinnati, Ohio

Randall M. Everts, MHSA
Assistant Administrator
Coliseum Medical Centers
Macon, Georgia

Carol Hill, RN, BSN, CCRN
Clinical Nurse II
Children's Hospital Medical
Center
Cincinnati, Ohio

Jon B. Klein, MD, PhD
Co-Director of Transplantation
University of Louisville School of
Medicine
Louisville, Kentucky

Sally Kohl, RN, BSN
Program Specialist
University of Wisconsin Hospital
and Clinics
Madison, Wisconsin

Becky Jo Lekander, MSN, RN,
CCRN, CS
Clinical Nurse Specialist
University of Minnesota Hospital
and Clinic
Minneapolis, Minnesota

Geri LoBiondo-Wood, PhD, RN
Associate Professor, Chair,
Parent-Child Nursing Program
University of Nebraska
College of Nursing
Omaha, Nebraska

Ruth S. Lutze, RN, BS
Senior Outreach Program
Manager
University of Wisconsin–
Madison, School of Nursing
Madison, Wisconsin

Diana Peters, RN, BSN, CNA
Assistant Director, Dialysis and
Related Services
University of Louisville Kidney
Disease Program
Louisville, Kentucky

Rachel I. Rhude, MSN, RN, CCRN
Critical Care Clinical Nurse
Specialist
Franciscan Health System of
Cincinnati, Inc.
Cincinnati, Ohio

Byers W. Shaw, Jr., MD
Professor of Surgery
University of Nebraska Medical
Center
Omaha, Nebraska

Joyce A. Slusher, RN
Clinical Nurse II
Children's Hospital Medical
Center
Cincinnati, Ohio

George P. Smith III, BS, VD, LLM
Professor of Law
The Catholic University of
America
The Columbus School of Law
Washington, DC

Elaine Snyder, RN, BSN
Nursing Supervisor I
University of Wisconsin Hospitals
Madison, Wisconsin

Mary L. Stoeckle, RN, MSN,
CCRN
Critical Care Instructor
Mercy Hospital Anderson
Cincinnati, Ohio

Robert J. Stratta, MD
Assistant Professor of Surgery
University of Nebraska Medical
Center
Omaha, Nebraska

Thomas A. Traill, MRCP, MD
Associate Professor of Medicine,
Cardiology
Johns Hopkins University School
of Medicine
Baltimore, Maryland

Margarite (Peggy) Worden,
RN, BSNA
Executive Director
Cincinnati Eye Bank for Sight
Foundation, Inc.
Cincinnati, Ohio

James J. Wynn, MD
Assistant Professor of Surgery
Medical College of Georgia
Augusta, Georgia

Contents

Chapter 8. PANCREAS TRANSPLANTATION 145

Marilyn Groshek, RN, BSN
Victoria L. Smith, RN, MSN

Chapter 9. THE PEDIATRIC TRANSPLANT PATIENT: DONOR AND RECIPIENT 169

Laurel Williams, RN, MSN
Mary Anne House, RN, MSN
Carol Hill, BSN, CCRN

Chapter 10. IMMUNOSUPPRESSIVE THERAPY 199

Patricia D. Weiskittel, RN, MSN, CNN

Chapter 11. FOLLOWUP CARE OF THE TRANSPLANT PATIENT

Joan Miller, RNC, MSN

Chapter 12. PATIENT EDUCATION: A RECIPIENT PERSPECTIVE

Tina Haberer-Weiss

History of Transplantation

Mary Anne House, RN, MSN

Although the replacement of human body parts was probably done in the first century, it has only been in the last few decades that organ and tissue transplantation has emerged as a successful and clinically applicable therapy for the treatment of end-stage organ and tissue disease. Currently, the lives of some 21,000 Americans are held in limbo by the need for an organ transplant. Of those, approximately 17,500 need kidneys, 1700 need hearts, 1000 need livers, 250 need combined heart and lungs, 400 need a pancreas, and another 100 wait for a single- or double-lung transplant (UNOS, 1990). For those awaiting kidney transplantation, the wait averages 18 months; half of those needing hearts, lungs, or livers will die without ever having the opportunity for a second chance at life.

The history of organ and tissue procurement and transplantation is a long one (Table 1–1). Since the time of the ancient Egyptians, people have been keenly interested in the replacement of parts of the human body. The idea that deficient or diseased tissues might be replaced by donations from another individual was clearly expressed in the 13th century legend of Saint Cosmos and Saint Damien, a story that tells of the act of transplanting the leg of a recently deceased Moor onto the body of a devoted church member whose own leg was afflicted with gangrene. The transplant was said to be successful providing what is, perhaps, the earliest record of clinical transplantation (Kahan, 1981).

Table 1-1. Historical Highlights

1682— First reported bone transplant — Meekren
1881— First reported skin transplant
1905— Introduction of corneal transplantation — Zirm
1902— First kidney transplant in the goat model — Ullman
1938— Isolated organ perfusion — Carrel and Lindbergh
1943— Hemodialysis machine developed — Kolff
1954— First successful kidney transplant in U.S. — Murray
1962— Introduction of Imuran
    — First successful cadaver kidney transplant — Murray
1963— First successful liver transplant — Starzl
    — First successful lung transplant — Hardy
1966— Introduction of arteriovenous fistula — Brescia
1967— First successful pancreas homograft — Lillehei
    — First successful heart transplant — Barnard
1969— Establishment of South-Eastern Organ Procurement Foundation
1980— Introduction of cyclosporine
1981— First successful heart-lung transplant — Reitz
1984— Incorporation of United Network for Organ Sharing (UNOS)

PROCUREMENT AND TRANSPLANTATION OF TISSUES

Successful tissue transplantation was achieved many years prior to successful organ transplantation. Church history records the first bone transplant as having been performed by Meekren in 1682. At that time, he used a piece of dog skull to correct a defect in the skull of a Russian soldier. Today, bone transplantation is the most common transplant procedure performed. Approximately 200,000 bone grafts are performed annually in the treatment of many neurosurgical, orthopedic, reconstructive, and dental problems.

Skin transplantation was reported in the medical literature as early as 1881. Now, some two dozen skin banks in the United States provide skin for an estimated 100,000 temporary replacement grafts each year. It is estimated that if five times the amount of skin were available, it would be used to shorten the wound healing time for the many thousands of individuals severely burned each year.

Eduard Zirm, an Australian ophthalmologist, performed the first successful corneal transplant in 1905. Annually, almost 40,000 corneal transplants are performed using donor tissue provided through the network of some 100 eye banks across the nation.

RENAL PROCUREMENT AND TRANSPLANTATION

The Development of Dialysis

The first attempts at dialysis may go back to the days of the Roman baths, but it was not until in the 1860s that Thomas Graham developed what is considered the forerunner of dialysis treatments. His machine used a hoop dialyzer made of wood casings. Dr. Wilhelm Kolff, working in the Netherlands during World War I, developed the predecessor to today's modern machines. His machine was made from sausage casings and wooden lathes with a small motor (Flye, 1989).

With the development of the Scribner shunt in 1960, dialysis became a technically practical tool for treatment of acute renal failure. Prior to that time, glass cannulas were inserted into the vessels, allowing for only one treatment. The reusable shunt greatly improved dialysis, and in 1966 the introduction of the arteriovenous fistula made chronic dialysis a reality.

In 1954, Dr. John Merrill established the world's first dialysis unit at the Peter Bent Brigham Hospital in Boston (Starzl, 1981). Even though the procedure for dialysis was then technically practical, there were major obstacles from the standpoint of cost. Death committees were established to decide who received treatments. People were dialyzed only if grants were available or if the patient could pay. The End Stage Renal Disease Medicare Amendments of 1972, however, made it possible for any patient desiring dialysis to receive it.

Transplantation

The first kidney transplant in the world was reported in a goat model in Vienna in 1902 (Ullman, 1902). It was not until December 23, 1954, that the first successful *human* kidney was transplanted in the United States. The operation was performed by Dr. Joseph Murray and Dr. Hartwell Harrison at the Peter Bent Brigham Hospital. The donor and recipient were identical twins (Merrill, 1956). No effort was made to preserve the donated kidney, which functioned promptly despite 82 minutes of warm ischemia time. The recipient lived with normal renal function for 7 years, dying of a myocardial infarction at the age of 29 years (Merrill, 1979).

Immunosuppression

The work of Sir Peter Medawar in the 1940s demonstrated the immunological process involved in graft rejection. Drugs were not used exclusively for immunosuppression until 1962, when the first successful cadaver-donated kidney transplant was performed by Dr. Joseph Murray in Boston (Moore, 1980). Sir Roy Calne and Dr. Murray used an analog of 6-mercaptopurine to immunosuppress the recipient and control rejection, resulting in a functioning graft for 21 months (Merrill, 1979). Azathioprine (Imuran) is a derivative of 6-mercaptopurine that was subsequently developed and widely adopted for use in transplantation. The addition of corticosteroids to the Imuran regimen became the standard baseline immunosuppression until the introduction of cyclosporine (Sandimmune) in the early 1980s. Additional methods used in attempts to manage rejection of the transplant organ include the administration of cyclophosphamide, antilymphocyte serum or antilymphocyte globulin, monoclonal antibodies, total lymphoid irradiation, and surgical procedures such as thoracic duct drainage and splenectomy.

Well over 80,000 kidney allografts have been performed in the last quarter century, and organ procurement has become a respected component of the clinical armamentarium for the treatment of end-stage renal disease. Today, 218 renal transplant centers serve the citizens of the United States, and there are 73 federally designated organ procurement organizations established to provide organ procurement services to transplant centers of all types (UNOS, 1989).

EXTRA-RENAL DONATION AND TRANSPLANTATION

Although extrarenal transplantation came to the forefront in the 1980s, it had its beginning more than 25 years ago. Pioneers in extrarenal transplantation did not give up even though survival rates were poor, but directed their research toward perfecting the procedures. With the introduction of cyclosporine in the early 1980s, graft survival rates began to increase significantly, making it possible to perform these transplants on a more routine basis. Surgical techniques and preservation methods have continued to be modified over the past 9 years, providing even greater success for some of the transplants.

Liver

In 1963, Dr. Thomas Starzl performed the first human liver transplant at the University of Colorado. Dr. Starzl, now Professor of Surgery at the University of Pittsburgh, has led the world in liver transplantation. Currently some 73 transplant centers have liver transplant programs. Overall, one-year graft survival rates have risen from 25% in 1979 to greater than 70% (Shaw, 1980).

Lungs

The first lung transplantation procedure was performed in 1963 at the University of Mississippi by Dr. James D. Hardy. Although the recipient lived for only 18 days, this was the beginning of more study on the process of lung transplantation. In the United States today, 39 centers have designated lung transplantation programs (UNOS, 1989). Active research to improve the surgical technique and preservation methods continues.

Pancreas

Although pancreas transplantation from animal to human was reported in 1893, 29 years before the isolation of insulin, it was not until 1967 that a successful procedure was performed. Dr. Richard C. Lillehei at the University of Minnesota performed the first successful pancreatic transplant in a 32-year-old woman, who received a combined kidney-pancreas transplant. Fewer than 1000 pancreas transplants have been performed worldwide. Although success rates waver around 50% one-year graft survival, many professionals still consider the procedure experimental. While decisions regarding the best method of surgical implantation (whole pancreas, partial pancreas, islet cells only) still remain to be determined, the outlook is promising (Sutherland, 1986).

Hearts

In 1967, Dr. Christiaan Barnard performed the world's first successful heart transplant in Capetown, South Africa. He used techniques pioneered in the United States at Stanford University by Drs. Norman Shumway and Richard Lower. Although the recipient lived only 18 days, this transplant was followed by a sudden flurry of increased interest in cardiac transplantation. Because graft survival statistics were low (approximately 22% one-year survival), this boom soon diminished and was revived only with the advent of cyclosporine. Today, one-year graft survival approaches 80%, and better than half of the recipients can be expected to live for at least 5 years (Flye, 1989). There are 148 heart transplant programs currently designated in the United States (UNOS, 1989).

Heart-Lung

The first successful heart-lung transplant was performed at Stanford University by Dr. Shumway and Dr. Bruce Reitz in 1981. The recipient, a 45-year-old Arizona woman, lived approximately four years. To date, around 200 such transplants have been performed. The longest survival is now 7 years post-transplant. Sixty-three transplant centers are currently recognized as heart-lung programs (UNOS, 1989). The one-year graft survival is approximately 50% (UNOS, 1989).

INFLUENCES ON THE ORGAN PROCUREMENT PROCESS

There have been many influences on the organ procurement process over the past decade that have assisted us in meeting the challenges of donation and transplantation. In regard to most of these innovations, it is impossible to recognize any one group as primarily responsible for its development. These influences include:

1. Standards for donor selection have broadened and have become increasingly uniform.
2. Brain death declaration has become widely accepted as a customary and usual practice.
3. Organ exchanges between widely separated regions of the United States and, in fact, the entire world have become commonplace.
4. The techniques of organ excision for kidneys have evolved toward the *en bloc* nephrectomy as the most widely accepted mode of surgical removal.
5. Extra-renal teams are now comfortably invited into local hospitals to recover hearts, lungs, pancreata, and livers for transplantation.
6. Emphasis has been placed on aggressive support of the potential donor so that all organs may be in an optimally functional state.

BRAIN DEATH

The impetus for defining death on the basis of irreversible loss of total brain function was initiated by Beecher in 1968. A report of an ad hoc committee at Harvard Medical School examined the definition of brain death and published the first widely accepted guidelines for clinical management of the medically and ethically complex circumstances surrounding brain death. Today, the Uniform Determination of Death Acts serve as a guide in the United States. A resolution of the American Association of Neurological Surgeons in 1988 demonstrated support from neuroscience specialists.

UNIFORM ANATOMICAL GIFT ACT

The Uniform Anatomical Gift Act (UAGA), passed by all 50 states in the late 1960s and early 1970s, has been an important advance upon which organ and tissue donation is built. In addition to the various state

Anatomical Gift Acts, additional legislation currently known as *required request* or *routine referral*, has resulted in significant changes within hospitals regarding identification, referral, and documentation of potential donors.

PRESERVATION

The rapid progress of clinical transplantation in the last decade has greatly renewed interest in organ preservation. Although the notion of artificial perfusion of organs was expressed by LeGallois more than 150 years ago, optimal perfusion and preservation of organs remains extremely complex. Great strides in preservation have been made since the 1930s when Alexis Carrel and Charles Lindbergh devised the first organ perfusion apparatus (Shaw, 1980).

The length of time for preservation of organs and tissues varies. Most transplant material is currently preserved using some method of cold storage. Maximum storage time for kidneys is 60 to 72 hours, livers 12 to 24 hours, pancreata 24 hours, and hearts or lungs 4 to 6 hours. All techniques have one main goal: to provide preservation of a specific organ for a sufficiently long interval to permit optimal donor-recipient matching and preparation of the recipient for transplantation.

DISTRIBUTION

The distribution of all organs has rapidly expanded over the past 10 to 15 years. For kidneys, biological requirements and preferences for matching have become more elaborate. To avoid waste, regional exchanges of organs are now commonplace. The founding of the South-Eastern Organ Procurement Foundation (SEOPF) in 1969 was the beginning of regionalization. The incorporation of the United Network for Organ Sharing (UNOS) in 1984 and its establishment of elaborate computer matching systems have significantly facilitated the sharing not only of kidneys but of all organs.

Increased public awareness of the need for transplantation and the shortage of organs and tissues led to a national governmental study of the field of organ and tissue procurement and transplantation. A Presidential task force was established out of the National Transplant Act (P.L. 99-507). The legislation also created the National Organ Procurement and Transplantation Network (OPTN), a federal contract awarded to UNOS. The OPTN is responsible for coordinating national policy on organ distribution.

THE FUTURE

During this century, the biological phenomenon of transplantation has emerged gradually. Clinical transplantation is at an extraordinarily interesting stage. Attempts have been made to transplant many different organs and tissues. A great deal has been achieved, yet much remains to be accomplished. The high ground represented by the technological achievements of cornea, kidney, liver, and heart transplantation has been conquered. We now know that all of these organs and tissues, when transplanted, can function normally in their recipients. Advances in the transplantation of other organs such as the lungs and pancreas also offer hope for those potential recipients. As medical research establishes new therapies involving transplantation, the list of recipients will undoubtedly increase. Improvement in one-year graft survival rates (which for kidneys, hearts, and livers now exceeds 70%) will widen the indications for transplant therapy. This will substantially expand the need for specific organs that are currently being transplanted. It is hoped that new or improved preservation methods for extra-renal organs will promote an increase in their transplantation. Growing public awareness and the support by the transplant community for organ and tissue procurement programs will increase the supply of organs and tissues available. The role of all healthcare providers in expediting the identification, evaluation, and procurement of organs and tissues from the multiple-organ and tissue donor will be central to this process over the next decade.

Many more donors exist than are actually referred. It is clear that dealing with potential donors and their families involves certain emotional risks, in addition to the extra time and effort involved in donor evaluation and management. A nurse's obligation to patients and their families is twofold. First, there is an obligation to those patients awaiting transplantation to do everything possible to identify potential donor organs and tissues for them. Second, there is an obligation to potential donors and their families to offer the opportunity for donation and to support them in whatever decisions they make. As healthcare providers, the challenge is ours.

Bibliography

Downing, R: Historical review of pancreatic islet transplantation. World J Surg 8:137–142, April, 1984.

Flye, MW: Principles of Organ Transplantation. WB Saunders, Philadelphia, 1989.

Griepp, RB: A decade of human heart transplantation. Transplant Proc XI(1):285–292, March, 1979.

Kahan, B: Cosmos and Damien in the 20th century. N Engl J Med 305:280, 1981.

Merrill, JP: A historical perspective of renal transplantation. Proceedings of the Clinical Dialysis and Transplant Forum 9:221–225, 1979.

Merrill, JP, et al: Successful homotransplantation of the human kidney between identical twins. JAMA 160:277, 1956.

Moore, FD: Transplantation — A perspective. Transplant Proc XII(4):539–550, December, 1980.

Shaw, R and Stubenbord, WT: Alexis Carrel, M.D.: Contribution to kidney transplantation and preservation. NY State J Med (August, 1980):1438–1442.

Starzl, TE: The succession from kidney to liver transplantation. Transplantation Proc (Suppl 1)XIII(1): , March 1981.

Sutherland, DER, et al: Pancreas transplantation. Surg Clin North Am 66:557, 1986.

Ullman, E: Experimentelle Nierentransplantation, Wienklin. Wchnschr 15:281, 1902.

United Network for Organ Sharing (UNOS), Public Relations Department, Richmond, Virginia, July, 1989.

United Network for Organ Sharing (UNOS), UNOS update:6:30, 1990.

CHAPTER

The Organ Donor

Robert M. Duckworth, BS,
CPTC (ARTC)
M. K. Gaedeke Norris, RN, MSN

The current growth and development in the field of organ transplantation are attributable to progress in the science of immunosuppression; the improvements in organ preservation, which enable long-distance procurement; and the refinement of surgical techniques. However, the major limiting factor in the continued growth of transplantation is the shortage of donor organs. A report issued by the Task Force on Organ Transplantation estimated that there are 17,000 to 26,000 potential organ donors annually in the United States, yet in 1984, for example, only about 12%–20% of these potential donors actually donated organs (United States Department of Health and Human Services, 1986). Several factors have consistently been identified as contributing to the gap between potential and actual donors. These factors include both the lack of awareness among healthcare professionals concerning identification and referral of potential donors, and a reluctance on their part to approach families to offer the option of donation.

Nurses can be a critical factor in changing the discrepancy between the number of potential and actual donors. Frequently nurses are the first healthcare professionals to recognize a potential organ donor. Identifying a patient as a potential donor and then contacting the local organ procurement agency according to their hospital's policy are two simple steps nurses can take to significantly improve the number of organs available.

Offering the option of organ or tissue donation to families is truly a nursing role. A major role function for the professional nurse is that of

11

patient advocate. Every family has the right to be informed of donation as a choice they may make concerning their loved one's death. This is a decision they have the right to make, just as decisions are made regarding autopsy and funeral arrangements. It is the nurse's responsibility to act as an advocate for the family by making them aware of the opportunity. This is especially relevant considering that donor families overwhelmingly describe their decision to donate as a positive one — one that helped them in their grieving process (Bartucci, 1987).

Nurses can make a tremendous contribution toward increasing the number of organs available for transplantation. By identifying and referring potential donors, they can increase the number of organs available to recipients who might otherwise die without them. Through such efforts, nurses can make a positive difference in how a grieving family deals with the loss of a loved one. To maximize availability of donor organs, healthcare professionals must be knowledgeable regarding the recognition of potential donors, mechanisms for obtaining consent for donation, the referral process to the organ procurement organization, and donor management.

There are two major groups into which organ donors are categorized. The first is the cadaveric vascular organ donor. This donor is most frequently a previously healthy person less than 60 years of age who is alive upon arrival at the treatment facility. The patient has suffered a serious insult to the brain, frequently a result of a traumatic accident, and deteriorates to brain death despite massive intervention and advanced life support.

Organs can also be obtained from living donors, who comprise the second type of organ donor. These donors offer several advantages, including availability and usually a close genetic relationship to the recipient (Ascher, 1984). Living donors, who are generally members of the recipient's family, are carefully screened, both medically and psychologically. These candidates are assessed to assure minimal impact upon their health and life expectancy as well as their true motivation to donate. The clinical nurse specialist and primary nurse play critical roles in evaluating the potential response of the living donor to the process of donation. The practice of using living-related donors is still the source of a significant number of transplants in many centers.

THE CADAVERIC VASCULAR ORGAN DONOR

Applying Brain Death Criteria

Brain death can often be a difficult concept for families, and even healthcare professionals, to grasp. A pulse and heart rhythm march across the monitor. The patient's skin is warm to touch and has a normal color. A ventilator, moving the chest up and down, gives the appearance of normal breathing. Even the sound of the ventilator moving air sounds like breathing, confusing the picture of death.

Cessation of cardiopulmonary function is obviously not a criterion in itself as evidenced by patients who survive an arrest through resuscitation efforts. Still other patients are maintained on cardiopulmonary bypass during surgery and as emergency management and surely are not considered dead. They are not dead because their brains remain alive. Brain death occurs when blood flow is lost to both the brain *and* brain stem, resulting in cellular death. Whether from severe trauma, an intracranial bleed, or an intracranial growth, swelling occurs inside the skull, which stops blood flow to the brain and results in death. No one survives brain death. Because both the brain and brain stem are dead, these patients quickly lose the ability to maintain a blood pressure, temperature, and pulse. This loss of the ability to regulate or maintain vital functions makes brain death different from a coma. Brain death quickly leads to cardiac arrest because of the loss of the ability to maintain vital functions.

The nurse caring for the cadaveric heart-beating donor must intellectually and emotionally understand brain death as death. Brain death is not "essentially dead," "clinically dead," or "for all practical purposes dead." Neither are these terms used when talking to donor families. The brain-dead patient is simply dead. No one has ever been resuscitated from brain death. The nurse helps the family understand the difference between a coma, irreversible vegetative state, and brain death. By explaining to the family that all "thinking" portions of the brain as well as the brain stem of these patients are destroyed, the nurse helps the family understand the physiological differences. It is clearly conveyed to the family that because the brain stem, which controls blood pressure, temperature, respirations, and other vital functions is dead, even artificial support cannot keep the heart and circulation functioning indefinitely. Cardiovascular demise is imminent in the brain-dead patient, but not necessarily in the patient who is comatose with a functioning brain stem. A clear understanding of brain death by the nurse is critical both to offering the option of donation and to supporting the family in their grief.

Recognizing the special difficulties in legal and ethical issues surrounding brain death, criteria were proposed in 1981 by the President's Commission for the Study of Ethical Problems in Medicine and Biomedical and Behavioral Research that led to the Uniform Determination of Death Act (Medical Consultants on the Diagnosis of Death, 1981). Supporters of these criteria include the American Bar Association, the American Medical Association, the American Academy of Neurology, and the American Electroencephalographic Society. The statute states:

An individual who has sustained either (1) irreversible cessation of circulatory and respiratory function or (2) irreversible cessation of all functions of

Table 2 – 1. **Clinical Criteria for Brain Death***

Criterion	Assess for
Absence of hypothermia	Body temperature >90°F (35°C)
Negative drug screens for central nervous system depressants	
Cause of coma is known	
No response to external stimuli	Absence of response to pain, noise, environment
No reflex activity unless of spinal cord origin	Absence of decerebrate, decorticate posturing
No pupillary response to light	Absence of pupillary constriction with direct light bilaterally
No oculovestibular reflex	Absence of nystagmus or other eye movement when the ear canal is irrigated with iced solution (verify the presence of an intact tympanic membrane first)
No oculocephalic reflex	Absence of doll's eye reflex (hold the eyelids open and rapidly turn the head side to side); note absence of eye movement from the midline
No spontaneous respirations	Absence of respirations when patient is removed from the ventilator after being pre-oxygenated with 100% and pCO_2 levels are elevated to promote a hypoxic drive
No corneal reflex	Absence of blink reflex by applying wisp of cotton to cornea
No other cranial nerve reflexes	Absence of yawning, swallowing, gag reflex, and vocalization

*Confirmatory studies (i.e., electroencephalogram, carotid arteriography, radionuclide blood flow scans) are **optional** and **not** required by law.

the entire brain including the brain stem is dead. Determination of death must be made in accordance with accepted medical standards.

Table 2-1 lists specific criteria that are necessary for a diagnosis of brain death by accepted medical standards.

Identifying the Donor

The nurse identifies a potential organ donor by recognizing a patient who meets brain death criteria as well as the general criteria for vascular organ donors. This situation is most often recognized by the critical care nurse. The nurse refers the potential donor to the appropriate organ procurement agency to further evaluate the donor. To avoid a conflict of interest, the donor team does not participate in the care of the potential donor prior to the pronouncement of death. By law, the donor team cannot make the determination of death. Nonetheless, the team is able to provide guidelines for declaring a person brain dead, and is responsible for assuring that the diagnosis is correct. The critical care nurse may be assured that no inappropriate interference in patient care will result from early referral of a potential organ donor.

The referral of a potential donor to the organ procurement agency does not represent a commitment for donation on the part of the health-care team. Rather, it helps prevent a needless approach to the family if the donor is unsuitable and also places the process into the support network supplied by the recovery program. Table 2-2 provides an organ donor referral form that may assist the nurse in providing key information to the transplant coordinator. The recovery team evaluates the potential donor based on a history of the injuries, hospitalization, and other data such as age, blood group, and vital signs. If the recovery program concurs with the nurse's assessment of the potential donor, the process of obtaining consent begins.

Obtaining Consent for Donation

The basis for the success of the organ procurement system in this country is the attitude of the American people. Many studies have demon-strated the high level of public support for organ donation and transplan-tation. For example, the Gallup survey of 1985 indicated that 93% of Americans report they have heard or read something about organ trans-plants (Gallup, 1985). Of those aware of organ transplants, 73% say they are very likely to give permission to have the organs of a loved one donated after death. In recent years, between 70% and 75% of all families asked have granted permission for organ donation (Prottas, 1985). Table 2-3 shows the results of another study of the public's willingness to donate organs and tissues (Manninen and Evans, 1985).

The largest obstacle to obtaining enough organs for transplantation is not the public's unwillingness to donate, but rather the reluctance of nurses and physicians to present the option to the family. Consequently, the consent process itself is the largest stumbling block from the perspec-tive of the healthcare professional. Many healthcare personnel are reluc-tant to offer this opportunity to the family of a potential donor based upon personal fears and misconceptions, as well as a common human refusal to deal with the issue of their own mortality. In reality, organ donation may well be the only positive event experienced by the family during this period of grieving and loss and can provide the family with positive feelings regarding the opportunity to help save the life of another human

Table 2-2. Organ Donor Referral Checklist

A Nursing Tool

PATIENT:

Name _____ Age: _____

    Cause of Death _____

    Brain Death Declared ____/____/____   ____:____
                       date   time

    Primary Nurse _____

    Primary Physician _____

Height _____ Weight _____ (lbs) ___ (kg) ___

PAST MEDICAL AND SURGICAL HISTORY:

_____

_____

_____

_____

_____

LAB DATA:

Date _____ Time _____		Date _____ Time _____	
BUN _____		Serum Osmo. _____	
Ser. Creat. _____		Glucose _____	
Na^+ _____		Creat. Clear. _____	
K^+ _____		Ca^{++} _____	
Cl^- _____			

VITAL FUNCTIONS:	Highest	Lowest	Average
Blood Pressure	_____	_____	_____
Mean Art. Pressure	_____	_____	_____
Pulse Rate	_____	_____	_____
Temperature	_____	_____	_____
Urine Output (cc/hr)	_____	_____	_____

Table 2–2. Organ Donor Referral Checklist (*Continued*)

CONSENT:

Nearest Relative _____

Relationship _____

Permission granted from: relative: ☐ yes   ☐ no

coroner ☐ yes   ☐ no

CURRENT MEDICATIONS:

Drug	Dose

---

being. Studies have shown organ donation is a positive part of the normal grief process and is viewed by the next of kin as the highest form of charity (Bartucci, 1987).

By the end of 1987, 45 states had implemented required request laws relating to routine inquiry. These laws mandate that all families whose loved ones meet the donor eligibility criteria be given the opportunity to donate their organs and tissues. Additionally, it is mandated that all Medicare-participating hospitals (Public Law 99-509) have policies and procedures in place for the identification and referral of potential donors. The premise of the law is that all families have the right to make their own decisions about donation. If healthcare professionals do not offer this opportunity, they are in effect making the decision against donation for the family. Coupled with the public's growing belief that donation is the right of a citizen, these legislative mandates provide a powerful incentive for the healthcare professional. More importantly, the vast majority of families (greater than 85% in many areas) will respond positively to this opportunity, and express happiness and relief that a tragic loss can bring health and possibly life to others. Many families will seek out the nurse

Table 2-3. Differences in Attitudes toward Organ Donation by Sociodemographic Characteristics of Individuals

Sociodemographic Characteristic	Currently Carry Organ Donor Card, %	Willingness to Donate, %				
		Relative's Organs	Own Kidneys	Own Corneas	Own Heart	Own Liver
Age*						
18-24	14.5	50.2	56.7	44.7	49.5	50.4
25-34	20.9	56.7	54.7	51.8	51.5	52.1
35-44	25.4	63.0	57.0	55.3	54.7	56.0
45-54	18.1	52.9	49.9	48.7	46.5	48.7
55+	17.5	46.4	38.7	37.2	35.3	35.6
Sex						
Male	20.3	52.6	49.8	47.8	47.0	47.5
Female	18.3	53.0	49.5	44.9	44.9	46.0
Race*						
White	29.8	54.6	52.3	49.4	48.9	49.4
Other	12.9	41.6	35.0	27.8	28.3	31.1
Education*						
Less than high school graduate	10.7	41.0	36.1	32.7	32.8	32.6
High school graduate	15.3	51.0	50.4	46.5	45.8	47.2
More than high school graduate	26.4	62.4	57.7	54.6	54.4	55.2
Income, $*						
<10,000	17.9	41.6	36.6	32.2	32.8	32.4
10,000-14,999	15.8	48.2	50.9	42.7	48.4	48.8
15,000-19,999	15.2	57.4	47.2	41.6	41.9	44.9
20,000-24,999	16.1	56.6	58.6	53.4	54.8	53.5
25,000-29,999	21.0	60.9	52.6	50.7	49.3	51.3
30,000-34,999	23.4	63.9	61.5	60.1	61.7	60.2
35,000-39,999	28.6	73.6	65.2	66.2	62.7	64.8
40,000+	30.1	70.5	62.4	64.3	59.4	60.9
Don't know	12.7	39.6	43.3	39.7	38.5	41.2

*Difference between groups was significant at the .05 confidence level using one-way analysis of variance.

Reprinted with permission from Manninen and Evans: Public Attitudes and Behavior Regarding Organ Donation. JAMA 253(21):3114, June 7, 1985. Copyright 1985, American Medical Association.

and initiate the discussion in order to ensure that this opportunity is not overlooked. However, the family cannot be expected to initiate the idea of organ donation during this stressful time. It is the responsibility of the nurse not only to identify the potential donor but also to act as an advocate of the patient and family by assuring that the right to consider donation has been offered to them.

Each family is assessed carefully regarding a request for organ donation. If a religious or moral conflict exists, the nurse uses judgment and discretion in making the request. The nurse and procurement coordinator must be aware of their own attitudes related to donation and how they may influence the request to the family. The nurse provides accurate information, anticipates and answers the family's questions, clarifies misconceptions, and assures them that their loved one will be respected during the procurement procedure. Under no circumstances are pressure, coercion, dishonesty, or guilt to be used in order to elicit a positive response from a family. The nurse who offers the opportunity for donation is acting as an advocate of the family.

In many cases, the nurse is the healthcare professional dealing with the family regarding consent for donation. However, the nurse must recognize the importance of involving other members of the healthcare team. Physicians, the hospital chaplain, social workers, the family's personal pastor or priest, and the organ recovery coordinator are integral team members providing support and comfort to the family by complementing other members of the team.

The grieving process plays an important role in the issue of consent. Elisabeth Kubler-Ross and others have written that a family experiencing the loss of a loved one proceeds through several well-defined stages while moving toward acceptance. While the nurse recognizes that this process will vary with individual families, certain common points may influence the method for offering the possibility of donation to a family. Timing the request is crucial to sensitive and effective offering. Only after the physician conveys to the family the hopelessness of the clinical condition and the family has had time to assimilate this information does the nurse initiate the request process (Bartucci, 1987). If the request is made prior to the family's acceptance of their loss, they will often respond negatively. Only after they have begun to accept and acclimate to their loss can the nurse expect the family to come to terms with certain realities.

The discussion takes place in a nonthreatening, private environment. A small conference room, consultation room, or empty patient room may be appropriate. The nurse does not discuss the topic at the patient's bedside, in the waiting area, or in open public places. The nurse talking with the family is at ease with the concept of organ donation and provides compassionate, honest care for the family members.

The nurse may begin the conversation with a simple inquiry into the family's interest in donation. A family with misgivings about donation will frequently express them at this time. Reluctance may stem from a variety of factors. A lack of knowledge or understanding of the processes utilized to determine death or of the donation process itself are some examples. The nurse may have the answer to questions, or may refer the family to a representative from the transplant or procurement agency. Written information is helpful for the family during the decision-making process. Many procurement agencies and transplant programs have prepared materials specifically for this purpose. Ensuring that the family has a basic understanding of brain death, and further that the family comprehends that it will be necessary to continue the mechanical support processes through the surgical organ recovery procedure, is important. The family must understand that this continuation of support does not represent a hope for recovery of their loved one or an attempt to create an opportunity for the premature donation of organs before death has occurred. The nurse reinforces the fact that despite continuing cardiovascular and ventilatory support, the donor is neurologically, legally, and biologically dead. At no time is such support referred to as "life-support," which can confuse the family.

The consent form utilized specifies the organs and tissues that the family wishes to be recovered and transplanted. Appendix F exemplifies a consent form that includes the essential information for proper permission. The nurse counsels the family that all possible efforts will be made to successfully recover and transplant the organs and tissues for which they have consented and that no other organs or tissues will be recovered. The family is clearly informed that they can limit the recovery to specific purposes such as transplantation and/or medical therapy, or exclude recovery of tissue for research if they so desire.

Many families are hesitant to raise the topic of financial responsibility. Families need assurance that the costs associated with the donation will be the responsibility of the agencies that recover the organs and tissues, not their own. No financial reward is given for donation nor are funeral or burial costs reimbursed. The removal of organs or tissues is carried out as a surgical procedure and will not interfere with funeral or burial services. Knowing that these may be common areas of misunderstanding, the nurse ensures that these areas are carefully addressed.

The family is informed by the nurse that the confidentiality of the recipient is also protected. The donor family will be informed that their gift has been utilized and may receive certain generic information regarding the transplant recipient(s). Donation is in most cases an act of anonymity.

The concept of "informed consent" is applicable in this situation. The nurse ensures that the family has a well-founded understanding of the process to which they are consenting. Continued reassurance and support by the nurse are provided. The nurse must accept and support the family's decision not to donate as well.

Evaluating the Vascular Donor

The organ donor is evaluated in the same manner as any patient being admitted to the hospital's emergency or special care area. General and organ-specific criteria (Table 2-4 and Table 2-5) are applied and the status of the organ systems is evaluated. A thorough history that includes current injuries, diseases, treatments, familial health, and social habits is determined from the patient's chart, the primary nurse, the attending physician, and the family. This knowledge helps determine the existence of any pathology such as history of chronic renal impairment or drug abuse that may preclude organ donation. The nurse performs a physical assessment, observing for old surgical scars, needle track marks, congenital anomalies, injuries, and the placement and adequacy of intravenous access. Blood cultures, as well as venereal disease research laboratory (VDRL), human immunodeficiency virus (HIV), hepatitis (antibodies and antigens), and cytomegalovirus serology, are performed. Liver function and cardiac enzyme tests are performed, and serum creatinine and blood urea nitrogen levels are assessed to monitor organ function. Of importance is the accurate measurement of height and weight, which provides information for matching extra-renal organs to a recipient of corresponding body size.

Managing the Organ Donor

Clinical care of the potential organ donor is not in conflict with the care of a patient in the intensive care unit. The nursing priorities of donor management are summarized in Table 2-6. Nursing diagnoses may be applied in meeting these objectives; these are listed in Table 2-7.

Table 2-4. **General Donor Criteria***

- Brain death present or imminent
- No history of diseases affecting organs of interest
- No history of extracranial malignancy
  except basal cell carcinoma of the skin, excised and recurrence free for one year
- No current systemic infections or diseases
- No transmissible diseases
- Intact cardiovascular functioning

---

*NOTE: Criteria may differ among transplant centers. These criteria serve as guidelines only.

Table 2–5. **Organ-Specific Criteria***

Liver
- Age newborn to 70 years
- Meets general criteria
- Donor size (height/weight) compatible with anticipated recipient
- Ideally donor blood group compatible with anticipated recipient
- No prolonged hypoxia (PO_2 <70 mmHg)
- No prolonged high-dose vasopressor support
- Normal or acceptable direct, indirect, and total bilirubin levels
- Normal or acceptable aspartate transferase, alanine transferase, lactic dehydrogenase levels
- Normal or acceptable clotting studies

Heart
- Age: male <55 years   female <60 years
- Meets general criteria
- Cardiology consult within normal limits
- No trauma to heart
- No cardiac disease
- ECG, chest x-ray, blood pressure all satisfactory
- Donor size (height/weight) compatible with recipient
- Ideally dopamine <10 μg/kg/minute during maintenance
- No prolonged hypoxia (PO_2 <70 mmHg)

Heart-Lung
- Age: <50 years
- Meets general and heart criteria
- Arterial blood gases acceptable to recipient transplant center
- No history or presence of:
  ∘ pulmonary disease
  ∘ pulmonary infection
  ∘ aspiration
  ∘ pulmonary edema
  ∘ trauma

Lung
(as with heart/lung above)

Pancreas
- Age: newborn to 50+ years
- Meets general criteria
- No history of diabetes mellitus
- No prolonged hypoxia (PO_2 <70 mmHg)
- Blood glucose, serum amylase acceptable to recipient transplant center

Kidney
- Age: 6 months to 75 years
- Meets general criteria
- Renal function within normal limits for present status
- No history of:
  ∘ significant uncontrolled hypertension
  ∘ renal disease
  ∘ long-term insulin-dependent diabetes
- Urinalysis within normal limits for present status
- Dopamine <25 μg/kg/minute during management

*NOTE: Age and other criteria may differ among transplant centers. These criteria serve as guidelines only.

Table 2 – 6. **Nursing Priorities**

• Maintain adequate organ perfusion to prevent ischemic injury.
• Maintain adequate tissue oxygenation to prevent hypoxic injury.
• Prevent or treat complications that may occur secondary to the initial injury or during the course of hospitalization.
• Maintain patent airway.
• Maintain normothermia.
• Prevent infection.
• Maintain adequate hydration.

SUPPORTING CARDIOVASCULAR FUNCTION

The autonomic nervous system fails in brain death. Consequently, the functional regulatory mechanisms no longer operate and the sympathetic nervous system often becomes inactive. This has serious systemic hemodynamic and thermodynamic effects for the brain-dead patient. There may be an initial increase in blood pressure from the increased intracranial pressure and sympathetic discharge, but the subsequent failure of the

---

Table 2 – 7. **Potential and Actual Nursing Diagnoses for the Organ Donor**

Health Perception – Health Management
• Infection, potential for, possibly related to
 ◦ altered respiratory pathways secondary to intubation and mechanical ventilation
 ◦ breaks in skin integrity secondary to invasive therapeutic and diagnostic lines

Nutritional-Metabolic
• Body temperature, altered: potential (hypothermia or hyperthermia), possibly related to
 ◦ loss of thermoregulatory function
 ◦ infection
• Fluid volume deficit: actual or potential, possibly related to
 ◦ loss of hormonal regulatory function of fluid conservation
 ◦ fluid restrictions secondary to intracranial pressure monitoring

Activity-Exercise
• Cardiac output, altered: decreased, possibly related to
 ◦ volume deficit
 ◦ poor vasomotor tone
• Airway clearance, ineffective/breathing pattern, ineffective, possibly related to
 ◦ loss of gag and cough reflexes
 ◦ loss of spontaneous respirations
• Tissue perfusion, altered: renal, cardiopulmonary, hepatic, and pancreatic, possibly related to
 ◦ inadequate circulating volume
 ◦ poor vasomotor tone

---

sympathetic nervous system results in arterial vasodilation with a loss of vasomotor tone, usually culminating in a dramatically decreased blood pressure. Hypotension may also be related to pre-existing fluid deficits in patients who have received diuretic agents in an earlier attempt to reduce cerebral edema. Preload is inadequate, systemic vascular resistance is decreased, venous pooling occurs, and cardiac output is insufficient to adequately perfuse vital organs.

Due to this hemodynamic instability, the nurse monitors cardiac rate and rhythm, arterial blood pressure, central venous and pulmonary artery pressures, fluid intake, and urine output hourly or more frequently, if indicated. If hypotension is recognized, the nurse reports the assessments and initiates treatment to maintain adequate perfusion of donor organs. Initial management includes rapid infusion of intravenous fluids to restore cardiac filling pressures, and placing the patient in Trendelenburg position as needed. The response to the administration of plasma volume expanders and crystalloid intravenous fluids, such as lactated Ringer's solution, is monitored closely and documented. It is not uncommon to infuse fluids at rates of 1000–1500 ml/hour in order to replace fluid losses from the common complication of diabetes insipidus and to deliver an additional amount each hour to correct insensible losses.

When fluid alone is unable to maintain an adequate blood pressure, vasopressor agents, primarily dopamine 5–10 μg/kg/minute, may be used to maintain systolic blood pressure greater than 100 mmHg pressure and urine output greater than or equal to 1 cc/kg/hour. Large doses of vasopressors such as aramine, levophed, epinephrine, and neosynephrine are avoided because the drug-induced vasoconstriction enhances acidosis and hypoperfusion of organs and tissues.

Dysrhythmias may be a problem in the brain-dead patient. Etiologies include electrolyte disturbances, hypoxemia, hypercapnia, and metabolic acidosis. Cardiac function may also be compromised secondary to chest trauma, pulmonary edema, hypothermia, or inotropic drug use. The nurse assesses for the underlying causes, and identifies and collaboratively treats them. Continuous ECG monitoring is indicated, with serial 12-lead ECGs frequently requested. A cardiac echocardiogram or cardiac catheterization, or both, is indicated prior to consideration of heart donation when cardiac problems are encountered.

During early management, tachycardia is usually a result of increased sympathetic discharge; later, it is most often associated with hypovolemia. The nurse assesses for the etiology and appropriate interventions are applied because heart rates greater than 150 beats per minute are usually poorly tolerated. The result is a decrease in stroke volume and cardiac output. Bradycardias may be seen in the later stages of increased intracranial pressure and are an ominous sign indicating decreased cardiac output and overall cardiovascular instability.

SUPPORTING PULMONARY FUNCTION

Because the brain-dead patient does not have spontaneous respirations, intubation and mechanical ventilation are necessary to maintain a patent airway and promote respiratory gas exchange. Neurogenic pulmonary edema may develop with rapid onset after injury to the central nervous system. Chest x-rays often reveal alveolar infiltrates, which cause severe disturbances in gas exchange. The nurse performs an assessment to monitor the effectiveness of mechanical ventilation and the status of gas exchange and acid-base balance. Breath sounds are auscultated and the expansion of the chest is observed. The color, consistency, and amount of sputum is documented and aggressive pulmonary toilet is utilized, including frequent suctioning and turning. Sputum cultures and gram stains are routinely done with antibiotic therapy utilized either specifically or prophylactically. Examining for cyanosis of the nailbeds and mucous membranes, and checking for subcutaneous emphysema complete the nurse's assessment.

SUPPORTING THERMODYNAMIC FUNCTION

Temperature regulation is a function of the central nervous system involving the hypothalamus, brain stem, and spinal cord. Loss of temperature regulation occurs with brain death and may cause either hypothermia or hyperthermia. Relative normothermia is required to make the diagnosis of brain death and to preserve the viability of the donor organs. Thus, aggressive treatment is imperative. Collaborative and independent management of hypothermia involves using warming blankets, extra bed clothes, and warmed intravenous solutions. Hyperthermia may be secondary to neurological injury, but it must not be assumed that the temperature rise is only due to a neurological basis — the potential for an infectious cause must also be considered. A cooling blanket, acetaminophen suppositories, tepid sponge baths, and removal of excess bed linen may be used by the nurse to manage hyperthermia. Medications are administered to control shivering and seizures as well.

PREVENTING INFECTIONS

Any patient in the special care unit is at increased risk of developing nosocomial infections. Invasive procedures and devices used for monitoring or therapeutic purposes alter host defense mechanisms and provide microorganisms an entry into the body. Respiratory infections in the donor may be related to intubation or tracheostomy, which bypass the natural upper airway defense mechanisms. This is also complicated by immobility of the patient. Dehydration decreases the activity of the macrophages in the lower respiratory system, making the mucus thicker and more difficult for the cilia to move out of the respiratory tract. Compounding this is an absent cough reflex. The nurse assures proper care of ventilator equipment and that only sterile technique is used in suctioning. The nurse monitors proper hand washing by all those coming in contact with the donor to help reduce infections.

Urinary tract infections comprise the majority of hospital-acquired infections and are the major source of gram-negative septicemia. The nurse utilizes sterile technique with catheter insertion, maintains a closed drainage system, and provides daily meatal care to prevent infections of the urinary tract.

Maintenance of overall skin cleanliness, frequent changes in position, and use of protective devices such as sheepskins and egg-crate or flotation mattresses are important nursing interventions. These will maintain skin integrity, supporting the body's first line of defense against invasion by pathogens.

Infection control is dependent on close observation, physical assessment, and monitoring of white cell and differential counts, temperature, and routine cultures of sputum, blood, and urine. The nurse provides this care in collaboration with the physicians, transplant coordinators, and infection control specialists.

MAINTAINING FLUID BALANCE

Regulation of body water depends upon the formation and release of antidiuretic hormone (ADH) from the pituitary gland. This hormone is formed in the supraoptic nuclei of the hypothalamus and transported to the anterior portion of the gland for storage. Damage to the hypothalamus and inadequate ADH production result in the excretion of copious amounts of dilute urine. Output may be as high as 3000 cc/hour, which can quickly lead to hypovolemia and electrolyte imbalance. This clinical syndrome is known as diabetes insipidus. Treatment is directed at replacing the lost water and decreasing the urinary output. Many centers recommend the administration of aqueous pitressin to replace the ADH normally produced. The nurse performs hourly assessments of urine output, and assesses the donor for dehydration. Monitoring of central venous pressures, pulmonary artery pressures, cardiac output, peripheral venous filling, and skin turgor are important components of the assessment and evaluation of fluid therapy.

Recovering Vascular Organs

The removal and successful transplantation of donated organs requires the surgical skills and efforts of one or more transplant centers and many surgeons. In previous years, before the era of multi-organ transplantation, many of the cadaveric kidneys utilized for transplantation were surgically removed by nonphysicians or organ procurement coordinators. Today, the complexity of the recovery procedures requires the entire professional surgical team, headed by transplant surgeons. In some communities and transplant programs, local surgeons are successfully employed as nephrectomy surgeons.

A single donor may donate several organs and tissues. For example, a young, previously healthy individual may meet the criteria for donation of all vascular organs — heart, lungs, liver, pancreas, and kidneys. However, anatomy and practicality may limit which organs may be concurrently donated. For example, many transplant programs prefer not to recover both total pancreas and liver from the same donor because of the anatomical juxtaposition of the arterial blood supplies of these two organs although new regulations now encourage recovery of both. Most multiorgan donors are donors of two to three organ systems. Commonly these are heart/kidneys, liver/kidneys, heart/liver/kidneys, heart/pancreas/kidneys, heart/lungs/pancreas/kidneys, heart/lungs/liver/kidneys.

Two or more organ recovery teams may be involved with a single donor. In many cases, at least one of these teams will travel from their distant transplant hospital to participate in the recovery procedure. Thus, the organ procurement organization and its staff are crucial in the coordination of timing and logistics.

There are two requirements prior to admission of the donor to the operating room. The donor's medical record must contain an appropriate progress note documenting the date and time of the declaration of death, and a consent must be present for the recovery of organs. This permit is in compliance with the hospital's policy and procedure or, where defined, in compliance with state law. The presence and appropriateness of these two prerequisites are verified by the primary nurse on the unit and the circulating nurse prior to the start of the operative procedure. In addition to these two documents, many hospitals also require a signed death certificate.

The protocol for management of the donor is similar to that of any patient in the operating room. The responsibilities of the anesthesiologist include monitoring and managing the donor's airway and gas exchange continuously, and maintaining respiration, circulation, fluid and electrolyte balance, and renal function. Anesthesiologists also provide muscle relaxants as needed. Brain-dead patients often require a variety of pharmacologic interventions to maintain hemodynamic stability and adequate organ perfusion. Occasionally it may be necessary to temper reflex hemodynamic and muscle responses to surgical stimulation (Ascher, 1984.)

Most recovery programs prefer to work with the donor hospital's operating room staff. The recovery team(s) provide any unusual needs in the form of specialized instrumentation, solutions, and supplies for their procedure. The hospital's responsibilities typically include normal instrumentation, supplies, and support for a similar surgical procedure. The Uniform Anatomical Gift Act prohibits the donor's personal physician from participating in the recovery or transplantation of any of the organs or tissues. Operating times for the recovery procedure vary depending upon donor anatomy, organs recovered, and the skill and experience of the recovery teams, but an OR time of 2 to 4 hours is usually sufficient.

Preserving Organs

The concept of an "organ bank" with shelves filled with preserved organs awaiting transplantation is still a dream of the future. However, recovered organs must be preserved for any period of time that they are ischemic (without blood supply). Early attempts at organ preservation ranged from the very simple and moderately effective technique of perfusing the isolated organs with cold electrolyte solution (to remove blood and cool the organ) to immensely complicated methodologies involving attempts to supply the organ with a normal *ex vivo* environment.

While the preservation of all transplantable organs is of great importance, the preservation of extra-renal organs (heart, lung, liver, pancreas) is of critical importance. Those involved in renal transplantation have the ability to provide their patients with backup modalities (dialysis) that can be used to maintain the lives of their patients should a transplanted kidney fail to function. For the extra-renal transplants, immediate function of the implanted organ is of paramount importance. With the notable exception of the artificial heart and similar assist devices, there are no life-sustaining methods of supporting these patients in the face of total organ failure. Therefore, the methods of preservation chosen and the periods of time for which they are applied must allow for immediate, life-supporting organ function upon implantation. Several basic requirements for organ preservation can be found in Table 2–8.

During the early days of renal transplantation, the simpler methods of washout and immersion in cold solution were adequate. The few transplants that were performed involved minimal ischemic time as they were typically between relatives in adjoining operating rooms.

As knowledge of the immunological complications of renal transplantation became known, interest in tissue matching of donors and recipients grew. With the knowledge that few patients suffering from end-stage renal disease would have relatives amenable to and suitable for related kidney donation, interest in cadaveric renal transplantation grew. The need for tissue matching produced an acute need for time to perform this testing, and thus a more effective methodology for renal preservation was required.

The 1960s saw the first widely applicable techniques for long-term

Table 2–8. **Organ Preservation**

Basic Requirements for Organ Preservation

1. **Viability:** The methods chosen must maintain the viability of the organs.
2. **Immediate, life-supporting function:** In certain cases, nothing less is acceptable.
3. **Simplicity and reproducibility:** Procedures should be simple to allow for widespread application by persons with diverse backgrounds.
4. **Lack of harm to the recipient:** The preservation system should not contribute to the morbidity or mortality of the recipient.

Common Preservation Times*

Kidney	48–72 hours
Heart	4–6 hours
Lung	2–4 hours
Liver	6–30 hours
Pancreas	4–30 hours

*Preservation times vary by transplanting institution.

(24-hour) renal preservation. Preservation systems described by Humphries and colleagues (1962) and Belzer and colleagues (1967, 1968) involved recirculating a cold oxygenated plasma perfusate through the kidneys in a special circuit, an adaptation of earlier, more complicated systems. Previous long-term renal preservation attempts in Belzer's laboratory had failed. One morning, however, the lab technician realized that he had forgotten to place the frozen plasma for the day's experiment out to thaw. He rapidly thawed the frozen plasma in a 37°C water bath and was surprised to see a precipitate (composed of cryoglobulins) in the plasma bags. He filtered the plasma before preparing the day's experimental perfusate. Twenty-four-hour renal preservation was now a reality.

During the early 1970s, less complicated static preservation methodologies became available and gained wide acceptance. These techniques involved an initial cold washout of the organ with a specially formulated high potassium, hyperosmolar solution followed by subsequent storage of the organ by immersion in this same solution at 4°C (Collins, 1972; Sacks, 1973). Initially, this technique provided for only 8 to 12 hours' preservation. Later modifications of this solution (Euro-Collins) and increasing experience have improved the preservation capability to 48 to 96 hours. Maximum preservation times, however, are very dependent upon individual transplantation centers. The premise of these newer systems was that they "mimicked" the intracellular electrolyte concentrations of the very cells that they preserved. This formulation (the "intracellular" preservation solutions) helped to prevent the shift of water into the cells during the

Table 2 – 9. Electrolyte Concentrations of Intracellular Preservation Solutions (mEq/L)

Electrolyte	Collins Solution	Euro-Collins	Ringer's Lactate*
Na^+	10	10	130
K^+	115	115	4
Cl^-	15	15	109
PO_4^{-3}	100	100	0
HCO_3^-	10	10	0
Mg^{+2}	50	0	0
SO_4^{-2}	50	0	0
Glucose	25G	38.5G	0
pH	7.2	7.2	6.5
mOsm/L	330	375	280

*For comparison purposes.

storage period and thus the subsequent nonfunction that often resulted from less sophisticated preservation methods.

Currently, the Euro-Collins system is utilized for preservation of both kidneys and livers. However, most agree that this system limits effective preservation of the *ex vivo* liver to 6 – 8 hours. Table 2 – 9 offers solution formulas.

The availability of a new preservation system, the U/W solution from the University of Wisconsin (Table 2 – 10), promises to offer the capability for 24 to 40-hour preservation of the liver and pancreas. This is a much more complex static storage system. It relies upon the basic principles proven by earlier systems and also addresses higher order biochemical

Table 2-10. U/W Solution

K^+ Lactobionate	100 mmol
KH_2PO_4	25 mmol
$MgSO_4$	5 mmol
Raffinose	30 mmol
Adenosine	5 mmol
Glutathione	3 mmol
Allopurinol	1 mmol
Hydroxyethyl starch	50 G%
Insulin	100 units
Dexamethasone	8 mg
Penicillin	40 units

Table 2–11. **Stanford Cardioplegia Solution**	
Glucose	50 grams
Mannitol	12.5 grams
KCl	30 mEq/L
NaHCO$_3$	44 mEq/L
H$_2$O	1 liter

functions thought to be important to the preservation of more complex organs such as the liver and the pancreas.

Preservation of the excised heart utilizes similar systems. Most cardiac teams prefer to recover the heart after arrest is pharmacologically induced by infusion of high concentrations of potassium in a cold solution known as cardioplegia. There are a variety of formulas for these solutions, usually containing elements that raise the osmolarity to at least 300 mOsm/L. Many contain additional substances such as high energy phosphates (ATP) or precursors of these energy-rich compounds. There is general agreement that these systems limit effective preservation of the heart to 4 to 6 hours. Table 2–11 describes the Stanford cardioplegia formula.

Preservation methodologies for heart-lung blocs and single lungs are variable and less well standardized. However, the common thread in all currently utilized methods of preservation of all organs is hypothermia — the application of low temperatures to reduce metabolic activity and thus metabolic requirements for relatively short periods of time.

SUMMARY

The role of the nurse in identifying and referring potential organ donors can make a great deal of difference in decreasing the gap between the number of potential donors and actual donors. By meeting the challenge of this role, nurses can not only be advocates for the thousands of patients awaiting transplantation, but can also assist the grieving family by making the positive option of donation available to them.

Bibliography

Ascher, NL, et al: Multiple organ donation from a cadaver. In Simmons, RL (ed): Manual of Vascular Access, Organ Donation, and Transplantation. Springer-Verlag, New York, 1984.
Bartucci, MR: The meaning of organ donation to donor families. ANNA Journal 14(6):369, 1987.

Belzer, FO, Ashby, BS, Gulassy, PF, and Powel, M: Successful seventeen hour preservation and transplantation of human cadaveric kidneys. N Engl J Med 278:608, 1968.

Belzer, FO, et al: 24-hour and 72-hour preservation of canine kidneys. Lancet p 536, September 9, 1967.

Belzer, FO and Southard, JH: Principles of solid organ preservation by cold storage. Transplantation 45(4):673–676, April, 1988.

Collins, GM, Bravo-Shugaram, MD, and Terasaki, PI: Kidney preservation for transplantation. Lancet 2:1219, 1972.

Gallup Survey: The US public's attitudes toward organ transplants/organ donation. The Gallup Organization, Princeton, NJ, 1985.

Humphries, R, et al: Successful implantation of the dog kidney after 24 hour storage. Surgical Forum 13:380, 1962.

Kubler-Ross, E: Living with Death and Dying. Macmillan, New York, 1982.

Manninen, DL and Evans, RW: Public attitudes and behavior regarding organ donation. JAMA 253(21):3111, 1985.

Guidelines for the determination of death: report of the medical consultants on the diagnosis of death to the President's Commission for the Study of Ethical Problems in Medicine and Biomedical and Behavioral Research. JAMA: 246:2184, 1981.

Prottas, J and Batten, HL: Professional attitudes toward organ donation (Part I). Brandeis University, Health Policy Center: Waltham, MA, 1985.

Sacks, S, et al: Canine kidney preservation using a new perfusate. Lancet p. 1024, May 12, 1973.

United States Department of Health and Human Services. Report of the Task Force on Organ Transplantation. Executive Summary, 1986.

The Transplant Candidate

Mary L. Stoeckle, RN, MSN, CCRN
Mary Anne House, RN, MSN

Due to advances in medical technology and surgical procedures over the last decade, organ transplantation has become an almost routine health-care option (Bouressa and O'Mara, 1987). In addition to advanced technology, another major element in the improved outcome has been the careful and precise evaluation of potential recipients. Thorough physical and psychological evaluation can assist the transplant team in identifying and eliminating conditions or situations associated with post-transplant complications, and thus decrease the incidence of graft rejection and possible death (Futterman, 1988; Krull and Hatswell, 1988; Miller, 1988).

THE TRANSPLANT TEAM

Only after having exhausted most available conventional medical and surgical therapies are patients with end-stage organ disease referred for transplantation (Futterman, 1988). The intense evaluation process requires coordination and input from a number of different disciplines. As transplantation has increased in both volume and complexity, the *team concept* has become more common. Unlike other forms of surgery, transplantation is not a referral from one physician to another for a single surgical procedure. Transplantation is a complex form of therapy often requiring a lifelong commitment from the transplant team, the referring physician,

33

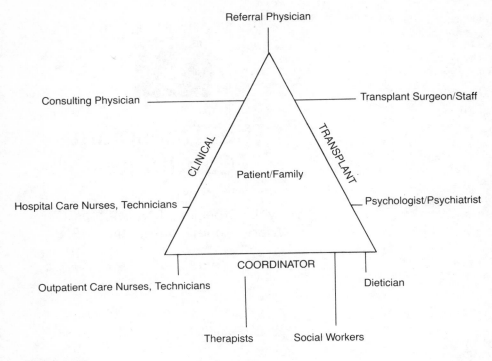

Figure 3-1

The transplant team.

and the recipient. Therefore, communication among the team members is vital to the success of the transplant.

Communication among the team members begins at the point of patient referral to the program and continues through the evaluation, transplantation, and followup. The clinical transplant coordinator establishes communication with the patient and family and acts as the nucleus for all care given (Fig. 3-1).

THE PROCESS

The evaluation process can become physically and emotionally taxing as the patient is subjected to numerous diagnostic procedures, examinations, and interviews by various members of the transplant team. The clinical transplant coordinator often meets first with the candidate and family unit, explains the evaluation process, and answers questions. The comprehensive evaluation includes clinical and diagnostic procedures to determine the medical suitability of the candidate, as well as a psychosocial and educational profile of both the candidate and the family.

Clinical Evaluation

The clinical evaluation and specific diagnostic studies vary from organ to organ and program to program. However, components of the clinical evaluation protocol usually include renal, hepatic, hematologic, and general metabolic lab studies (Becker, 1989; Futterman, 1988; Krull and Hatswell, 1988; Miller, 1988). Nurses must refer to the specific evaluation criteria for potential recipients at the center with which the patient is affiliated.

In the early 1970s, diabetes topped an extensive list of medical conditions considered to be contraindications for transplantation. However, increased graft survival due to advances in surgical technology and immunosuppression has dramatically eliminated many of these contraindications (Futterman, 1988; Krull and Hatswell, 1988; Dutten, 1987). Medical conditions felt to be acceptable for transplantation vary from program to program. Cancer, diabetes, extensive cardiovascular disease, and even acquired immune deficiency syndrome (AIDS) may be acceptable at one program and totally unacceptable at another. Informing the patient and family of the increased risks associated with a pre-existing medical condition, the possible effect on the outcome of the transplant, and the effect of immunosuppression on the disease process is of vital importance. The nurse's role is to validate and document the patient's and family's understanding since this information will serve as the foundation for ongoing education.

Psychosocial Evaluation and Psychological Management

Throughout time, research has shown that physical illnesses have psychological as well as physical effects (Hailey and Harden, 1988). These psychological effects include a variety of factors common to any individual and family with a chronic illness such as end-stage organ failure. Specific psychological effects have been identified with transplantation. Since the potential for psychological complications is inherent in transplantation, a psychological evaluation of both the transplant candidate and family has evolved as a standard procedure (Gharbieh, 1988; Dutten, 1987).

Individuals with chronic illness experience demands generated by such direct effects of the disease and its treatment as changes in social activities, loss of strength, fear of death, anger, denial, loss of self-esteem, and stress within the family unit (Woods, Yates, and Primomo, 1989). Moreover, families experience demands in dealing with the extended family, work or school environments, changes in internal processes such as decision making and family roles, and stress due to financial instability from healthcare costs and loss of income (Woods, Yates, and Primomo, 1989).

Psychological management begins with an unbiased discussion of transplantation as an option for the treatment of end-stage organ failure. The patient's ability to manage the stressors associated with transplantation, such as the constant threat of rejection, the dependency on and the side effects of immunosuppression, and the resumption of an independent role, are evaluated (Gharbieh, 1988). In addition to the daily stressors associated with end-stage organ failure, some families may experience feelings of anger, depression, and guilt if it becomes necessary to uproot the family in order to be near the transplant center to await transplantation (Woods, Yates, and Primomo, 1989). Psychological evaluation and counseling can assist the patient and family in coping with these feelings and stressors. The members of the transplant team have a responsibility to assist the patient and family throughout the transplant process.

THE LIVING-RELATED TRANSPLANT

To some extent, psychological management is dictated by the type of transplant performed (Gharbieh, 1988). In the case of living-related kidney donation, psychological evaluation of the donor is imperative to determine motivation for donation, the possibility of family coercion, and the donor's ability to handle the possibility of rejection of the donated kidney by the recipient (Gharbieh, 1988; Dutten, 1987). These factors are central to the acceptance of a potential living donor.

Living-related donor transplantation is an emotionally charged issue for the family involved, particularly the mother(s) and the spouses of the donor and recipient. Two family members undergo simultaneous surgery. One person, the donor, risks possible complications and death for the potential rehabilitation of the other. Because of the intense emotional investment, these families need information and emotional support throughout the transplantation process.

Living-related kidney recipients may experience feelings of guilt or indebtedness to the donor (Gharbieh, 1988). Nursing care specific to the recipient is directed at supporting the family unit, especially the donor-recipient relationship. Providing information regarding the donor and recipient's recovery and facilitating visits are useful interventions.

Waiting Period
for Cadaveric Transplantation

The waiting period is said to be the most difficult time of all. Factors that influence the length of time a patient may have to wait for an organ include the geographic location of the transplant center, the priority of the patient on the waiting list, and the availability of the needed organ (Futterman, 1988). Despite the technological advances in transplantation over the last decade, a serious imbalance remains between the number of transplant candidates and the number of available organs (Appendix D).

The emotional toll of a difficult and prolonged waiting period on the patient and family is a serious concern nurses must address. As weeks, even months pass, the focus of waiting patients often becomes their deteriorating health, family stress, and doubts about transplantation (Futterman, 1988). Interactions with other patients who have received similar transplants or other waiting patients and their families are beneficial during this difficult time. In addition, frequent contact with the transplant coordinator and transplant team members can redirect energies and often provide encouragement.

Financial Evaluation

The federal government, health insurance organizations, and general public are becoming increasingly aware of healthcare costs. Transplantation has received a large share of this attention due to the high cost associated with the procedure and immunosuppressive drugs (Marsden, 1988). The costs of transplantation are mandated by the individual transplant centers (Appendix D). During the first year of transplantation, these costs can be divided into the following categories:

1. pre-transplantation costs — the cost of caring for a patient with end-stage organ disease before transplantation referral;
2. evaluation costs — costs associated with the workup of a patient to determine suitability for transplantation;
3. costs incurred while awaiting a donor;
4. transplantation costs; and
5. post-transplantation costs — costs from the time of discharge including outpatient charges, treatment for complications, and immunosuppressive therapy (Futterman, 1988).

Since 1973, renal transplantation has been covered by Medicare under the End-Stage Renal Disease Program. Patients who are eligible for this coverage receive 80% of all transplant costs, as well as immunosuppression costs for the first year (Marsden, 1988).

The 1986 limited funding approval by Medicare for cardiac transplantation changed the status of this procedure from experimental to accepted therapy. However, this funding is available only to those individuals who are normally eligible for Medicare and only at specific Medicare-approved centers (Marsden, 1988).

The majority of heart transplant candidates, and all liver, pancreas, and lung transplant candidates do not receive any federal funding. These patients must rely on private insurance, private funding, and in some cases, state medical assistance.

The financial evaluation is comprised of a thorough analysis of the patient's health insurance to determine the extent of coverage for the procedure, for the post-transplant followup care, and for medication. Knowledge of the healthcare coverage can alleviate at least one stressor for many recipients and their families. In cases where there is either inadequate or no coverage, assistance can be given to the patient and family regarding application for financial assistance or with fund-raising activities to cover the necessary costs.

Education

The interval between referral and the beginning of the clinical evaluation gives the patient time to consider the significance of organ transplantation. Information and education by the clinical transplant coordinator, clinical nurse specialist, and other members of the team allow the patient to make the ultimate decision to proceed with the evaluation and possible transplant. Patients must be given as much information as possible regarding the transplant process and post-transplant risks and complications in order to make an informed and legal consent with regard to transplantation. As with any medical or surgical procedure, the patient has the right to accept or decline this form of treatment, even if refusal of treatment may result in death.

PATIENT EDUCATION

Patient education regarding transplantation begins with the initial visit by the clinical transplant coordinator. At this time, written information explaining the transplant process is given to the patient. Written information is an important aspect of patient education as it allows patients to review the information at their leisure and to share the information with their families.

Although the written information is an important part of patient education process, it needs to be supplemented with individualized, personal contact with members of the team. This may be a short meeting to answer questions and clarify information given in the written material or a formal presentation with audiovisual material (Gharbieh, 1988). Whatever the protocol of the program, flexibility is important in the education process. The ability to adapt to the special needs of each patient is important to successful pre-transplant education.

FAMILY EDUCATION

The cooperation and support of the family is an important factor in the successful outcome of transplantation. However, in order to continue its support, the family must understand the entire transplant process. Therefore, the family needs to be included in the educational process of the patient. Additional written material is made available to the family, and family members are included in the question-and-answer sessions and formal presentation segments of the evaluation.

An important segment of family education involves the living-related donor. A complete understanding and knowledge of the donation process, risks and benefits, and long-term outcome are essential aspects of the evaluation for a potential living-related donor. The living-related donor must have as much information as possible prior to beginning the clinical evaluation. Only with this information can a living-related donor make a comfortable and educated decision regarding donation.

The primary goal in providing patient and family education during the evaluation is to inform them of the evaluation and transplant process, the risks and benefits to the patient, and to establish lines of communication that will continue throughout the transplant process. In addition, a precedent for patient and family involvement is established that prepares them for the transition to post-transplant teaching.

ORGAN ALLOCATION

The National Transplant Act (Public Law 98-507) created the National Organ Procurement and Transplant Network (OPTN). This government-contracted agency is responsible for overseeing organ distribution and data collection on donation and transplantation. The United Network for Organ Sharing (UNOS) successfully bid for the contract and currently is the agency serving as the OPTN.

The UNOS Board of Directors has struggled with developing the best methods to distribute donated organs. Many changes in the system have been made in an effort to ensure equitable distribution of available organs. Nurses may always contact their local organ procurement organization (OPO) for more information about the latest distribution system. The current method for matching donated organs with recipients varies with

each organ. Three separate sharing plans exist for the following categories:
1. kidneys
2. hearts
3. livers, pancreata, lungs, and combined heart-lung blocs.

Kidneys

With regard to the sharing of kidneys, six antigen matches and phenotypically identical kidneys are mandatorily shared between centers by UNOS regulations. Except in the instance of a six-antigen match, blood type O kidneys must go to ABO-identical recipients. The remainder of potential recipients are given a point-value ranking based on several other factors. Although the system continues to evolve, time waiting, quality of antigen match, and cytotoxic antibody level are examples of the factors that influence the selection of a potential recipient. The OPO that is retrieving the organ(s) enters specific donor data such as age, sex, and HLA antigens into the national computer system. The computer first provides a list of local recipients for the OPO's service area. Next, a regional list is compiled, according to the UNOS region in which the OPO is located. Finally, a national list is also generated, Some centers belong to a special sharing system known as categorical sharing. For those centers, a special sharing of O kidneys between centers is printed.

Hearts

For potential heart recipients, there are only two categories of urgency: status I and status II. In addition to medical urgency, time waiting and logistical factors influence how patients are listed by the computer. Using zones defined by concentric circles of 500 miles each, the UNOS system matches first local donors with local recipients, then donors with recipients within 500 miles of the donor hospital, 1000 miles, and finally greater than 1000 miles. Priority is given first to placing a donor heart with any local status I patient who has a compatible blood group type, and then to a local status II patient first with ABO-identical or second with ABO-compatible blood types. After local matches, the system then lists status I recipients within the first 500 miles followed by status II recipients within 500 miles. Other potential recipients are listed similarly at distances of 1000 miles and greater than 1000 miles.

Extra-Renal Organs (Other Than Heart)

Allocation of extra-renal organs varies. Histocompatibility testing is not generally taken into consideration. Size of the donor in comparison with the recipient and ABO type are most important in pairing organs with recipients.

For liver, pancreas, lung, and combined heart-lung donors, specific information is entered into the matching system. The primary nurse often serves as a source of this information, and can anticipate the need to have this data available to the transplant coordinator. Awaiting recipients are then matched with available donor organs, taking into consideration these matching factors in addition to factors such as the time the patient has been on the waiting list, medical urgency, and distance from the donor and transplant centers. The OPO first assesses local transplant center needs, then regional, and finally national lists as they are provided by the computer system.

Equitable Sharing

The centralized waiting list maintained by UNOS is designed to assure equitable organ distribution to each transplant candidate. All transplant centers and organ procurement organizations must be UNOS members. Every donor must be entered into the computer. For kidneys, the match must be run within 15 hours of organ recovery to decrease the chances an organ would be wasted. Non-UNOS members may not access the system. Centers must be specifically approved for each type of organ transplant they perform. This method of sharing helps ensure selection of patients for transplantation based on waiting time as well as medical and scientific criteria. Discrimination shall not occur because of race, sex, political influence, or financial advantage.

SUMMARY

Solid organ transplantation is a complex, multidiscipline system requiring extensive communication and coordination among a variety of healthcare professionals, the patient, and the family. A vital part of this system is the process by which a chronically ill patient becomes a transplant candidate. Therefore, transplant evaluation requires a detailed yet flexible program to ensure the best selection and preparation of the transplant candidate and a successful outcome.

Bibliography

American Association of Critical Care Nurses: Roles and Responsibilities of Critical Care Nurses in Organ and Tissue Transplantation. AACN Position Statement. June, 1986.

American Council on Transplantation: U.S. Transplant Stat Sheet. Lifesource, Summer, 1989.

Becker, S: The risks and rewards of pancreatic transplant. RN (July, 1989): 54–57.

Bouressa, G and O'Mara, RJ: Ethical dilemmas in organ procurement and donation. Critical Care Nurse Quarterly 10:37–47, 1987.

Crowder, E: A new nursing role: Transplant coordinator. Texas Nursing (October, 1987): 13.

Dutten, M: Transplantation. Nursing 87: 641, 1987.

Futterman, LG: Cardiac transplantation: A comprehensive nursing perspective. Part 1. Heart Lung 17:499–510, September, 1988.

Gartland, C: Organ transplants. Nursing Times (February, 1987): 24–28.

Gharbieh, PA: Renal transplant: Surgical and psychologic hazards. Critical Care Nurse 8:58–71, 1988.

Hailey, BJ and Harden KN: Perceptions of seriously ill patients: Does diagnosis make a difference? Patient Education and Counseling 12:259–265, 1988.

Hamilton, D: Kidney transplantation: A history. In Morris, PJ (ed): Kidney Transplantation: Principles and Practice. WB Saunders, Philadelphia, 1988.

Keogh, A: The role of the transplant coordinator. Nursing Times (March, 1987); 48–49.

Krull, K and Hatswell, E: Single-lung allograft: A nursing perspective. Critical Care Nurse 8:35–57, 1988.

Marsden, C: Ethical issues in cardiac transplantation. Journal of Cardiovascular Nursing 2:23–30, 1988.

Miller, HD: Liver transplantation: Postoperative ICU care. Critical Care Nurse 8:19–31, 1988.

Pate, JA: Transplant nursing in the '80s. Texas Nursing (October, 1987): 11–12.

Woods, NF, Yates, BC, and Primomo, J: Supporting families during chronic illness. Image 21:46–50, Spring, 1989.

CHAPTER

Kidney Transplantation

Peggy Schreck Pattella, RN, BSN
Patricia D. Weiskittel, RN, MSN, CNN

In 1936, the first human kidney transplant was performed in the Ukraine by the Soviet surgeon Voronoy (Hamilton, 1988). None of the six transplants performed achieved substantial function. Renewed interest in transplantation occurred in the 1950s. The first successful kidney transplant in the United States was performed by Murray and Harrison in Boston in 1954 (Hamilton, 1988). This transplant, between identical twins, increased the confidence that kidney transplants could be technically and safely performed.

The early attempts at immunosuppression to increase graft survival utilized total body irradiation. In 1961, azathioprine became available for human use. However, azathioprine alone did not offer prolonged graft survival. Murray and his colleagues in 1962, as well as Starzl and his colleagues in 1963, used the combination of azathioprine and prednisolone (Hamilton, 1988). Success with this drug combination encouraged the practice of kidney transplantation throughout the world. The advances in surgical techniques and the improved understanding of the immune response have increased the success rate of kidney transplantation and created a viable alternative treatment for patients with end-stage renal disease.

Patients with end-stage renal disease face a complex decision regarding treatment options available to them. In order to make this decision, patients and their families must be provided with current and accu-

43

rate information from the nurse about the available treatment modalities. The available treatment options are:

1. In-center hemodialysis
2. Home hemodialysis
3. Continuous ambulatory peritoneal dialysis
4. Conservative management
5. Kidney transplantation

Ideally, the educational process begins in the pre-dialysis period. During this time period the nurse, patient, and family have adequate time to discuss all the options and consider which treatment option will best meet the needs of the patient.

Most patients who choose the transplantation option are already being maintained with dialytic therapy. It is, however, possible that a patient may choose transplantation as a primary option. Transplantation is a possible primary option for those who have a family member who wishes to donate a kidney. The decision to pursue transplantation must be based on accurate information about the advantages and disadvantages associated with transplantation. The potential benefits of successful transplantation include:

1. Freedom from dialysis
2. Increased sense of well-being
3. More flexible life-style
4. Greater employment potential

The symptoms associated with renal failure and dialysis such as nausea, vomiting, anemia, headaches, pruritus, decreased libido, infertility, and poor appetite are usually eliminated following a successful renal transplant.

The major risk factors following transplantation include rejection, infection, and the side effects of the specific drugs utilized. The potential side effects of immunosuppressive therapy can be life threatening. (These side effects are discussed in Chapter 9.) The nurse's responsibility is to assist the patient and family to make an informed decision by having an adequate understanding of the risks and benefits associated with transplantation.

Applied Pathophysiology

End-stage renal disease (ESRD) is a term used to describe irreversible renal failure. Treatment with dialysis or transplantation is needed to maintain life. Residual renal function is less than 15% of normal at this stage. It is characterized by severe impairment of excretory, regulatory, and hormonal functions, causing the body's failure to maintain homeostasis. Homeostatic functions are decreased to the extent that the kidneys can no longer meet the usual metabolic demands of the body. Chronic abnormalities in fluid, electrolyte, and acid-base balance result in a series of signs and symptoms known as the uremic syndrome. Uremia, or the accumulation of uremic toxins, causes many pathophysiological changes that eventually affect all body systems.

Laboratory Evaluation of Renal Function

BUN, or blood urea nitrogen, becomes elevated as renal failure progresses. Urea nitrogen is an end-product of protein metabolism. Urea production is not constant, and is formed as a result of metabolism of amino acids not used for protein synthesis. As more amino acids are metabolized by the liver, more urea is produced. Increased urea production can occur with a high-protein intake; catabolism (increased tissue breakdown) occurring as a result of trauma, burns, or gastrointestinal bleeding; or during corticosteroid administration. Normal BUN levels are approximately 10–20 mg/dL (Rose, 1987). Manifestations that may be observed in patients with a progression in BUN elevation are anorexia, nausea, vomiting, headache, and fatigue. Not all patients with an elevated BUN will manifest all of these symptoms (Thompson and colleagues, 1986).

Creatinine is a by-product of muscle metabolism. It is released into the plasma at a constant rate. Plasma creatinine level is fairly constant, and creatinine is freely filterable across the glomerulus. Serum creatinine is the most reliable indicator of renal function. The amount of creatinine produced depends upon the patient's muscle mass. Men tend to run higher creatinine levels than women as a result of the difference in muscle mass. Normal serum creatinine in males ranges from 0.8 to 1.3 mg/dL; and in females 0.6–1.0 mg/dL (Rose, 1987). Creatinine clearance is the method utilized to determine the filtering capacity of the kidneys. To measure creatinine clearance, all urine is collected for 24 hours and the creatinine is measured. Utilizing the serum creatinine and urinary creatinine levels, the clearance is calculated. Normal values for creatinine clearance are:

1. 120–125 mL/minute in men
2. 95–115 mL/minute in women
3. Clearance declines with age, approximately 1 mL/minute each year over the age of 40 (Rose, 1987).

Treatment with dialysis or transplantation is necessary when the creatinine clearance falls below 10 mL/minute (Lancaster, 1984). The most common causes of ESRD are found in Table 4–1 (Luckmann and Sorensen, 1987).

Table 4-1. Causes of End-Stage Renal Disease (ESRD)

- Glomerulonephritis
- Diabetic nephropathy
- Nephrosclerosis and renal vascular disease
- Congenital or hereditary kidney disease
- Chronic pyelonephritis
- Others and unknown etiology

CLINICAL SIGNS AND SYMPTOMS OF END-STAGE RENAL DISEASE

Integumentary Manifestations

Pruritus is probably the most common problem seen in renal failure patients. Possible causative factors of the dry itching skin include:

1. Atrophy of sweat glands
2. Decreased activity of oil glands
3. Deposition of phosphate or calcium crystals
4. Elevated parathyroid hormone (PTH) levels

This pruritus may lead to relentless scratching, which can result in excoriated or infected skin as well as an irritable, restless, and frustrated patient. Nursing interventions include:

1. Bathing with lanolin-based soaps
2. Keeping fingernails short and clean
3. Applying emollient after bathing
4. Giving antipruritic medications as ordered (Jacobsson, 1986).

Skin color changes that occur are a result of retained urochrome pigment and carotene. This creates a yellowish cast over the pallor created by the anemia.

Metabolic Manifestations

Acidosis occurs in the patient with ESRD due to the kidneys' inability to excrete hydrogen ions, its inability to produce ammonia, and the loss of bicarbonate in the urine. As the glomerular filtration rate falls, phosphate retention occurs, and phosphate is used as a hydrogen acceptor. Approximately 40% of the acid buffering occurs from bone salts. This contributes to bone dissolution (Jacobsson, 1986).

Fluid retention is a common problem for patients with ESRD. As the glomerular filtration rate decreases, the kidney loses its ability to excrete salt and water. Patients can accumulate large amounts of fluid between dialysis treatments, resulting in fluid overload, which may lead to congestive heart failure or pulmonary edema. Sodium and fluid restrictions are necessary in conjunction with ultrafiltration during dialysis to avoid the complications of pulmonary edema, uremic pneumonitis, and congestive failure (Lancaster, 1984).

Hyperkalemia becomes a potentially fatal complication as renal function decreases. In severe renal failure, the hyperkalemia results from decreased secretion of potassium, acidosis, excess dietary intake, blood transfusions, bleeding, or ingestion of potassium-containing medications. Hyperkalemia may be silent or manifest itself with muscle weakness, flaccid paralysis, or cardiac dysrhythmias. Common ECG changes include peaked T waves, ST segment depression, and widened QRS complex and P – R interval. Severe hyperkalemia is life threatening and may be treated with IV infusion of hypertonic glucose, insulin and bicarbonate infusion, sodium polystyrene sulfonate (Kayexalate), or with dialysis. If untreated, this may progress to asystole or ventricular fibrillation (Jacobsson, 1986).

Other metabolic abnormalities that occur in ESRD are abnormal carbohydrate metabolism, hyperinsulinism, abnormal lipid metabolism, and protein metabolism. Cholesterol levels tend to remain normal but triglyceride levels are elevated and may account for the accentuated atherosclerotic disease in this population. Protein-restricted diets (0.5 gm/kg) are used to contain rising BUN levels. However, severe restriction of protein intake, particularly in patients with increased loss of protein in the urine, may lead to hypoalbuminemia (Luckmann and Sorensen, 1987).

Cardiovascular Manifestations

The majority of deaths that occur in ESRD patients result from cardiovascular complications. The most frequent cardiovascular manifestation is hypertension. Fluid and sodium retention resulting in volume overload, and renin-angiotensin system dysfunction are two fundamental causes of hypertension in renal patients (Luckmann and Sorensen, 1987). Hypertension, advanced arteriosclerotic disease, and vascular volume overload cause ESRD patients to be at high risk for cerebral vascular accidents and congestive heart failure.

Pericarditis is another cardiac complication, caused by inflammation of the pericardial sac from uremic toxins. The nurse assesses for the following clinical signs and symptoms: pericardial friction rub, fever, hypotension, pulsus paradoxus, distended neck veins, tender enlarged liver, and tachycardia. Pericarditis can lead to pericardial effusions and cardiac tamponade. These life-threatening conditions are caused by bleeding or fluid collection into the space between the visceral and parietal layers of the pericardium (Lancaster, 1984). Chronic congestive heart failure that is unsuccessfully managed with salt and water restrictions and dialytic therapy may lead to a myocardiopathy. Dysrhythmias that occur are usually a result of increased serum potassium or decreased serum calcium levels (Jacobsson, 1986).

Hematologic Manifestations

Anemia is the primary hematologic complication of renal failure. It is caused by reduced erythropoiesis, hemolysis, decreased life span of red blood cells (RBCs), capillary fragility, clotting abnormalities, gastrointestinal bleeding, and blood loss occurring during hemodialysis. The use of androgen therapy (testosterone or nandrolone decanoate [Deca-durabolin]) may improve the anemia by stimulating erythropoiesis through acting directly on the bone marrow to increase the RBC precursors. However, androgens have major side effects, which include hirsutism in women and priapism in men. Nutritional deficiencies cause iron and folate depletion, which also contribute to the anemia. Replacement of folic acid and vitamin B_{12} are essential to the formation of RBCs.

Thrombocytopenia, decreased platelet adhesiveness, and decreased platelet factor 3 may cause prolonged bleeding time and manifest through bruising, nose bleeds, bleeding gums, and gastrointestinal bleeding. When bleeding disorders occur, dialytic therapy is rapidly instituted (Jacobsson, 1986).

Erythropoietin deficiency is considered the major cause of anemia in the ESRD population. The production of recombinant human erythropoietin (r-HuEPO) is a recent breakthrough made possible through modern gene technology. This product has been used successfully in clinical trials to correct anemia (Zehnder and Blumberg, 1989). This drug has recently been FDA approved, but the cost and reimbursement mechanisms are not yet in place.

Gastrointestinal Manifestations

The entire gastrointestinal system is affected by renal failure from irritation of the mucous membranes by uremic toxins. Signs and symptoms of gastrointestinal involvement include nausea, vomiting, a bitter metallic taste in the mouth, and an ammonia-like smell of the breath. Oral hygiene care is included as a frequent intervention for these patients. These symptoms usually decrease when the patient is adequately dialyzed. Other common gastrointestinal problems include esophagitis, gastritis, indigestion, hiccups, colitis, duodenal ulcer disease, anorexia, diarrhea, and constipation. Ulcerations and gastrointestinal irritation cause renal patients to be at risk for major gastrointestinal bleeding. The nurse checks for and documents the presence of occult blood in the stool, emesis, and naso-gastric (NG) aspirate (Lancaster, 1984).

Skeletal Manifestations

Progression of renal failure to end-stage disease leads to major problems with calcium and phosphate balance. Uncontrolled hyperphos-phatemia and hypocalcemia lead to renal osteodystrophy. Decreased phosphate excretion and decreased absorption of calcium from the gas-trointestinal (GI) tract result in stimulating parathormone secretion. If this cycle continues, hyperparathyroidism will develop. Mobilization of cal-cium from the bone causes demineralization, progressing to bone disease and metastatic calcifications. The patient may experience bone pain, frac-tures, and erosions around the joint. Medications that bind dietary phos-phate in the GI tract to prevent absorption of phosphate, such as alumi-num hydroxide and calcium carbonate, are helpful in controlling hyperphosphatemia and subsequent bone demineralization. The use of phosphate binders is a frequent cause of constipation and leads to non-compliance, resulting in secondary hyperparathyroidism and renal osteo-dystrophy (Jacobsson, 1986).

Muscle cramps, atrophy, and weakness also occur in the ESRD pa-tient. Causative factors include increased potassium-calcium ratio in the cerebrospinal fluid, increased phosphate levels in the cerebrospinal fluid, decreased magnesium levels, increased levels of urea, and tissue hypoxia. Alterations in vitamin D metabolism result in changes in muscle contrac-tion and relaxation. Changes in mobility, neurological changes, and low serum albumin leading to a catabolic state may contribute to increased muscle weakness and atrophy (Jacobsson, 1986).

Neurological Manifestations

All patients with ESRD experience some nervous system problems. Signs and symptoms of neurological involvement may manifest as changes in mentation, behavior, or as peripheral neuropathy. In addition to the psychosocial problems caused by chronic illness, uremia can cause meta-bolic encephalopathy and contribute to decreased attention span, mem-ory loss, confusion, stupor, insomnia, fatigue, and sleep disturbances. With advancing uremia, gait abnormalities, asterixis (flap), myoclonus, slurred speech, seizures, and coma occur. Behavioral changes can run the gamut from mild depression and agitation to full-blown psychosis. Neuropathy affects the lower extremities and is caused by a slowing of peripheral nerve conduction. This condition is manifested by ascending numbness and burning and by "restless legs" syndrome. Restless-legs syndrome is usually nocturnal and causes painful prickling sensations and cramps that can be relieved by movement (Lancaster, 1984).

Sexual Manifestations

The sexual dysfunctions are physical, psychological, and iatrogenic. Infertility is seen in both men and women with ESRD, although successful pregnancies have been reported (Rickus, 1987). Impotence in men, amenorrhea and cessation of ovulation in women, and absent or decreased libido are common. Sexual function is affected by the extreme stress of a chronic, life-threatening disease and the subsequent change in body image. Sex-related problems involve many aspects of a person's life, including reproduction, sensuality, intimacy, and identity-related issues (Dailey, 1983).

Endocrine Manifestations

Some patients with chronic renal failure have excess amounts of pituitary hormones such as prolactin and growth hormone. However, despite the presence of excess growth hormone, children with renal failure have severely stunted growth. Hypothyroidism is another common finding among the ESRD population. There is also delayed insulin production and utilization impairment caused by resistance of peripheral tissues to insulin (Luckmann and Sorensen, 1987). This results in an increased half-life of insulin. Diabetics approaching ESRD may mistakenly believe their diabetes is improving because they require less insulin therapy. The nurse must emphasize that insulin requirements will decrease as renal failure progresses and severe hypoglycemia is a potential life-threatening problem. Blood glucose monitoring is very helpful with insulin regulation as renal failure progresses.

Immune System Manifestations

Patients with ESRD manifest decreased cell-mediated immunity, diminished delayed hypersensitivity, abnormal neutrophil function, and increased susceptibility to infection. Patients must be assessed frequently for the signs and symptoms of viral, fungal, and bacterial infections (Jacobsson, 1986). Table 4 – 2 lists possible nursing diagnoses for the pretransplant renal patient.

Table 4–2. Common Nursing Diagnoses for the Pre-Transplant Renal Patient

Health-Perception — Health Management
- Health maintenance, altered
- Health seeking behaviors
- Noncompliance

Nutritional — Metabolic
- Fluid volume, altered: excess
- Infection, potential for
- Nutrition, altered: less than body requirements
- Nutrition, altered: more than body requirements
- Oral mucous membranes, altered

Elimination
- Bowel elimination, altered: constipation
- Urinary elimination, altered patterns

Activity — Exercise
- Activity intolerance
- Cardiac output, altered: decreased
- Diversional activity deficit
- Home maintenance management, impaired
- Gas exchange, impaired
- Fatigue

Sleep — Rest
- Sleep pattern disturbance

Cognitive — Perceptual
- Comfort, altered
  - Chronic pain
  - Pruritus
  - Nausea
  - Vomiting
- Knowledge deficit
- Decisional conflict
- Thought processes, altered

Self-Perception — Self-Concept
- Anxiety
- Fear
- Hopelessness
- Powerlessness
- Self-concept, disturbance in: body image; personal identity; self-esteem

Role — Relationship
- Family process, altered
- Self-concept, disturbance in: role performance
- Social interaction, impaired
- Social isolation

Sexuality — Reproductive
- Sexual dysfunction
- Sexuality patterns, altered

Coping — Stress Tolerance
- Adjustment, impaired
- Coping, ineffective individual
- Coping, ineffective family: compromised

PRE-TRANSPLANT MANAGEMENT

Not every patient is a suitable candidate for transplantation. The patient's healthcare status and psychological stability are important considerations. The requirements (Table 4 – 3) have become less restrictive in the past few years because of improved patient and graft survival. Age limits are flexible and risks are relative to other factors. Every transplant center has selection criteria that are examined through an evaluation and selection process. This process serves two purposes: to identify risk factors and to correct or stabilize conditions that may lead to complications following transplantation (Hanson, 1987) (Table 4 – 4). Some major high-risk factors for transplantation are active infection, current malignancy, or positive human immunodeficiency virus (HIV) test with Western blot confirmation. Transplantation can be potentially fatal in these patients because the normal surveillance activity of the immune system is impaired by the immunosuppressive drugs. After active infection has been successfully treated, transplantation workup may proceed.

When a patient has a positive purified protein derivative (PPD) test, the possibility of reactivation or progression of the tuberculosis is a significant risk following transplantation. Therefore, patients who have active tuberculosis are usually treated with the appropriate drug therapy for at least 6 months prior to transplantation; this drug therapy is continued post-transplant for as long as the patient is immunosuppressed.

Pre-Transplant Workup

The pre-transplant workup commonly includes urine cultures (if the patient still voids) to rule out infection and a voiding cystourethrogram to rule out the presence of reflux or other lower urinary tract abnormalities. A patient may require a prostatectomy, urethroplasty, ileal conduit, or bilateral nephrectomy to correct existing abnormalities before transplantation can be considered a reasonable choice of treatment. In recent years, bilateral nephrectomy has been performed only in the presence of reflux;

Table 4 – 3. **Indications for Renal Transplantation**

- Chronic renal dysfunction progressing toward ESRD
- End-stage renal disease
- Potential related donor
- Potential for successful outcome
- Patient desires a transplant
- Loss of previous transplant due to chronic rejection

Table 4-4. **High-Risk Factors for Renal Transplantation**

- Malignancy (except dermal)
- Acquired immune deficiency syndrome (AIDS)
- Progressive liver disease
- Extensive vascular disease (peripheral, cardiac, cerebral)
- Chronic infection — unresponsive to treatment
- Severe uncorrectable urinary tract abnormalities
- Severe chronic respiratory disease
- Obesity
- Refractory cardiac failure
- Severe mental retardation
- Psychosis, alcoholism, drug abuse
- Dialysis dementia
- Active tuberculosis or positive PPD treated for less than 6 months

uncontrolled hypertension; or bleeding, infected, or space-occupying polycystic kidneys. Whenever possible, the patient's native kidneys are not removed because of the benefits of their erythropoietin production, blood pressure control, and prostaglandin production and synthesis. Other health problems that affect the patient's eligibility for transplant are gastric ulcer disease, coronary artery disease, gallstones, and diverticulosis.

Radiology workup pre-transplant is designed to rule out any of the above stated problems. Routine x-rays may include: upper GI series, barium enema, gallbladder ultrasound, and voiding cystourethrogram.

An active ulcer in a patient who is immunosuppressed can be fatal because the anti-inflammatory effects of steroids mask the early warning signs of gastrointestinal bleeding such as increased pulse and abdominal pain. Barium enemas are often required in patients over 40 to rule out diverticular disease or malignancy. A colectomy may be necessary pre-transplant if the patient has extensive diverticular disease. Identification of patients at risk from cardiovascular disease may require a stress thallium test, computerized tomographic (CT) scan, Doppler studies, ECG, and MUGA (multiple gated [image] acquisition [analysis]) scan with special attention to ejection fraction. Patients who are at greater cardiac risk may need coronary arteriography with subsequent coronary artery bypass surgery prior to transplantation.

It is necessary to correct all existing abnormalities that may prove life threatening following transplantation. Generalized immunosuppression and the anti-inflammatory effects of steroids may mask active ulcer disease, ruptured diverticuli, acute cholecystitis or major infection post transplantation. The pre-transplant workup attempts to insure that each recipient is in optimal condition to receive a transplant.

All patients should have routine dental exams to rule out potential abscess formation and to correct other dental problems prior to immuno-suppression. Female recipients should have a gynecological exam, Pap smear, and mammogram if recommended by the gynecologist.

Other added risk factors to be addressed in the pre-transplant workup period are obesity, previous history of alcohol or drug abuse, and chronic noncompliance. Compliance with healthcare regimens and medications is crucial for graft and patient survival after transplantation.

All donors and recipients are further screened for the presence of certain viruses. Routine screening for hepatitis, HIV, cytomegalovirus (CMV), and Epstein-Barr virus (EBV) is common pre-transplant.

Prior to transplantation, most centers still require blood transfusions. Opelz's and Terasaki's data showed that graft survival improved by approximately 20% in cadaver-donated transplant recipients who received blood transfusions.

The immunologic mechanisms of this phenomenon are not clearly understood, but the increase in graft survival has prompted many centers to utilize pre-transplant transfusions. There are, however, risks attached to this practice, which include potential transmission of hepatitis and the development of multiple antibodies in the recipient (Kottra-Buck, 1986).

Donor Evaluation

Once the potential recipient has been accepted as a transplant candidate, donor sources must be evaluated. Traditionally, success rates with living-related donors have been superior to results obtained using cadaveric donors. There are several advantages in receiving a related-donor transplant:

- The degree of tissue matching is greater.
- Immediate graft function is attained.
- Elective scheduling of the procedure when the recipient is in optimum condition and the time is convenient for the donor.
- Advantageous for the recipient due to the demand exceeding the supply of cadaveric organs.

With the improved results from donor-specific transfusions and the use of cyclosporine, some centers have increased their donor pool to consider living-unrelated but emotionally related volunteers (i.e., spouses).

Donor workup begins with obtaining ABO type and tissue typing results. Donor and recipient must be ABO compatible and preferably a good tissue match. ABO compatibility for transplantation is the same as for blood transfusions:

Recipient	Donor
O	O
A	A or O
B	B or O
AB	A, B, O, AB

The Rh factor is not important for organ transplantation, but does become a factor if donor-specific transfusion is utilized. If the recipient is Rh-negative and the donor is Rh-positive, the "buffy coat" rather than packed red blood cells are transfused as part of the donor-specific transfusion process.

The body's ability to accept or reject a kidney depends on its response to the antigens in the donor organ. Therefore, the similarity in antigens between the donor and recipient will enhance graft acceptance.

Tissue typing, or the antigen combination of donor and recipient, can be determined from a blood sample. The human leukocyte antigens (HLA) are found on the surface of white blood cells. The HLA antigens are inherited in pairs from each parent. Three antigen loci on the sixth chromosome have significance for transplantation. The A, B, and DR loci contain two antigens each. Each individual inherits a set of antigens (one haplotype, i.e., an A, B, and DR antigen) from their mother and a second set (one haplotype) from their father. Therefore, parents are a one-haplotype or "half-match" for their children, and siblings may be a two-haplotype (identical), one haplotype (half-match), or a no-haplotype match (Kottra-Buck, 1986).

During the initial tissue-typing workup, a white-cell or cytotoxicity crossmatch is also performed. This test mixes the recipient serum with donor lymphocytes to determine the presence of preformed cytotoxic antibodies to the donor antigens. A positive white-cell crossmatch precludes transplantation; therefore, the donor cannot be used.

If an identical match is not found in the tissue-typing workup, but equal matches exist between the recipient and all donors screened, a mixed lymphocyte culture is helpful in choosing the best donor. This test takes approximately 5 to 7 days to complete and consists of mixing donor and recipient lymphocytes to determine the reactivity between donor and recipient. The donor with whom the lowest response or the lowest percentage of cell death occurs is the preferable donor.

The evaluation for a potential donor is extensive. The donor must be in excellent health in order to give one of his or her kidneys to a relative. When one normal kidney is removed, the remaining normal kidney enlarges and increases its function to compensate. Studies indicate there is no significant risk to the health of the living donor (Irwin, 1986). The search for a donor within the family unit often results in many emotional conflicts for individual family members. Parent-to-child donation is often the least stressful situation because parents are expected to sacrifice for their children. The selection process among siblings can generate feelings of ambivalence, guilt, fear, and anxiety. The donor may experience a conflict between obligation to the birth family and responsibility for marital family (Thompson, 1987). Private meetings between the transplant team and the potential donor may help to assure that a donor is not being coerced into donation by family members.

Cadaveric Kidney Crossmatching

The majority of patients (approximately 60%–70%) are not fortunate enough to have the opportunity for a living-related transplant and must wait for a cadaveric kidney (Rivers, 1987). Recipients of an unrelated or cadaveric kidney may receive a kidney with zero to six antigens in common. Current sera are maintained on all patients on the cadaveric waiting list and a final white-cell crossmatch is performed to determine compatibility just prior to transplantation. The test requires T and B lymphocytes from both the donor and potential recipient; results are usually available in 4 to 6 hours. A crossmatch determines if the potential recipient has a preformed antibody directed at the HLA antigens on the donor kidney. At some centers, patients may be called in for current sera and must wait for the crossmatch to determine if they will receive the kidney. Psychological and emotional support provided by the nurse is paramount for the often anxious and fearful recipient and family during this time.

Reducing Anxiety

Many dialysis patients are ambivalent about transplantation. This is because they are in a comfortable, known, and safe environment. The dialysis center can be a second home for these patients. They learn to trust the nursing and medical staff of their dialysis center. The dialysis unit provides the opportunity for socialization. Another factor is the uncertainty associated with transplantation. There is no guarantee the transplant will be successful. The future is uncertain, whereas on dialysis the patients may believe they know what to expect from day to day. The unknowns of transplantation can be very threatening to the security of the dialysis patient. The nurse can help allay this by establishing a trusting relationship, which can influence a patient's decision to become a candidate for transplantation. It will also facilitate adjustment to transplantation postoperatively (Thompson, 1987).

During the preoperative preparation of the kidney recipient, it is often necessary to assist the patient in formulating realistic expectations. It is stressed that transplantation is not a cure, but another form of treatment for ESRD patients. The nurse assures that the patient and family thoroughly understand the risks and limitations of transplantation. While kidney recipients often have improvement or reversal of dialysis-associated complications, the patient frequently develops new health problems from the side effects of immunosuppression and the medications used to prevent rejection (see Chapter 9). Patients with hypertension frequently remain hypertensive after transplantation and continue to require antihypertensive therapy. Diabetics have more difficulty controlling their blood sugar because of the high-dose steroid therapy initially post transplantation. Long-term graft survival varies and recipients of cadaveric kidneys are counseled for the possibility of loss of their kidney. The patient can experience loss of graft due to mechanical problems, severe acute rejection, chronic rejection, recurrence of original disease, or other long-term complications. The emotional impact of this loss may result in a long grieving process.

The use of denial as a method of coping with anxiety and apprehension is sometimes helpful for the patient and family. However, patients need to express some understanding and be able to openly discuss realistic concerns about the risks associated with transplantation before they are accepted as transplant candidates. Patients may be fearful of rejection, death, and their ability to function outside the sick role (Thompson, 1987). Some patients are concerned with cosmetic changes caused by the surgical scar and the side effects of steroids and cyclosporine (Sandimmune). As the patient awaits cadaveric transplantation, there is the stress of being "on call" 24 hours a day. The patient has no control over the timing of an event which will alter his or her life completely.

INTRAOPERATIVE MANAGEMENT

The kidney is generally placed in the right or left anterior iliac fossa. A right or a left donor kidney can be grafted to either side. The left kidney is higher because of a longer renal vein. This surgical technique is more advantageous than placing the graft in the normal anatomical position for several reasons:

- the peritoneal cavity is not entered, resulting in less postoperative pain;
- there is a reduced chance of paralytic ileus; and
- there is easier access to the graft for biopsy or any re-operative procedure.

The kidney is, therefore, superficial and can be easily palpated and auscultated to help diagnose postoperative complications, including rejection. Another advantage of placement in the iliac fossa is the closer approximation to the major recipient blood vessels and urinary bladder. Most commonly, the renal artery and vein are anastomosed to the hypogastric or the iliac artery and vein. After the kidney has been revascularized, the urinary tract is restored by the creation of a submucosal tunnel in the recipient's bladder wall for implantation of the donor ureter. An important feature of the ureteroneocystostomy is that it acts as a one-way valve. This prevents the reflux of urine to the transplanted kidney, thereby preventing the potentially devastating complication of infection. The surgery itself lasts 2 to 3 hours. A longer operative period may be necessary for multiple donor vessels, diabetics with atherosclerosis, and repeat transplants (Kottra-Buck, 1986).

Generally, the surgery is followed by a stay in the postanesthesia care unit or the special care unit for 1 to 3 days. Immediately postoperatively, the recipient requires constant monitoring of fluid and electrolyte balance and blood pressure control. Patients are told upon awakening from anesthesia that they will have a Foley catheter, central venous line, one or more peripheral intravenous lines, and a cardiac monitor. The usual length of hospital stay is 7 to 14 days, but it is contingent on renal function, potential postoperative complications, and the patient's ability to manage regimens at discharge. The surgical stitches or staples are removed approximately 14 days postoperatively unless the patient is obese, diabetic, or having wound complications.

POSTOPERATIVE MANAGEMENT

Renal function may be immediate or delayed. As soon as the kidney is revascularized, urine flows from the not yet implanted ureter. When the transplant recipient has immediate function, there is usually a rapid and progressive fall of serum creatinine and urea nitrogen. The phosphorus, calcium, and potassium levels normalize. Patients may feel much better and dialysis is no longer necessary. However, patients may experience a temporary period of delayed function that can last from several days to weeks. This is frequently caused by acute tubular necrosis (ATN). ATN is a reversible condition caused by physiological changes in donor kidneys due to oxygen interruption during the renal procurement, prolonged preservation period while a recipient is being located, or the transplant surgery itself. Cold and warm ischemic times are contributing factors to ATN. Cold ischemic time is the length of time the kidney is being preserved on ice and is increased with long-distance procurement sites due to travel time. Warm ischemic time is the amount of time from cessation of renal circulation until adequate hypothermia of the organ is achieved. Some centers include anastomosis time in total warm ischemia time. Anastomosis of the renal artery and vein normally takes 20 to 30 minutes. Surgical complications such as multiple renal arteries or hypovolemia increase anastomosis time. To complicate matters, ATN can be superimposed by a rejection episode. The patient may experience nonoliguric or high-output ATN where there is normal or greater than normal urine output without evidence of clearance of nitrogenous wastes. The patient with ATN is usually oliguric or anuric. Dialysis and/or fluid and electrolyte restrictions are necessary while awaiting resolution of ATN.

Other causes of delayed function or absence of function in the postoperative period include vascular anastomotic failure, thrombosis, infarction, obstruction of urine flow, extravasation of urine, and rejection. It is necessary to rule out these conditions before assuming the oliguria or anuria is secondary to ATN. Renal ultrasound or sonogram is a simple diagnostic test that is commonly done in concurrence with a renal scan as a baseline within the first 24 hours after surgery. The ultrasound can diagnose ureteral obstruction by demonstrating enlargement of the renal pelvis and calices. It may show evidence of hematomas, urinomas, abscesses, or lymphoceles surrounding the kidney. The renal scan involves injection of a radioactive material into a peripheral vein. It is performed to evaluate vascular supply and perfusion to the kidney. After the injection, there should be good uptake of radioactive material by the kidney from the iliac arteries. The functioning kidney should then excrete the radioactive material to the bladder via the ureter. A urinary leak is obvious if the radioactive material is visualized outside the urinary tract (Kottra-Buck, 1986). Ultrasounds and scans are repeated at various time intervals following transplantation. These radiologic tests not only are useful in diagnosing surgical complications but also can aid in the diagnosis of rejection of the kidney. Kidney biopsy is often a necessary diagnostic procedure for determining the cause of renal dysfunction. It is used to determine the type and severity of rejection and the presence of vascular or tubular changes. The procedure is done under fluoroscopy, ultrasound, or CT scan with local anesthesia. The patient is usually placed on bedrest for at least 6 hours following this procedure. The nurse observes the patient for signs of bleeding, tachycardia, hypotension, pain over the graft, falling hemoglobin and hematocrit, hematuria, or decreased urine output following the biopsy.

Rejection

Hyperacute Rejection

Hyperacute rejection occurs after the kidney is surgically implanted and causes immediate, irreversible damage. The donated kidney is incompatible with the patient's immune system and is immediately attacked by preformed cytotoxic antibodies. These pre-existing anti-HLA antibodies are developed by the patient's immune system from a previous exposure to foreign antigens. Total tissue infarction and necrosis occur and the graft must be removed. Due to advances in immunology, this type of rejection is rarely seen. Routine monthly assessments of circulating antibodies and crossmatching the donor and recipient before transplantation detect the preformed antibodies. Accelerated rejection is a term given to hyperacute rejections that occur between the second and fifth day following transplantation. The likelihood of a successful reversal of a rejection episode of this type is small (Williams, 1984).

Acute Rejection

Acute rejection is the most common type of transplant rejection and usually occurs within 24 months of the transplant. If the rejection is treated promptly, reversal is likely. The success of treatment is dependent on the length of time from onset of rejection to the initiation of treatment. Treatment may consist of intravenous steroid pulses, anti-lymphocyte sera, or monoclonal antibodies. All patients undergoing transplant are prepared for the possibility of rejection (Hopper, Sweeney, and Pierce, 1984).

Chronic Rejection

Chronic rejection is characterized by a gradual decline in glomerular filtration and permeability of the glomerulus to protein. The most common signs of chronic rejection are hypertension, proteinuria, edema, gradual rise in BUN and creatinine levels, and decreased creatinine clearance. This is a subtle process of antibody destruction of the graft progressing to end-stage failure over a period of months to years. Chronic rejection cannot be reversed and careful management of azathioprine to avoid leukopenia is necessary due to declining renal function (Williams, 1984). Adjusting medicines, diet and fluid restriction, and emotional support are provided by the nurse during the transition to chronic dialysis or re-transplant.

Assessment of renal function during the immediate postoperative period is crucial to the success of the transplant. Parameters used to evaluate renal function are serum creatinine, blood urea nitrogen, total urinary output, creatinine clearance, blood pressure, weight, and presence or absence of edema. The Foley catheter is usually left in place for 3 to 7 days. This allows for continual urine flow to avoid stretching the bladder wall, which can cause suture breakdown of the ureteral anastomosis. Common postoperative complaints are bladder spasms and urethral discomfort from the indwelling catheter. Male patients often state that this is more painful than the surgical incision. Bladder relaxants such as belladonna and opium suppositories are useful in treating the painful spasms. A thorough pain assessment by the nurse helps to differentiate between the various causes of pain in order to select the proper intervention. The catheter is removed as soon as it is deemed surgically safe. At this time, a urine specimen is sent for culture and sensitivity.

The patient often has a small bladder from a pre-transplant state of anuria or oliguria. This condition is aggravated by the use of diuretics and initially some patients need to void every 15 to 30 minutes. The nurse prepares the patient that retraining of the bladder muscle may take months. As the muscle tone improves and bladder capacity increases, the patient will have less urinary urgency and frequency. The diabetic patients have large bladders and bladder neuropathy and may have difficulty with complete emptying of the bladder. It may be necessary to prescribe medications to increase bladder tone and muscle function to enhance emptying.

Immediate Followup

Preventing Infection

Infections are the leading cause of morbidity and mortality after renal transplantation (Cohen, Hopkin and Kurtz, 1988). Any evidence of infection is thoroughly investigated. The immunosuppressive agents that protect the patient from rejection are also responsible for causing the patient to be extremely vulnerable to infection. The potential problem is most severe during the first 3 months post transplantation. Early signs of infection are often masked by the use of steroids. The infections can be bacterial, viral, fungal, or parasitic. Bacterial infections commonly involve the urinary tract, wound, lung, or IV catheter sites.

Opportunistic pathogens such as cytomegalovirus, *Pneumocystis carinii, Candida albicans,* and *Aspergillus* are life threatening in the immunocompromised host (Rivers, 1987). It may be necessary to reduce or discontinue immunosuppressive therapy in order to control infection and save the life of the patient. This can, of course, jeopardize the survival of the graft (Luckmann and Sorensen, 1987). The nurse plays an important role in the prevention of infectious complications. During the inpatient hospital course, nursing personnel use strict aseptic technique during dressing changes. The nurse caring for the newly transplanted patient avoids contact with other patients who have known communicable diseases. Strict adherence to good hand washing techniques between patients is imperative. Invasive lines such as intravenous or Foley catheters require strict asepsis. Aggressive discharge planning by the nurse can facilitate early discharge from the hospital and result in fewer nosocomial infections.

Due to a compromised immune system, the transplant recipient is

---

Table 4–5. Signs of Infection

•Fever
•Pain or achiness in chest, back, bladder, kidney
•Urinary frequency, urgency, or burning
•Cough (productive or nonproductive)
•Drainage from any wound
•Chills
•Sweating
•Generalized flu-like symptoms

---

constantly vigilant against opportunistic infections. Patients are taught to recognize the signs of infection before discharge from the hospital. They are instructed to call the transplant center if they have fever, achiness, pain, sweating, swelling, chills, productive cough, and urgency, frequency, or burning with urination (Table 4–5).

Chest x-rays are obtained if the patient has any signs of an upper respiratory tract infection. Patients are advised to avoid people who are obviously ill. If a family member becomes ill, the patient should use separate drinking glasses and practice frequent hand washing. Herpes simplex and zoster infections are common and need to be treated promptly. Patients are informed to contact the transplant center for any signs of cold sores or shingles. Acyclovir (Zovirax) is used as a treatment for both of these conditions. To prevent the overgrowth of Candida albicans, the patients are instructed to rinse their mouth with mycostatin suspension after each meal and at bedtime. The suspension is held in the mouth for 5 minutes and then swallowed. Dentures are removed before using this medication. Patients are also instructed to examine their mouth daily for the presence of yellow patches on the tongue and/or inflammation or sores in the mouth or on the tongue.

It is also important, particularly in female transplant recipients, to teach preventative measures to avoid urinary tract infections (Table 4–6).

Promoting Positive Self-Concept

There are reports of improvements in self-esteem and body image following a successful transplant (Thompson, 1987). It is not unusual for patients with functioning transplants to report feeling better within days following surgery. Patients offer comments such as "I didn't know how bad I felt," or "It has been so long since I've felt good that I didn't remember what it was like." With a successful transplant, the patient experiences an increased sense of well-being with more energy, increased appetite, and a hopeful outlook. This generalized sense of well-being can be attributed to the steroid treatment as well as to the restoration of renal

Table 4-6. **Preventive Measures to Avoid Urinary Tract Infections**

- Empty bladder every 2-4 hours
- Wash after each bowel movement
- Do not take bubble baths
- Avoid tight-fitting pants or jeans
- Void before and after sexual intercourse
- Change tampons frequently
- Take showers rather than baths
- Do not use perfume in the genital area
- See gynecologist promptly to receive treatment for vaginal discharge
- Drink 2 liters of fluid daily
- Avoid use of chlorine bleach in laundering clothes
- Follow prophylactic antibiotic therapy if previous infections have occurred

function. The emotional response is individualized and nurses must recognize that patients may experience a wide range of rapidly changing emotions following transplantation. Along with the improvements in quality of life, there exist many potential problems and new psychosocial issues that the patient must face.

Patients must live with the constant threat of rejection, infection, and other complications. Changes in physical appearance that occur as side effects of some of the immunosuppressive medications can cause low self-esteem and withdrawal from social contact. Increased responsibilities for patients include following a new healthcare regimen, seeking employment, and coping with the added medical expenses not covered by Medicare or insurance (Porter and Dreyfus, 1987).

Hopper, Sweeney, and Pierce (1984) describe the transplant psychological process in three phases: *anticipation, actualization,* and *reconciliation.* In the anticipation phase, the patient decides that transplant is a worthwhile alternative to dialysis. While awaiting transplant surgery, the patient experiences worry, fear, and conflict over the decision as well as elation and hope. After the transplant occurs, patients undergo the actualization stage, where they incorporate a new organ into their body image. This integration involves changes in the body image, coping with feelings about the donor, and the complexities of rejection. During the final or reconciliation phase, the patients and their families successfully adapt to their new existence. Realistic goals and expectations result from an understanding and acceptance of the unpredictable and fragile nature of transplantation. Patients' premorbid personalities and family structures determine the level of adjustment to the transplant process (Thompson, 1987). Potential nursing diagnoses for the post-renal transplant patient are found in Table 4-7.

Table 4–7. **Common Nursing Diagnoses for the Post-Transplant Renal Patient**

Health-Perception — Health management
- Health maintenance, altered
- Health seeking behaviors
- Infection, potential for
- Noncompliance

Activity — Exercise
- Activity intolerance
- Diversional activity deficit
- Fatigue
- Home maintenance management, impaired

Sleep — Rest
- Sleep pattern disturbance

Cognitive — Perceptual
- Decisional conflict
- Knowledge deficit
- Thought processes, altered

Self-Perception
- Anxiety
- Body image disturbance
- Chronic low self-esteem
- Fear
- Hopelessness
- Powerlessness

Role — Relationship
- Family process, altered
- Role performance, altered
- Role performance, altered
- Social interaction, impaired
- Social isolation

Sexuality — Reproductive
- Sexuality patterns, altered

Coping — Stress tolerance
- Adjustment, impaired
- Coping, ineffective individual
- Coping: compromised, ineffective family

Sexual Function

Following a successful transplant, fertility and libido improve for the majority of patients. Patients are instructed to resume sexual activities as soon as it is comfortable after the surgery. The patient is reassured by the nurse that sexual intercourse cannot harm the kidney. The renewed fertility status warrants birth-control counseling before the patient leaves the hospital. Condoms or diaphragms in conjunction with spermicides are the safest methods of contraception. Birth-control pills are not recommended because of the adverse side effects (Rickus, 1987a). Female patients are advised to avoid pregnancy for at least 1 to 1½ years after successful transplantation. There is no evidence of increased incidence of teratogenic effects related to the immunosuppressive therapy (Williams, 1984). Males can safely father children at any time after transplantation.

Long-Term Followup

After the patient's recovery from the surgery, the healthcare team works with him or her to monitor potential complications and provide prompt evaluation and management of these complications. Long-term, continuous followup care is vital to the life of the patient. Prevention, recognition, and early treatment of complications can be accomplished with a learning/teaching program that involves the nurse, the patient, and the family. Patient and family participation are vitally important components of a successful transplant program. Specific guidelines regarding self care are provided to the patient and family before discharge from the hospital. These guidelines are also reinforced in the outpatient setting. The teaching plan includes the following topics:

Rejection: Rejection is the most common complication in the first 3 months following transplant. The majority of rejection episodes occur during this period. The patient must learn the cardinal signs of rejection before leaving the hospital (Table 4–8). Prompt treatment of rejection can prevent graft loss. The chances of acute rejection occurring decrease the longer the patient has the kidney. This can be a comforting piece of information for the patient approaching or passing the 2-year mark. Severe acute rejections rarely occur after the first 2 years following transplant. The patient is also reassured that most rejection episodes are reversed and that this complication usually does not result in graft loss.

Activity: Most surgeons restrict driving for 4 to 6 weeks and heavy lifting for 3 months after the transplant. Contact sports, such as football

Table 4–8. **Signs of Rejection**

- Swollen, tender, hard kidney
- Elevated temperature
- Flu-like symptoms
- Fluid retention (swollen feet, ankles, hands, or face)
- Elevated blood pressure
- Decreased urine output
- Sudden weight gain

Table 4-9. **Nursing Priorities for the Renal Transplant Recipient**

- Monitor renal function
- Assess for rejection
- Promote normal urinary elimination patterns
- Prevent infection
- Promote maximum independence and restoration of activities of daily living
- Foster return to normal sexual functioning

and soccer, are discouraged because of the risk to the kidney from an accidental blow. An exercise program to prevent muscle wasting from long-term steroid therapy is instituted as soon as possible. Walking, biking, and swimming are good exercises to strengthen quadriceps muscles, an area particularly weakened by long-term prednisone use.

Dental Care: The patient is encouraged to practice good dental and oral hygiene after transplantation and visit the dentist every 6 months. Due to the risk of sepsis, prophylactic antibiotics are given before any dental work.

Eye Care: All patients should have a routine eye exam yearly. Patients on long-term steroid therapy may develop cataracts.

Gynecological Care: All female patients should have an exam and Pap smear every year. Immunosuppressed females have an increased risk of developing malignancy.

SUMMARY

Medicare has covered the cost of renal transplantation since 1972. Medicare protection ends 36 months after transplantation. Since 1986, Medicare has covered 80% of the cost of outpatient cyclosporine (Sandimmune) and azathioprine (Imuran) for the first 12 months following transplantation. Coverage under insurance companies, health maintenance organizations, and preferred provider organizations varies.

Renal transplantation offers nurses an exciting role as key providers of long-term care. The evaluation of candidates, pre- and postoperative teaching, and participation in long-term followup care are vital roles for the professional nurse. Table 4-9 lists the goals of nursing care for this population. Nurses have a major impact on the success of the transplant and subsequent rehabilitation of the transplant recipient. The opportunity to watch patients regain their health and return to an active life is truly a rewarding experience.

Bibliography

Cohen, J, Hopkin, J, Kurtz, H: Infectious complications after renal transplantation. In Morris, P (ed): Kidney Transplantation Principles and Practice, ed 3. WB Saunders, Philadelphia, 1988, pp 533–573.

Dailey, A: Clinical observations on renal failure and sexuality. Peritoneal Dialysis Bulletin Suppl 3(4):12–15, 1983.

Hamilton, D: Kidney transplantation: A history. In Morris, PJ (ed): Kidney Transplantation: Principles and Practice. WB Saunders, Philadelphia, 1988.

Hanson, P: Current concepts in renal transplantation. American Nephrology Nurses Association Journal 14(6):367–368, 415, 1987.

Hopper, SA, Sweeney, JT, Pierce, PF: The patient receiving a renal transplant. In Lancaster, L (ed): The Patient with End-Stage Renal Disease. Wiley Medical Publications, New York, 1984, pp 254–274.

Irwin, BC: Ethical problems in organ procurement and transplantation. American Nephrology Nurses Association Journal 13(6):305–310, 1986.

Jacobsson, PK and McNutt, GE: Holistic nursing of the client with end-stage renal disease. In Richard, C (ed.): Comprehensive Nephrology Nursing. Little Brown & Co, Boston, 1986, pp 229–245.

Kottra-Buck, C: Renal transplantation. In Richard, C (ed.): Comprehensive Nephrology Nursing. Little Brown & Co, Boston, 1986, pp 409–422.

Klein, J: Natural History of the Major Histocompatibility Complex. John Wiley & Sons, New York, 1986, p 17.

Lancaster, L: End stage renal disease: Pathophysiology assessment and intervention. In Lancaster, L (ed): The Patient with End-Stage Renal Disease. Wiley Medical Publications, New York, 1984, pp 1–21.

Luckmann, J and Sorensen, K: Medical Surgical Nursing: A Psychophysiological Approach, ed 3. WB Saunders, Philadelphia, 1987, pp 1222–1228, 1235–1239.

Porter, A and Dreyfus, K: Renal transplantation psychosocial issues. Life Cycles (Summer, 1987):13.

Rickus, M: Pregnancy in dialysis and transplant patients. American Nephrology Nurses Association Journal 14(3):189–190, 1987a.

Rickus, M: Sexual dysfunction in the femal ESRD patient. American Nephrology Nurses Association Journal 14(3):184–187, 1987b.

Rivers, R: Nursing the kidney transplant patient. RN (August, 1987):46–53.

Thompson, D: Stress in kidney recipients and their families. In Hansen, JC (ed): Family Stress. Aspen Publishers, Rockville, Maryland, 1987, pp 19–31.

Thompson, JM, et al: Clinical Nursing. CV Mosby, St Louis, 1986, pp 1031–1037.

Ting, A: HLA matching and crossmatching in renal transplantation. In Morris, P (ed): Kidney Transplantation Principles and Practice, ed 3. WB Saunders, Philadelphia, 1988, pp 183–210.

Williams, GM: Clinical course following renal transplantation. In Morris, P (ed): Kidney Transplantation Principles and Practice, ed 2. Grune & Stratton, Orlando, 1984, pp 342–346.

Zehnder, C and Blumberg, A: Human recombinant erythropoietin treatment in transfusion dependent anemic patients on maintenance hemodialysis. Clinical Nephrology 31(2):55–59, 1989.

CHAPTER

Heart Transplantation

Jo Ann I. Lamb, MSN, RN-C

Scarcely 25 years ago cardiac transplantation was viewed by the public and medical world alike as a science fiction dream. Today, it has become almost routine in many open heart surgery centers in this country and around the world.

After the first human heart transplant was performed in December, 1967, in Capetown, South Africa, transplantation efforts were slow, and only periodically successful. The first flurries of enthusiasm soon gave way to skepticism and negativism. Over the following 10 years, cardiac transplantation was pursued and improved in only a handful of centers worldwide.

By 1977, however, a cautious resurgence was beginning. In the last decade, this has been spurred by improvements in drug therapies (new immunosuppressives, monoclonal antibodies, antibiotics, antivirals), the development of the endomyocardial biopsy technique, and a better understanding of the rejection process. Concurrently, new advances in cardiac medications and techniques such as angioplasty have provided prolongation of cardiac effectiveness in failing hearts. Modern diagnostic techniques such as radionuclide tracer imaging and echocardiography have enabled physicians to correctly determine disease etiologies and refer patients earlier and more appropriately for transplantation. In 1987, according to the Office of Health Technology of the Department of Health and Human Services, 1512 heart transplants were done in the United States.

The goal of cardiac transplantation is to return terminally ill patients to an active and productive life-style. This has become a reasonable patient goal.

APPLYING PATHOPHYSIOLOGY OF CARDIAC FAILURE

Anything that interferes with the normal functioning of the heart can precipitate cardiac disease. Weakening of the cardiac muscle because of excessive stretching (dilatation) or thinning (e.g., an aneurysm), scarring of the muscle wall, inflammation (myocarditis), or anoxia-induced cell death after infarction may prevent normal contraction and pumping. Heart valves can weaken and prolapse, allowing regurgitation of blood, or they may become calcified and noncompliant (stenosed), impeding forward flow. The coronary artery walls may become thickened, with narrowing or occlusion of the lumen due to arteriosclerosis. This leads to cellular oxygen deprivation. Rhythm disturbances of many types may prevent the myocardium from contracting properly and may lead to life-threatening dysrhythmias and death. Congenital defects may cause immediate or eventual left ventricular insufficiency that may also lead to transplantation.

The result of any of these problems is the inability of the heart to perform adequately as a pump. The outcome is lowered cardiac output that is insufficient to meet the body's needs. Consequently, stagnation or backup of blood occurs in all parts of the body.

Many cardiac conditions can be worsened by poor health practices. Smoking, drinking alcohol, excessive weight, sedentary living, and a diet high in salt and fats can weaken the heart muscle and lead to heart failure. Hypertension and diabetes also have deleterious effects on the heart. Patient teaching should stress the elimination of risk factors and encourage adherence to diet and medication regimens. Because a healthy heart life-style, cardiac medications, and invasive and noninvasive treatments can prevent terminal heart disease in most people, cardiac transplantation is a relatively rarely indicated mode of therapy.

ASSESSING FOR CLINICAL SIGNS AND SYMPTOMS

Because of poor blood flow to the brain, viscera, and extremities, patients in heart failure usually complain of profound fatigue, shortness of breath, and swelling of the ankles when giving a health history. The nurse's assessment includes these signs and symptoms. Angina may be present due to coronary ischemia. The patient may describe poor memory, mood swings, dyspnea, and chronic cough. The client may also describe abdominal enlargement as ascites develops and loss of weight and abdominal pain from intestinal ischemia. As the heart attempts to compensate, there may be tachycardia and dysrhythmias. The patient may complain of "palpitations" or "skipped" beats.

When performing a physical assessment, the nurse may find a rapid and irregular pulse, jugular vein distention from backup of blood due to right-sided heart failure, and rales and rhonchi due to left-sided heart failure. Examination of the heart may reveal the point of maximal impulse (PMI) dislocated to the left, and an S3 or S4 gallop may be detected on auscultation. The nurse may assess for an enlarged liver and abdominal tenderness due to congestive pressure from the right side of the heart. Pitting edema may be found in the legs and feet. The nurse recognizes severe, terminal failure by extreme cachexia, ascites, jaundice, tachypnea, tachycardia, and dysrhythmias.

SELECTING THE RECIPIENT

Selection of appropriate recipients for heart transplantation is crucial to the achievement of satisfactory results. Cardiac transplantation is considered a procedure of last resort. This implies that the failure of the heart is untreatable by any other medical and surgical approaches. These treatments may have been attempted without lasting success. Patients requiring cardiac transplantation have suffered severe end-stage congestive failure (New York Heart Association [NYHA] class IV) that may have been caused by many conditions (Table 5–1).

Table 5–1. **Indications for Heart Transplantation**

- Congenital malformations
- Valvular heart disease
- Arteriosclerotic coronary artery disease
- Cardiomyopathy:
  - Viral
  - Ischemic
  - Idiopathic
  - Familial
  - Postpartum
- Ventricular aneurysm
- Primary cardiac tumor
- Inability to wean from cardiopulmonary bypass

Patients who are referred for transplantation may have had trials of various medications, diagnostic catheterization, pacemaker insertion, or heart surgery to repair aneurysms or perform coronary artery bypass grafting. Transplantation is usually not done unless the heart has significantly deteriorated. Patients who are advised to undergo this procedure are generally considered to have less than a year to live.

The definition of significant risk factors for cardiac transplantation varies from one institution to another. Some still adhere to the stringent criteria that were applied during the early years of cardiac replacement. These prohibited surgery for patients over 50 years of age, or those with a history of insulin-dependent diabetes, severe hypertension, peptic ulcers, neoplasms, peripheral vascular disease, pulmonary hypertension, cardiac cachexia, or other signs of end-stage failure. Such patients were felt to be at further high risk related to treatment with steroid drugs postoperatively, or for not surviving the surgical insult. With recent advances in immunosuppression, and better organ preservation and postoperative support mechanisms, transplantation is now offered to some carefully selected patients who may have pre-existing conditions (Table 5–2).

At some centers, pediatric cardiac transplantation is still considered experimental or ill-advised. However, it is being attempted more frequently with growing success. Neonatal cardiac transplantation is also being applied cautiously in a few centers with remarkably good results (Bailey, 1988). However, the future for these forms of transplantation is yet to be determined.

MANAGING THE PRE-TRANSPLANT PATIENT

Selecting the Recipient

Most cardiac illnesses are first diagnosed by the patient's local doctor or a consulting cardiologist in the home community. The patient may be admitted to his or her regional hospital for preliminary diagnostic workup following either an acute cardiac event or gradual increase in cardiac symptoms. Subsequent admissions will often occur as the disease progresses and the staff of the coronary care unit or cardiac medical-surgical unit will become well acquainted with the patient and his or her family. As the cardiac illness progresses, successive admissions, diagnostic procedures, medication trials, or surgery will probably each fail to provide much lasting relief for the patient. Patient and family teaching and support by the nursing staff help lead to acceptance of the terminal nature of the disease and preparation for transplantation, if possible, or death.

Referral of the patient for transplantation may herald new emotional stressors for the patient and family as well as the staff. They must under-

Table 5-2. **Risk Factors for Cardiac Transplantation**

- Age over 65 years.
- Insulin-requiring diabetes mellitus
- Systemic diseases (e.g., active neoplasms) or co-existing terminal entities
- Marked obesity
- Irreversible dysfunction of extracardiac organ systems including renal, hepatic, pulmonary, central nervous
- Severe peripheral vascular disease
- Recent or unresolved pulmonary embolism or infarction
- Unresolved substance abuse or psychiatric disorder
- Active infectious process

stand that all other therapies have been futile and that this seemingly radical approach is their only hope. Some patients refuse to be evaluated for transplantation through ignorance or fear, or because they feel their emotional reserves have been exhausted. Many more patients and families readily accept the potential option that transplantation may offer. Still others refuse transplantation because they do not see it as having potential for improving their quality of life.

After the patient accepts referral and is admitted to the transplant center, he or she may be filled with additional apprehensions. The transplant center may be in a distant city where the patient has no friends or support. Becoming acquainted with a new health team adds stress.

Nurses at the transplant center will introduce the patients to their new environment and try to facilitate the adjustment. In addition, nurses provide teaching and emotional support for the newly admitted patients and describe the procedures that will be done as part of the transplant workup.

Evaluating the Candidate

The evaluation of the prospective transplant candidate is usually done in the hospital because most patients are too ill to endure repeated visits to the center. The patient's personal physician may be willing to perform many of the evaluative tests. Completion of the workup is then done at the transplant center. This has the advantage of requiring less travel and stress for the ill client (Table 5-3).

At the transplant center, the patient and family members are usually seen in consultation with the various members of the transplant team. This may include personnel from cardiology, surgery, nursing, social service, psychiatry, physical therapy, neurology, pastoral care, and dietary divisions. All of these consultants evaluate the patient from their special

---

Table 5 – 3. **Evaluation of the Potential Cardiac Transplant Recipient**

- Complete medical history
- Physical examination
- Laboratory studies:
  - Biochemical electrolyte and metabolic profiles, liver function tests, triglycerides, cholesterol, urine analysis
  - Hematologic: completed blood count (CBC), platelet count, prothrombin time (PT), and partial thromboplastin time (PTT)
  - Immunologic: ABO type and antibody screen, donor-specific lymphocyte toxicity (random panel)
  - Chest x-ray
  - Virologic and microbiologic: cytomegalovirus (CMV), Epstein-Barr virus (EBV), human immune deficiency virus (HIV), rapid plasma reagent (RPR), *Aspergillus*, toxoplasmosis, *Candida*, hepatitis antigen and antibody, purified protein derivative (PPD)
- Pulmonary function testing (if indicated)
- Cardiac catheterization (right, left, or both) with endomyocardial biopsy and angiography as indicated
- Electrocardiogram

---

perspective and create a plan of care depending on the patient's needs. This may include referral for transplantation.

Most cardiac transplant centers have nurse coordinators, clinical nurse specialists, or nurse practitioners who facilitate the myriad needs of each patient as he or she proceeds through the transplant process. Because a thorough understanding of each patient's needs and compulsive medical and nursing followup is essential to long-term success for cardiac transplantation, most centers find these team members indispensable for coordinating and facilitating care.

Patients who are found acceptable for transplantation and are clinically stable may be referred back to their local physician while awaiting identification of a suitable donor heart. A patient who lives many miles from the transplant center may decide to relocate nearby and be followed at the transplant clinic. These practices will vary depending on geographical considerations and the policies and capacity of the transplant center. If the patient is found to be an unsuitable candidate for transplantation, care will also be transferred back to the local physician.

Nursing Support While Awaiting Transplantation

Patients who are accepted for cardiac transplantation are placed on the waiting list for a suitable donor heart. Patients are grouped according to clinical status and blood type, and donor hearts are chosen for them according to blood type compatibility, size, and other factors that may

Table 5–4. A Typical Waiting List for Heart Transplantation

Blood Group	Name	Wks on List	Dx	Age (yrs)	Weight (lbs)
A	Smith	20	CAD	45	160
A	Maloney	10	ICM	52	140
A	Charles	1	CAD	49	120
AB	Droop	40	ICM	30	138
B	Brown	35	CAD	55	166
B	Murphy	18	ICM	29	122
O	Peacock	12	ICM	33	136
O	Feldman	9	ICM	39	112
O	Anderson	8	CHD	22	188
O	Jones	5	ICM	44	155
O	Diaz	1	CAD	60	179

CAD = coronary artery disease; ICM = ischemic cardiomyopathy; CHD = coronary heart disease.

vary from center to center. These include degree of illness, length of time on the waiting list, age, previous chest or open-heart surgery, and presence and degree of pulmonary hypertension. Donor/recipient compatibility may need to be determined by direct crossmatching for certain recipients. Table 5–4 shows a typical waiting list for cardiac transplantation. Prospective recipients are also listed on the computer system of the United Network for Organ Sharing (UNOS) as described in Chapter 1.

The waiting period has often been described as the most difficult and stressful time of the entire transplant process by patients and family members alike. During this time of active candidacy, the patient's disease progresses and may be only minimally controlled by medications, diet, fluid and salt restriction, and decreased activity. Patients may require frequent rehospitalization for treatment of worsening failure, readjustment of medications, diuresis with intravenous cardiotonic drugs, and increased rest. Patients may be disappointed by false alarms when donors are found to be unacceptable, or when other patients on the list are transplanted ahead of them. They and their families often suffer alternating feelings of hope and despair. Indeed, the patient may be one of those who die on the waiting list while awaiting a suitable heart. It is not uncommon for patients to wait weeks to months for a donor that is compatible. Invariably, some patients die while awaiting transplantation. This varies depending on the length of the list, season of the year, and the donor supply in any given geographical area. A list of common nursing diagnoses for the pre-transplant patient is presented in Table 5–5, and a list of possible pre-transplant complications is presented in Table 5–6.

When a suitable donor is identified, the prospective recipient waiting outside of the hospital is notified by phone or beeper. This may occur at

Table 5–5. Common Nursing Diagnoses for the Pre-Transplant Heart Patient

Health Perception — Health Management
- Health maintenance, altered, possibly related to
  - denial of illness
  - inadequate energy
  - depression
- Health seeking behaviors
- Infection, potential for, possibly related to
  - debilitated state
  - cachexia
- Noncompliance (potential for)

Nutritional — Metabolic
- Fluid volume, altered: excess
- Nutrition, altered: less than body requirements, possibly related to
  - decreased appetite
  - malabsorption

Activity-Exercise
- Cardiac output, altered: decreased, possibly related to
  - increased preload
  - decreased afterload
- Home maintenance management, impaired
- Mobility, impaired physical
- Self-care deficit: total
- Tissue perfusion, altered, possibly related to
  - decreased cardiac output

Sleep — Rest
- Sleep pattern disturbance, possibly related to
  - paroxysmal nocturnal dyspnea (PND)
  - angina
  - nocturia
  - anxiety

Self-Perception — Self-Concept
- Anxiety
- Fatigue
- Fear
- Hopelessness
- Powerlessness
- Self-concept, disturbance in: body image, possibly related to
  - chronic illness
  - weight loss
  - hair loss

Role — Relationship
- Family process, altered
- Grieving, anticipatory
- Self-concept, disturbance in: role performance
- Social interaction, impaired

Table 5–5. Common Nursing Diagnoses for the Pre-Transplant Heart Patient (*Continued*)

Sexuality — Reproductive
• Sexual dysfunction

Coping — Stress Tolerance
• Adjustment, impaired
• Coping, ineffective individual, possibly related to
  ◦ denial
• Coping, ineffective: compromised

Value — Belief
• Spiritual distress

Table 5–6. Potential Complications for the Preoperative Heart Transplant Patient

Gastrointestinal — Hepatic
• Hepatorenal syndrome
• Hyperbilirubinemia
• Ascites

Metabolic — Immune
• Negative nitrogen balance
• Electrolyte imbalance
• Sepsis
• Acidosis/alkalosis
• Anasarca

Neurologic — Sensory
• Stroke
• Paresis/paresthesia

Cardiovascular
• Dysrhythmias
• Congestive heart failure
• Cardiogenic shock
• Thromboemboli
• Peripheral vascular insufficiency
• Anemia

Respiratory
• Atelectasis/pneumonia
• Pulmonary embolism
• Pleural effusion
• Ventilator dependency

Renal — Urinary
• Renal failure

any hour of the day or night and the patient has to be constantly available. The patient needs to be given sufficient time to get to the hospital, and is usually asked not to eat or drink anything after being called in. He or she is reminded that a decision regarding the acceptability of the donor heart will not be made until the recovery surgeons have actually seen the heart at the donor hospital. The patient knows that the transplant may be cancelled at any time up until the actual removal of the heart from the donor. Because the donor heart has to be transplanted in the recipient within about 4 hours of removal, the recipient and the donor surgery have to proceed at the same time. Therefore, the recipient surgery may be aborted even after the recipient has been taken to the operating room if the donor heart is not perfect. Nothing that is surgically irreversible is done to the recipient until the donor heart is found to be acceptable and is ready for transplantation.

Physical preoperative preparation includes routine blood tests and a chest x-ray. The chest may be shaved or just washed with a cleansing solution. A preoperative dose of immunosuppressive drug(s) will often be given just prior to sending the patient to the operating room, depending on the institutional procedure.

Preoperative teaching involves a description of the operating room, the personnel the patient will meet, and the clothing they wear. The anesthesiologist and nurses will explain each step of the anesthesia procedure, including placement of intravenous lines, arterial line, and central pressure monitoring catheters, and the administration of anesthesia. The patient is told what to expect on awakening in the intensive care unit. They are taught that they will have an incision, bandages, chest tubes, and an endotracheal tube that will be attached to a ventilator which will not allow them to talk. Reassurance is given that the nurses will anticipate most of their needs. Patients are told that they will be able to write messages if their wishes are not understood. The patients are also taught that they may feel drowsy and have a sensation of heaviness in their arms and legs until the anesthesia wears off. Numerous intravenous lines, tubes, and catheters can be expected, and there may be strange sights, sounds, and smells that are all normal parts of the ICU environment. The nurse explains that the patient will not be able to eat or drink for the first 24 to 48 hours. They are assured that they will be given sufficient medication to alleviate pain and to permit them to cooperate with chest physiotherapy and leg exercises. These measures help decrease anxiety and promote patient compliance. Patients who have had previous open heart surgery may be more relaxed because they know what to expect. Conversely, a bad previous experience may exacerbate apprehension. Finally, the isolation policies and visiting rules that will vary from hospital to hospital are explained to the patient and family.

MANAGING THE PATIENT INTRAOPERATIVELY

The cardiac transplant procedure is done in an unmodified open heart surgery operating room. The usual open heart team can be used, including anesthesiologists, nurses, and cardiopulmonary technicians. The surgery is done through a median sternotomy and the patient is placed on cardiopulmonary bypass. Usually an intravenous dose of steroids is given at the beginning of the case. The recipient's ventricles and anterior atria are removed, leaving the posterior atria as cuffs for the implantation of the donor heart.

The donor and recipient surgery proceed at the same time. If the donor hospital is distant from the transplant center, tight coordination is required to see that the donor heart arrives in the recipient operating room just as the explanted (diseased) heart is removed.

The posterior atrial walls of the donor heart are anastomosed to the remnant cuffs of the recipient atria and the aorta and pulmonary artery are anastomosed end-to-end. Figure 5–1 represents an orthotopic heart transplant. The blood is slowly rewarmed through the cardiopulmonary bypass circuit. As the heart is gradually allowed to fill and stretch, a spontaneous rhythm often begins. If not, low-voltage defibrillation is used to initiate a regular beat. Occasionally, pacing wires are left in place for several days if the heart function is not vigorous and regular.

Heterotopic heart transplantation involves the implantation of a donor heart beside the native heart while leaving the latter in place. The posterior atria of donor and recipient are connected together and the aorta and pulmonary artery of the donor heart are attached in end-to-end fashion to the recipient's vessels. This procedure provides auxiliary pumping in the case of patients who have pulmonary hypertension that is too high to allow the orthotopic transplantation procedure described above. (The patient's native right ventricle becomes hypertrophied in order to deliver blood to the hypertensive lungs. A normal donor right ventricle does not have enough strength to provide this propulsion and abruptly fails.) After transplantation, the native heart continues to provide most of the right ventricular function while the heterotopic donor left ventricle often provides most of the left ventricular flow. The four ventricular chambers may gradually equilibrate over time. It has also been suggested that heterotopic transplantation is the procedure of choice for patients with intractable angina or active myocarditis that might heal over time (Barnard, 1981). These patients require anticoagulation due to sluggish flow in the native left ventricle and to the danger of emboli. While this procedure can work well, most transplants today are orthotopic procedures.

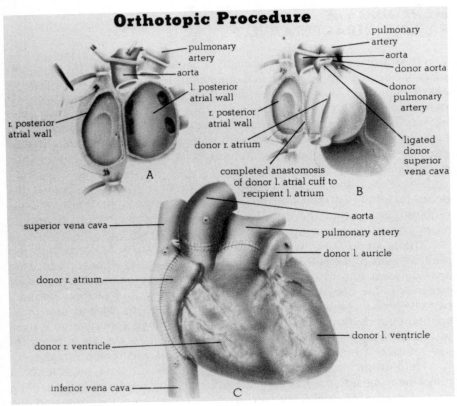

Figure 5-1

Orthotopic heart transplant procedure that replaces the recipient's anterior atria and ventricles completely. (From Herman, M: Heart Transplantation. Am J Nurs 80(10):1786, 1980, with permission.)

MANAGING THE POST-TRANSPLANT PATIENT

The First Forty-Eight Hours

The postoperative care of the cardiac transplant patient is similar in most respects to that required following conventional open heart surgery. The nurse will emphasize to the patient and family that the patient has a new, healthy heart, not one that has undergone repair. Therefore, full cardiac function can be expected soon after the anesthesia leaves the patient's system. The patient's preoperative ischemia or dysrhythmia problems will bother him or her no longer and, because the heart is denervated, angina will not occur. A thorough knowledge of the patient's related clinical problems is helpful as resolution may take time after normal perfusion is restored through the transplanted heart.

Routine aspects of postoperative open heart surgery nursing care include maintenance of adequate ventilatory function and acid-base balance. The nurse monitors cardiac function for any signs of failure, dysrhythmias, or ECG changes that may be due to ischemia caused by intraoperative cooling, perioperative infarction, or cardiac tamponade. Through hemodynamic monitoring, the nurse identifies hypertension, hypotension, and intracardiac or intrapulmonary pressure changes. Fluid and electrolyte balance is maintained with special attention to hemorrhagic output from the chest tube. Renal failure may be due to decreased cardiac output or renal perfusion. Emboli may occur in patients during or following cardiopulmonary bypass. Patients also need to be observed for normal recovery from anesthesia, including gradual return of consciousness, motor strength, and appropriate response to commands. The nurse needs to be aware of complications that may affect those patients who have undergone a transplant.

Because of the terminal nature of the disease, transplant patients may have greater end-stage organ failure than patients usually selected for open heart surgery.

Ventricular failure in the early postoperative hours may occur secondary to ischemia from prolonged donor organ transport time. Right-heart failure sometimes occurs in patients whose preoperative intrapulmonary pressures were relatively high. Sluggish forward flow of the right side of the heart often prevents prompt clearance of hepatic and lower extremity vessels. This leads to hepatic congestion, ascites, peripheral stasis, and extravasation of fluid in the lower extremities.

Assessment of renal function may reveal decreased output or anuria accompanied by an elevated blood urea nitrogen (BUN) and creatinine. This may be due to the patient's pre-transplant heart failure or failure of the donor heart. The most likely cause, however, is the immunosuppressive drug cyclosporine, especially if the BUN and creatinine have risen since surgery (Lamb, 1988).

Emboli may occur on the arterial side (to coronary arteries, brain, kidneys, periphery) due to a residual clot in the left atrial cuff. (A large, tightly adherent clot sometimes forms in massively dilated atria when low blood flow occurs due to profound pre-transplant failure.) Patients who undergo heterotopic (parallel) heart transplantation will also require anticoagulation.

Anticoagulation is necessary to prevent clot formation in the sluggish native left ventricle. The presence of Dacron grafts that may be used in vessel anastomoses also increases the risk of clot formation.

Myocardial infarction may occur due to intraoperative manipulation of the heart or prolonged transport time for the donor organ. A transplant recipient who suffers ischemia due to thrombosis or infarction will not have angina because the graft has been denervated. The diagnosis is made by observing ECG changes and rising cardiac enzymes. The nursing assessment includes signs and symptoms of diaphoresis, nausea and vomiting, and dysrhythmias.

Recovery from anesthesia may be much slower than usual in any patient who has had severe liver failure and cerebral hypoxia from poor heart function preoperatively. The nurse offers frequent reassurances to patient and family and attempts to reorient the slowly awakening patient.

Infection may occur, related to the immunocompromise that begins at the time of the transplant surgery. Strict aseptic technique is applied by all caregivers when adjusting tubes, intravenous or intra-arterial lines, and catheters. All lines, tubes, and catheters are removed as soon as possible. Routine antibiotics are administered for 2 to 3 days, as ordered, and care of the wound is fastidious. The nurse ensures that chest physiotherapy and leg exercises are performed routinely. The nurse carefully monitors the patient for signs or symptoms of infection, including fever, reddened or painful wounds, pulmonary or urinary tract distress, signs of pericarditis, or postcardiotomy syndrome. Fever may not be evidenced by the immunosuppressed patient. A pericardial friction rub may also be found in the early postoperative period. The nurse monitors its presence, effect on cardiac function, and resolution.

A list of common nursing diagnoses for the post-transplant patient is presented in Table 5–7, and a list of possible post-transplant complications is presented in Table 5–8.

Initial Rehabilitation Period

After the first 48 hours, the patient usually begins ambulation. The physiotherapist provides a program of increasingly complex activity for the patient.

During this time, the patient also begins to learn the new medication regimen. This usually requires frequent reinforcement and supervision by the nurse, with the goal of independence in self-medication before discharge.

Table 5-7 **Common Nursing Diagnoses for the Post-Transplant Heart Patient**

Health Perception — Health Management
- Noncompliance, possibly related to
  ◦ denial of post-transplant status
  ◦ fear of graft failure
  ◦ depression

Nutritional — Metabolic
- Infection, potential for, possibly related to
  ◦ immunosuppressed state
- Nutrition, altered: potential for more than body requirements, possibly related to
  ◦ steroids

Activity — Exercise
- Growth and development, altered, possibly related to
  ◦ steroids

Sleep-Rest
- Sleep pattern disturbance, possibly related to
  ◦ steroids
  ◦ nocturia

Self-Perception — Self-Concept
- Anxiety
- Fear
- Self-concept, disturbance in: body image, possibly related to
  ◦ moon face
  ◦ truncal obesity
  ◦ hirsutism
  ◦ scars and striae
  ◦ acne

Role — Relationship
- Family process, altered

Sexuality — Reproductive
- Sexual dysfunction

Coping — Stress Tolerance
- Adjustment, impaired
- Coping, ineffective individual, possibly related to
  ◦ denial
- Coping, ineffective family: compromised

Managing Rejection

Cardiac rejection is the largest individual threat to success in cardiac transplantation. Although several innovative diagnostic methods are under investigation, cardiac biopsy, first developed in 1962 by Sakaki-barra and Konno and made clinically applicable by Caves in 1973, remains the most sensitive method for the diagnosis of acute rejection. Patients

Table 5-8. Potential Complications for the Postoperative Heart Transplant Patient

Gastrointestinal — Hepatic
- Ascites
- Gastrointestinal bleeding

Metabolic — Immune
- Hyperglycemia
- Sepsis
- Diabetes
- Donor heart rejection
- Adrenal insufficiency

Neurologic — Sensory
- Stroke
- Seizures
- Meningitis
- Neuropathies

Cardiovascular
- Dysrhythmias
- Congestive heart failure
- Cardiogenic shock
- Thromboemboli
- Peripheral vascular insufficiency
- Hypertension
- Thrombocytopenia
- Anemia

Respirtory
- Atelectasis/pneumonia
- Pleural effusion

Renal — Urinary
- Renal failure

Musculoskeletal
- Osteoporosis

usually undergo their first biopsy within a week of transplant surgery and additional biopsies on a schedule of decreasing frequency over the subsequent months. The procedure is typically performed in the cardiac catheterization laboratory under fluoroscopy. A catheter introducer is placed in the right internal jugular vein and intracardiac and intrapulmonary pressures are measured with a central catheter. A bioptome is then introduced and advanced into the right ventricle, where tiny tissue samples are obtained. Figure 5-2 shows the endomyocardial biopsy technique. The pathologist or surgeon determines if rejection is present and determines the treatment regimen. The infiltration of white blood cells into the heart may herald the beginning of rejection. A low grade but persistent fever or malaise may also be early signs of rejection. Treatment of rejection usually

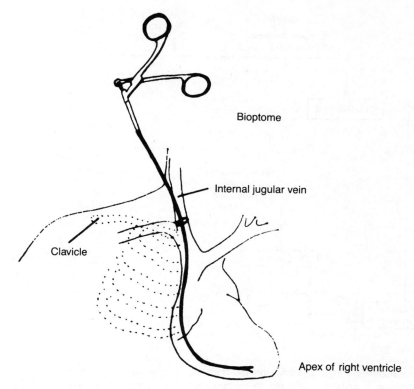

Bioptome

Internal jugular vein

Clavicle

Apex of right ventricle

Figure 5–2

Endomyocardial biopsy technique showing the bioptome in place in the right ventricle. (From Copeland, JG and Hinson, EB: Human Heart Transplantation. Current Problems in Cardiology 4(8):21, 1979, with permission.)

involves an increase in the oral prednisone dose or administration of intravenous steroids, monoclonal antibodies, or anti-lymphocyte preparations. Figure 5–3 is a decision-making algorithm for treatment of cardiac rejection.

Patient teaching during this stage of recovery is essential to long-term success. The nurse assures that the patient and care partner fully understand all of the post-cardiac transplant protocols and the reasons for each one. The patient and family will be required to verbalize the signs and symptoms of rejection and infection and the importance of reporting these to their healthcare providers. The most profound problems in the aftercare of cardiac transplant patients as well as causes of death have occurred when patients did not call for help.

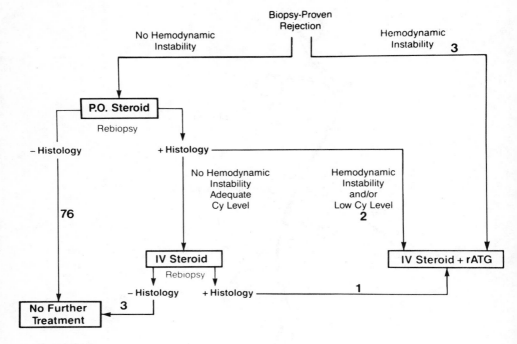

Figure 5 – 3

A decision-making algorithm for treatment of biopsy-proven cardiac rejection (Cy = cyclosporine; rATG = rabbit anti-thymocyte globulin). (From Michler, RE, et al: Reversal of cardiac transplant rejection without massive immunosuppression. Circulation 74(Suppl 3):68, 1986, with permission of the American Heart Association, Inc.)

Patient Education

It is not safe to discharge cardiac transplant patients from the hospital until they or their care partner have fully mastered the required medication regimen, diet, and exercise plan. Some patients may need extensive support from a relative, friend, or visiting nurse service. Most patients, however, will have returned to a state of moderate activity and independence with daily activities that is improved from the pre-transplant status.

The patient must know and understand the schedule of appointments, biopsies, lab tests, and how and when to contact the designated healthcare provider. Reinforcement is given to the patient regarding stress management and abstinence from drinking alcohol, smoking, and recreational drugs. Reduction of other risk factors for cardiac disease is also included. They are warned that the transition back into the family as a healthy, contributing member may not be smooth and that social workers, psychiatrists, or other counselors may be needed to assist with this change.

Both short- and long-term survival of patients undergoing cardiac transplantation are still improving. However, patients who do not have co-morbid conditions at the time of transplantation enjoy better than 95% operative survival, and over 80% one-year survival. While no one yet knows how long cardiac transplant patients can be expected to live, the numbers of patients being followed worldwide are growing rapidly and most centers achieve 65% or better survival beyond 5 years. The important fact, however, is that more than 97% of cardiac transplant patients regain NYHA class I activity level. Within a year or two, most patients are able to return to their previous activities whether these are full-time employment, household work, or attendance at school.

Rehabilitation and Outpatient Care

The extent of rehabilitation for the cardiac transplant patient usually depends on his or her degree of debility before the transplant. Many weeks or months of therapy may be required to return patients who had deteriorated significantly to full functioning. Some patients enroll in cardiovascular fitness programs in their home community after initial work with the cardiac transplant physical therapist. Eventual full recovery is expected in most cases.

Patients are followed as outpatients at the transplant center according to each center's policy. Some transplant centers follow the patients exclusively, in perpetuity, while others return responsibility for the patient to the referring physician. However it is done, it is essential that the cardiac transplant patient continue to have close medical supervision and immunosuppression monitoring.

Financial Aspects

In most areas of the country today, cardiac transplantation is covered by both private insurance and public assistance medical programs. Some Medicaid offices may also assist the patient with travel and living expenses during the waiting and post-transplant periods when the patient may be visiting the transplant center frequently. Medicare now covers cardiac transplantation at selected centers throughout the United States. Some transplant centers require a cash deposit before cardiac transplant patients can be evaluated. Historically cardiac transplantation has been very expensive, and reimbursement amounts have been inadequate to cover the expenses that are incurred.

Future Directions

Despite an increase in public awareness campaigns and professional education concerning identification of suitable donors and organ donation, the need for donor hearts still outweighs the supply. Research continues toward effective artificial hearts and heart assist devices, and progress can be expected in these areas over the next decade. Until the day that a heart can be taken off the shelf and implanted into a needy patient, organ donation remains our only hope. It is extremely important that healthcare providers educate themselves in the area of organ donor identification and recovery processes.

Bibliography

Barnard, CN, et al: The present status of heterotopic cardiac transplantation. J Thorac Cardiovasc Surg 81:433–439, 1981.

Bailey, Leonard, et al: Surveillance techniques in infant heart transplantation. In Heart and Heart/Lung Transplant Update. Uses Edizione Scientifiche, Florence, 1986.

Baumgartner, W, et al: Organization, development and early results of a heart transplant program: The Johns Hopkins experience. Chest 89(6):836–839, 1986.

Caves, PK, et al: Diagnosis of human cardiac allograft rejection by serial cardiac biopsy. J Thorac Cardiovasc Surg 66:461, 1973.

Funk, M: Heart transplantation: Postoperative care during the acute period. Critical Care Nurse 6:2, 1986.

Gibson, G: Harefield's choice. Nursing Times (July, 1987):368.

Lamb, J: Cardiac transplantation. In Johanson, BC, et al (eds): Standards for Critical Care Nursing, ed 3. CV Mosby, St Louis, 1988.

Lamb, J and Carlson, V: Handbook of Cardiovascular Nursing. JB Lippincott, Philadelphia, 1986.

Lough, ME, et al: Impact of symptom frequency and symptom distress on self-reported quality of life in heart transplant recipients. Heart Lung 16:2, 1987.

Rudolphi, D, Nagy, K, and Verne, D: Cardiac transplantation. AORN Journal 45:1, 1987.

Sakakibarra, S and Konno, S: Endomyocardial biopsy. Jpn Heart J 3:537, 1962.

CHAPTER

Heart-Lung and Single Lung Transplantation

Sharon M. Augustine, RN, MS, CANP

Combined heart and lung transplantation has progressed from an experimental procedure sporadically performed during the last three decades to an accepted option for selected patients with end-stage cardiopulmonary disease. Prior to the first successful heart-lung transplantation procedure by Reitz and associates in 1981 at Stanford University in a 45-year-old woman (Reitz, et al., 1982), patients with end-stage pulmonary vascular disease had limited therapeutic options. Early attempts at both unilateral lung transplantation and combined heart-lung transplantation were unsuccessful primarily due to lung infection and inadequate tracheobronchial healing secondary to steroid-based immunosuppression. Additionally, inadequate ability to recognize and treat rejection contributed to the overall dismal results.

HISTORICAL OVERVIEW

Successful heart-lung transplantation was initially accomplished in a small primate animal model (Reitz, et al., 1980). Primates did not exhibit abnormal breathing mechanisms associated with bilateral denervation (Castaneda, 1972) observed during the earlier canine experiments. The introduction of cyclosporine (Sandimmune) provided the necessary immunosuppression for successful transplantation (Reitz, et al., 1982). Since

89

that time, heart-lung transplantation has been performed in over 140 patients in the United States as well as in numerous recipients outside of the United States (Fragomeni and Kaye, 1988). Results are encouraging, with one-year survival of 60% to 70%, but not yet as good as for heart or kidney transplants. Survivors, however, usually experience a marked improvement in quality of life. Heart-lung transplantation has now become a realistic option for patients with end-stage pulmonary vascular disease.

ISOLATED LUNG TRANSPLANTATION

In recent years, the majority of clinical successes have been obtained with combined heart-lung transplantation in one bloc. Single lung transplantation, however, has also benefited from much experimental study. In 1963, Hardy and associates performed the first human lung transplantation using a single lung (Hardy, et al., 1963). Like heart-lung transplantation, discouraging results over the next few years led to a decline in the number of procedures performed. Recently, however, single and bilateral lung transplantations have been performed with higher predictability of results (Cooper, et al., 1987). It was suggested at one time that because of the apparent success, combined heart-lung transplantation was the optimal procedure in any patient requiring a lung transplant. This is no longer necessarily the best choice. Advantages for the combined procedure are better tracheal anastomotic healing and removal of all diseased or infected lung tissue from the thorax (Veith, et al., 1983; Reitz, et al., 1983). Today, with the use of cyclosporine, tracheal healing is no longer a major obstacle. Single lung transplantation, in the absence of pulmonary infection, has proven effective in the treatment of patients with interstitial fibrosis (Veith, et al., 1983; Cooper, et al., 1987; Goldsmith, et al., 1987). Since most patients requiring lung transplantation have advanced pulmonary vascular disease, any single lung graft must accept the major portion of pulmonary blood flow without overworking the right ventricle. Patients having pulmonary fibrosis are ideal candidates for unilateral lung transplantation. Poor compliance and increased pulmonary vascular resistance of the remaining native lung should ensure that ventilation as well as perfusion is directed to the transplanted lung (Toronto Lung Transplantation Group, 1986). Conversely, the alveolar air trapping in patients with emphysema may aggravate ventilation-perfusion mismatches and/or shifting of the mediastinum toward the transplanted lung (Toronto Lung Transplantation Group, 1986; Stevens, et al., 1970).

Bilateral lung transplantation offers a potential advantage to patients in whom single lung transplantation is not feasible but cardiac function is adequate. In addition to expansion of the precious donor pool, accelerated cardiac graft atherosclerosis is avoided in isolated double lung transplantation. Optimistic with success in animal models, Dark and associates proposed double lung transplantation for patients with pulmonary sepsis in the absence of cardiac involvement (i.e., bronchiectasis, cystic fibrosis, and emphysema) (Dark, et al., 1986). The future proposals for lung transplantation might be single lung transplantation for pulmonary fibrosis, double lung transplantation for diffuse lung disease, and heart-lung transplantation for pulmonary vascular disease. Donor limitations, however, currently preclude wide application of any of these procedures.

ANATOMY AND PHYSIOLOGY

Before discussing the major diagnoses leading to heart-lung transplantation, it is important to review briefly the determinants of pulmonary artery pressure. The key points of the determinants of pulmonary artery pressure are related to blood flow and resistance. The pulmonary circulation accommodates the entire right ventricular stroke volume. Blood flow, or cardiac output is the same for both the systemic and pulmonary circulations. However, the walls of the pulmonary arteries are much thinner (more elastic and less muscular) than systemic arteries, making the pulmonary vessels more distensible. Combined with the large capacity of the pulmonary vascular bed, the pulmonary circulation is normally a high capacitance/low resistance circuit so that the pressure is low and relatively constant despite fluctuations in blood flow. Typically, systolic pulmonary artery pressure is 20 to 25 mmHg. The pressure downstream in the left atrium and pulmonary veins is 8 to 10 mmHg (Traill and Michael, 1988). Pulmonary vascular resistance (PVR) is calculated to be the difference between the pulmonary artery mean pressure and the pulmonary capillary wedge pressure divided by cardiac output (CO):

$$(PVR = PAM - PCW/CO).$$

There are three general mechanisms of pulmonary hypertension (West, 1977).

1. Increase in left atrial pressure, as in mitral stenosis or left ventricular failure. In this situation, the resistance in the pulmonary circulation is not increased, but since the pressure downstream is elevated, the pulmonary pressure has to go up as well.
2. Increase in pulmonary blood flow, as occurs in congenital heart defects, causing a left to right shunt. Again, the resistance can be normal but the high flow raises the pressure.
3. Increase in pulmonary vascular resistance. This can occur as a secondary consequence of 1 or 2 above, or as the result of the diseases listed in Table 6-1.

Table 6-1. **Causes of Pulmonary Hypertension**

Downstream Obstruction
- Raised left ventricular filling pressure
- Mitral stenosis
- Left atrial myxoma
- Cor triatriatum
- Congenital pulmonary vein anomalies
- Pulmonary veno-occlusive disease

Communication Between Systemic and Pulmonary Circulation
- With left-to-right shunt (low resistance)
- Eisenmenger syndrome

Primary Pulmonary Hypertension

Thromboembolic Pulmonary Hypertension

Cor Pulmonale
- Chronic respiratory failure
  - Chronic obstructive lung disease
  - Sleep apnea
  - Kyphoscoliosis
  - Muscular dystrophy
- Obliterative parenchymal disease
  - Fibrosing alveolitis
  - Cystic fibrosis

(Adapted from Traill and Michael, 1988.)

APPLYING PATHOLOGY OF END-STAGE ORGAN FAILURE

Primary Pulmonary Hypertension — Etiology

Pulmonary hypertension, like systemic hypertension, can be classified as primary hypertension, having no identifiable cause, or as secondary hypertension, which can be caused by a variety of disorders or structural abnormalities (see Table 6-1). When pulmonary artery pressure is elevated (mean pressure greater than 15 mmHg) but pulmonary capillary wedge pressure remains normal, pulmonary vascular disease is present (West, 1977; Whitcomb, 1982; Fishman, 1982; Balchum, 1983). Primary pulmonary hypertension is characterized by extremely severe pulmonary vascular disease, high pulmonary vascular resistance, and pulmonary artery pressure elevated to levels that may be even higher than the systemic pressure, without a known cause and in the absence of antecedent heart, chronic lung, or thromboembolic disease.

Primary pulmonary hypertension is usually silent in its early stages.

Symptoms begin gradually and by the time of diagnosis, the disease is usually so advanced that expected survival is 2 to 3 years (Glanville, et al., 1987). Primary pulmonary hypertension affects women more than men, and may occur at any age but most frequently between 20 and 40 years. Since patients with pulmonary hypertension are often young and without previous thoracic surgery, they are particularly good operative candidates (Jamieson, et al., 1984). A typical chest x-ray of a 32-year-old patient with primary pulmonary hypertension referred for a combined heart-lung transplant is shown in Figure 6–1.

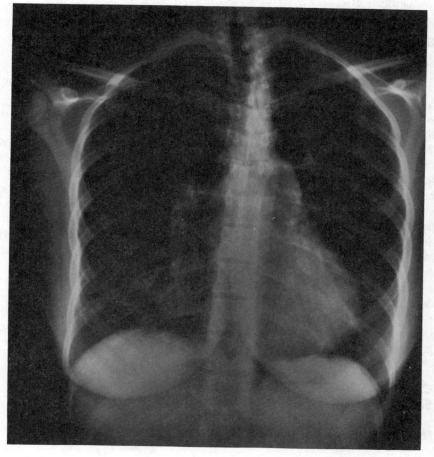

Figure 6–1

Chest x-ray of a 32-year-old patient with primary pulmonary hypertension referred for a combined heart-lung transplant.

Eisenmenger's Syndrome — Etiology

Eisenmenger's syndrome is defined as pulmonary hypertension due to a congenital heart defect. Often an atrial or ventricular septal defect or patent ductus allows increased blood flow to the lungs and with time, if uncorrected, may produce irreversible changes in pulmonary vascular resistance. Many patients with Eisenmenger's syndrome do well into early life but eventually decompensate. The current medical treatment and nursing management are primarily symptomatic and limited to management and avoidance of polycythemia, congestive heart failure, hemoptysis, infective endocarditis, and cerebrovascular accident or sudden death (McGregor, et al., 1986; Harvey, et al., 1988).

Cystic Fibrosis — Etiology

Cystic fibrosis is a generalized disorder of exocrine glands for which the basic defect has not yet been found. The clinical picture, although highly variable in the degree and type of involvement of different organs, is usually dominated by symptoms involving the lungs and pancreas. In the lungs, hypersecretion of viscid mucus, in addition to chronic bacterial infections, produces a progressive type of chronic obstructive airway disease which eventually leads to diffuse severe bronchiectasis. Respiratory secretions increase when a cystic fibrosis patient, typically chronically colonized with *Pseudomonas aeruginosa* or *Staphylococcus aureus*, develops a viral respiratory tract infection. Repeated episodes lead to a progressive bronchiectasis and/or atelectasis accompanied by a gradual and irreversible decrease in pulmonary function. As the pulmonary disease increases, patients with cystic fibrosis develop pulmonary hypertension and right-sided heart failure (Scanlin, 1988).

Because the use of synthetic pancreatic enzymes has become useful in controlling gastrointestinal disorders and because most patients with cystic fibrosis die of respiratory failure (Scanlin, 1988), heart-lung transplantation has recently become an option for certain patients with cystic fibrosis.

CLINICAL SIGNS AND SYMPTOMS OF END-STAGE ORGAN FAILURE

Integumentary Manifestations

Cyanosis and clubbing are very pronounced in Eisenmenger's syndrome. In primary pulmonary hypertension, clubbing is rare and cyanosis is mild. Right-sided heart failure is pronounced, leads to edema, and, if very severe, to jaundice secondary to venous congestion.

Cardiovascular Manifestations

Patients may complain of weakness, palpitations and exertional substernal or left chest pain (Whitcomb, 1982; Balchum, 1983). The nurse may observe signs and symptoms of right-sided heart failure including jugular venous distention, hepatomegaly, and peripheral edema. Right ventricular hypertrophy may cause a lift or heave over the left lower sternum and a palpable impulse may be noted over the region of the pulmonary artery. Murmurs of tricuspid and pulmonic insufficiency may be heard.

Hematologic Manifestations

Low-flow oxygen may be needed to prevent or reduce hypoxia. In Eisenmenger's syndrome, cyanosis causes secondary polycythemia and may require therapeutic phlebotomy.

Pulmonary Manifestations

Although the predominant changes are cardiovascular, pulmonary hypertension is accompanied by abnormalities in lung function tests. A restrictive ventilation defect with a decrease in vital capacity and total lung capacity, and reduced diffusing capacity may occur, causing alterations in respiratory function related to impaired gas exchange (Whitcomb, 1982). The patient chiefly complains of dyspnea on exertion, and the nurse assesses for effects on activities of daily living.

Gastrointestinal Manifestations

Hepatomegaly and splanchnic congestion lead to anorexia and early satiety. Progressive loss of dry weight, cardiac cachexia, is an ominous sign in these patients. Nursing measures are aimed at promoting optimal nutritional status.

Neurological Manifestations

Dizziness and syncope may occur and are usually related to exertion (Whitcomb, 1982; West, 1977). Ensuring the patient's safety and evaluating hazards of the environment during normal activities are nursing goals.

Sexual Manifestations

Patients may complain of sexual dysfunction related to physiologic limitations caused by limited oxygen reserve. Table 6 – 2 summarizes potential and actual nursing diagnoses for the patient awaiting heart-lung transplantation.

CRITERIA FOR TRANSPLANTATION

Indications

Selection criteria are similar to those used for heart transplantation, except for restrictions related to elevated pulmonary pressure, and are strictly applied for optimal patient survival, insuring maximal utilization of scarce donor organs (Baumgartner and Reitz, 1982; Borkon and Reitz, 1988; Shinn, 1985). In brief, potential recipients must have no other significant systemic disease, and must demonstrate good medical compliance, emotional stability, and excellent family support (Table 6 – 3).

High-Risk Factors

High-risk factors restricting the option of transplantation include active infection, malignancy, or insulin-dependent diabetes mellitus. A further risk factor is a history of previous thoracic or cardiac surgery. Intrathoracic adhesions may adversely affect the outcome of operation because of technical problems at the time of operation, including excessive collateral blood supply in the posterior mediastinum and difficulty in preserving phrenic and vagus nerves (Borkon and Reitz, 1988). See Table 6 – 4 for high-risk factors.

Evaluating the Recipient

PHYSICAL ASSESSMENT

There must be no known reversible cause of pulmonary hypertension. A thorough cardiopulmonary examination is performed to confirm the signs and symptoms of pulmonary hypertension and to exclude occult mitral valve disease or other lesions correctable by conventional treatment.

Table 6-2. Common Nursing Diagnoses for the Pre-Transplant Heart-Lung Patient

Health Perception — Health Management
- Health maintenance, altered
- Health seeking behaviors
- Noncompliance

Nutritional — Metabolic
- **Fluid volume, altered: excess**
- Nutrition, altered: less than body requirements
- Nutrition, altered: more than body requirements

Elimination
- Urinary elimination, altered patterns

Activity — Exercise
- Activity intolerance
- Airway clearance, ineffective
- Breathing pattern, ineffective
- Cardiac output, altered: decreased
- Gas exchange, impaired
- Home maintenance management, impaired
- Diversional activity deficit
- Fatigue
- Mobility, impaired physical
- Self-care deficit: total
- Tissue perfusion, altered

Sleep — Rest
- Sleep pattern disturbance

Cognitive — Perceptual
- Knowledge deficit
- Decisional conflict
- Thought processes, altered

Self-Perception
- Anxiety
- Fear
- Hopelessness
- Powerlessness
- Self-concept, disturbance in: body image; personal identity; self-esteem

Role — Relationship
- Family process, altered
- Grieving, anticipatory
- Self-concept, disturbance in: role performance
- Social interaction, impaired
- Social isolation

Sexuality — Reproductive
- Sexuality patterns, altered

Coping — Stress Tolerance
- Adjustment, impaired
- Coping, ineffective individual
- Coping, ineffective family: compromised

Table 6–3. Recipient Criteria: Heart-Lung and Single Lung

- See heart recipient criteria, Chapter 5
- No other significant systemic disease
- Demonstrated medical compliance
- Adequate cardiac function with isolated lung transplantation
- Irreversible cardiopulmonary disease

RADIOLOGY

The chest x-ray shows enlargement of the central pulmonary arteries (see Fig. 6–1).

ELECTROCARDIOGRAM

The electrocardiogram shows right ventricular hypertrophy.

ULTRASOUND

An echocardiogram is performed to confirm right ventricular and often right atrial enlargement, and to exclude left atrial obstruction as the cause of pulmonary hypertension.

CARDIAC CATHETERIZATION

Cardiac catheterization is not usually essential in making or confirming the diagnosis, but is often performed in order to absolutely rule out a treatable lesion and to assess the potential palliative role of vasodilators.

PSYCHOSOCIAL ASSESSMENT

Each patient is evaluated by a clinical nurse specialist, social worker, and in some centers also by a psychiatrist or psychologist to determine the patient's ability to cope with the lifelong potential for complications, such

Table 6–4. High-Risk Factors for Heart-Lung and Single Lung Transplantation

- Active infection
- Malignancy
- Insulin-dependent diabetes mellitus
- Previous cardiac or thoracic surgery
- Intrathoracic adhesions

as rejection and infection. Additionally, compliance is an extremely important issue since these patients are totally dependent on their immunosuppressive drugs, which must be taken each day without fail. This is especially trying for some patients because of the numerous side effects of their medications, which range from mild to severe. Financial issues are also of great concern; the cost of hospitalization and all professional fees, even if the patient has insurance, may not be covered because some insurance companies continue to view heart-lung transplantation as experimental. Additionally, the cost of medications is generally between $7000 and $10,000 the first year. If the patient resides elsewhere, living expenses for family members add to the financial burden. Unfortunately, heart-lung transplantation is not possible, or even the best choice, for all individuals. The psychosocial assessment is of prime importance in the overall evaluation of potential heart-lung transplant recipients, and provides a foundation for the continued nursing and medical management.

MANAGING THE HEART-LUNG DONOR

Donor availability has been the limiting factor in heart-lung transplantation for numerous reasons. Only 10% of possible donors are acceptable for heart-lung transplantation (Borkon and Reitz, 1988). Brain death is often accompanied by neurogenic pulmonary edema. Since many of the deaths are traumatic in etiology, pulmonary contusion and aspiration often occur. Furthermore, ventilatory support of cadaveric donors increases the risk of tracheobronchial infection or nosocomial pneumonia.

Potential heart-lung donors are usually less than 40 years of age, have no sign of pulmonary infection, and have thoracic volumes similar to the recipient as demonstrated by comparable x-rays. It may be necessary to treat the donor with antibiotics and vigorous pulmonary physiotherapy. Arterial PO_2 must be greater than 150 mmHg on an FIO_2 of 40%, with peak inspiratory pressure on the ventilator of less than 30 mmHg with normal tidal volumes. Donor management prior to heart-lung transplantation requires careful fluid management. The central venous pressure is maintained at less than 6 mmHg to decrease the chance of fluid overload and excessive lung water. Meticulous sterile technique and consistent attention to pulmonary toilet are essential in the nursing care plan. Tracheal aspirates are obtained for gram stains and cultures. High levels of inspired oxygen in the donor are avoided because the ischemic and denervated lung is more susceptible to oxygen toxicity (Borkon and Reitz, 1988; Baumgartner and Reitz, 1982; Jamieson, et al., 1984). ABO blood group compatibility and a negative lymphocyte crossmatch are required between donor and recipient.

Donor availability has also been limited by distant organ procurement. Until recently, distant procurement was accomplished only occasionally by a few centers with variable results. The University of Pittsburgh initially employed an autoperfusion system for heart-lung procurement (Hardesty and Griffith, 1987; Ladowski, et al., 1985; Robicsek, et al., 1985). An alternate technique of preserving organs using systemic cooling with cardiopulmonary bypass was used by the University of Pittsburgh (Hardesty and Griffith, 1985; Ladowski, et al., 1984) and Harefield Hospital, Harefield, England (Wahlers, et al., 1986) for on-site and distant procurement, respectively. Comparison of the autoperfused system versus hypothermia was examined in an experimental model by Adachi, et al. (1987). Adequate preservation was achieved with both methods, although core cooling was a less complex procedure. Recently, the development of a portable cardiopulmonary bypass device at The Johns Hopkins Medical Institutions has allowed this very effective core-cooling procedure to be accomplished at distant donor centers (Kontos, et al., 1987). Initial results of these distant procurement procedures (mean ischemic time = 281 minutes) demonstrated good lung function in each case. This method has also been advantageous for multiple organ procurement.

PREOPERATIVE NURSING CARE

Preparing for Surgery

Anxiety related to several causes is commonly seen in the patient waiting for heart-lung transplantation. In addition to psychosocial concerns common to any transplant patient (see Chapters 4, 5, and 7; Augustine, 1989 and Michalisko, 1989), potential heart-lung transplant recipients have fears related to several unique concerns. These concerns include finding a suitable donor in time to save their lives, the decrease in function they are experiencing during the lengthy wait for a donor (up to a year or more), as well as the operative procedure and recovery. The fact that survival rates for heart-lung transplantation, although improving, are not as high as those of isolated heart transplantation is not unknown to most patients.

A knowledge deficit related to heart-lung transplantation, regardless of age, background, education, or intelligence, is noted in all patients. Patients are given as much information as is appropriate about survival rates, functional ability after surgery, the operative procedure, recovery, potential setbacks, and medications and their side effects. The amount and detail of this information are tailored specifically to each patient. All patients do not want or require lengthy detailed instructions regarding postoperative procedures at this point. Their wishes are respected since readiness to learn varies depending on several factors including extent of deterioration, personality, and anxiety level. Although increasing knowledge alleviates anxiety to a point, beyond that, for some patients in the preoperative stage, massive facts and figures can increase anxiety and decrease comprehension and retention of information. In addition, an alteration in thought processes sometimes occurs secondary to decreased brain perfusion. Patients while waiting for a heart-lung transplant also experience an alteration in nutrition, almost always less than body requirements, disturbance in self-concept related to body image, role performance, personal identity, and a chronic disturbance in self-esteem. Impaired social interactions related to weakness and inactivity and feelings of powerlessness and hopelessness are common. All nursing interventions that may begin to reverse these deficits (i.e., patient repetition of instructions, realistic reassurances, small amounts of appropriate information, touching, assistance in personal hygiene and grooming, meeting other heart-lung transplant recipients) will add to the general fitness of the patients as they enter the operating room.

INTRAOPERATIVE MANAGEMENT

The operative procedure can be described only in brief here. In the recipient, the heart and lungs are removed, preserving both the phrenic and left recurrent laryngeal nerves. The trachea is divided one ring above the carina as shown in Figure 6 – 2. The donor heart and lungs are prepared and removed *en bloc* after core cooling and administration of cardioplegia to the heart. Reimplantation of the heart-lung graft is accomplished by sequential anastomoses of the trachea, followed by the aorta and then the right atrium.

POSTOPERATIVE NURSING CARE

Immediate

Admission to the designated critical care unit is similar to that for any cardiac surgery patient. Nursing responsibilities include a complete physical assessment: neurologic status, heart rate and rhythm, and systemic pressures. Cardiac output is assessed by the quality of peripheral pulses, capillary refill, skin temperature and color, and urinary output. Pulmonary artery catheters are not used routinely. Baseline pacemaker settings, electrolyte levels, arterial blood gas values, and amount of chest tube drainage are recorded as well as heart and respiratory sounds. Filling pressures and volume status require careful monitoring in the early postoperative period. Isoproterenol is usually administered to augment heart rate, increase cardiac output, and lower pulmonary vascular resistance. Patients are kept in

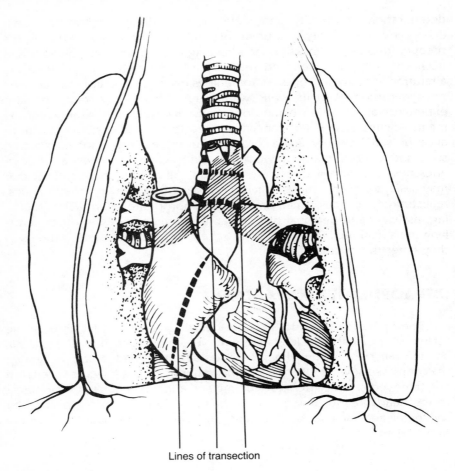

Lines of transection

Figure 6-2

Dissection of the recipient for heart and lung transplantation with preservation of the phrenic nerves on pedicles. Anticipated lines of transection are shown. (From Reitz, Pennock, and Shumway, 1985, with permission.)

negative fluid balance (fluid volume deficit) for the first 2 weeks (Jamieson and Oguannaike, 1986) to decrease interstitial edema. Renal function is monitored carefully. Therapeutic options may include adjustment of cyclosporine (Sandimmune) dosage, or infusion of low-dose dopamine to augment renal perfusion. If renal failure occurs, hemodialysis and/or ultrafiltration may be required.

Meticulous pulmonary care is essential as the lungs are the most frequent site of infection following both heart and heart-lung transplantation (Wilson, et al., 1985). Traditional nursing measures such as turning, suctioning, or coughing and deep breathing if extubated, are important to mobilize fluid and avoid congestion. Weaning from the ventilator is usually accomplished within the first 48 hours according to a standard protocol.

There are several areas of nursing care unique to the early postoperative period for heart-lung recipients. These include effects of denervation of the heart and myocardial dysfunction covered in Chapter 5 and in other sources (Augustine, 1989), reimplantation response, rejection, infection, nutritional status, physical therapy, psychosocial issues, and patient education. Table 6–5 lists actual and potential nursing diagnoses of the heart-lung transplant recipient in the postoperative period.

Table 6–5. Common Nursing Diagnoses for the Post-Transplant Heart-Lung Patient

Health Perception — Health Management
- Health maintenance, altered
- Health seeking behaviors
- Infection, potential for
- Noncompliance

Activity — Exercise
- Activity intolerance
- Diversional activity deficit
- Fatigue
- Home maintenance management, impaired

Sleep — Rest
- Sleep pattern disturbance

Cognitive — Perceptual
- Decisional conflict
- Knowledge deficit
- Thought processes, altered

Self-Perception
- Anxiety
- Fear
- Hopelessness
- Powerlessness
- Self-concept, disturbance in: body image
- Self-esteem, chronic low

Role — Relationship
- Family process, altered
- Self-concept, disturbance in: role performance
- Social interaction, impaired
- Social isolation

Sexuality — Reproductive
- Sexuality patterns, altered

Coping — Stress Tolerance
- Adjustment, impaired
- Coping, ineffective individual
- Coping, ineffective family: compromised

Supporting Respiratory Function

Unique to caring for heart-lung (or isolated lung) transplantation patients is the recognition and management of respiratory distress known as the reimplantation response. This phenomenon has been reported by many investigators in dogs, monkeys, and humans (Veith, et al., 1983; Jamieson and Oguannaike, 1986; Reitz, et al., 1980; Corris, et al., 1987; Trummer and Christiansen, 1965; Eraslan, et al., 1964). The response consists of radiologic and functional changes that occur in a transplanted lung as a result of surgical trauma, denervation, lymphatic interruption, and ischemia (Veith, et al., 1983). The reimplantation response is composed of an alveolar infiltrate due to fluid within the alveoli beginning centrally and extending peripherally (Siegelman, et al., 1973). This process may start 24 to 48 hours postoperatively, with maximal signs and symptoms being apparent by the third postoperative day. This is followed by variable improvement, with ultimate resolution occurring within a 21-day period (Siegelman, et al., 1973; Covner and Shinn, 1983; Baumgartner and Reitz, 1982). The patient may present with symptoms similar to adult respiratory distress syndrome manifested as defects in pulmonary gas exchange, compliance, and vascular resistance as well as an inability of the disrupted lymphatic system to clear interstitial fluid. Subjectively, the patient becomes very anxious and complains of shortness of breath. Objectively, examination of the patient reveals diffuse rales and a chest x-ray demonstrates pulmonary edema. Pleural effusions may also develop and may recur until lymphatic function returns. The incidence and severity of this complication seem to be decreasing, possibly due to better preservation techniques (Borkon and Reitz, 1988).

Treatment consists of vigorous diuresis, respiratory physiotherapy, and reintubation if necessary. Although extremely anxiety producing for the patient, management is usually routine with predictable improvement. Differential diagnosis includes rejection, infection, and reimplantation response. Distinguishing among these diagnoses is often difficult but essential to formulating a treatment and nursing care plan.

Preventing Infection

Assessing clinical parameters for signs of infection begins with observing the patient's vital signs. Due to immunosuppression, normal body temperature tends to be somewhat lower; therefore, even a small increase in temperature can be a harbinger of infection. Fevers greater than 38°C require prompt and aggressive workup. A primary nursing responsibility is overseeing the proper collection and delivery of specimens for culture (Gurevich, 1987). Persistent or productive cough with or without fever, or decrease in FEV_1, requires further investigation by chest x-ray and usually bronchoscopy.

Common opportunistic infections in heart-lung transplant patients tend to be cytomegalovirus (CMV) and *Pneumocystis carinii*. CMV infection can occur as a result of reactivation of a latent process in the recipient or transmission from donor organs or blood transfusion. Infection with this virus can be subclinically manifested by only a drop in white blood cell count or as a severe illness with associated leukopenia, fever, hepatitis, arthralgias, and pneumonia (Peterson, et al., 1980; Betts, et al., 1977). Disseminated CMV can contribute directly to mortality but can also predispose to superinfection with other organisms (Preiksaitis, et al., 1982).

The risks of infection by any organism are directly related to potency and duration of immunosuppression, donor selection, operating room technique and postoperative exposure to pathogens. Early infections tend to be nosocomial whereas late infections are more often caused by opportunistic pathogens (Garibaldi, 1983). Since most infections tend to be nosocomial during initial hospitalization, prevention is a major nursing goal at this time. It is routine practice at some institutions to use immunoglobulins and/or sulfamethoxazole/trimethoprim prophylactically against CMV and *Pneumocystis*. Thorough observation for signs and symptoms of infection, should prevention prove unsuccessful, is another important nursing care objective.

Monitoring for Rejection

Monitoring for rejection includes physical assessment, chest x-ray, simple pulmonary function testing and bronchoscopy with biopsy or in some centers bronchioalveolar lavage. In the early days of heart-lung transplantation, it was believed that there was a close concordance between the rejection status of the heart and of the lungs (Reitz, et al., 1983). However, this no longer appears to be the case, and lung rejection cannot be excluded by normal endomyocardial biopsy results (Prop, et al., 1985; Cooper, et al., 1986; McGregor, et al., 1985; Griffith, et al., 1985; Borkon and Reitz, 1988).

In rats, bronchus associated lymphoid tissue (BALT) is actively involved in the rejection process and may explain why lung allografts are more vigorously rejected than hearts (Prop, et al., 1985). At The Johns Hopkins Hospital, four out of nine heart-lung transplant patients have had one episode or more of lung rejection without associated heart rejection. The diagnosis of rejection must be made by total assessment of the patient.

Once infection has been ruled out, the presence of fever, respiratory insufficiency, and a diffuse pulmonary infiltrate after the first postopera-

Table 6-6. **Signs and Symptoms of Rejection for Heart-Lung and Isolated Lung Transplant**

- Fever
- Respiratory insufficiency
- Diffuse pulmonary infiltrate
- Decreased peak expiratory flow

tive week should be regarded as lung rejection. Even when infection is present, it is important also to look for evidence of rejection since the two processes may coexist or lead to one another. Recent changes have been made in protocols for rejection surveillance. After the first 3 months, endocardial biopsies may no longer routinely be performed. Biopsies may be done only at annual examination and when symptoms are suggestive of heart rejection. Instead, routine bronchoscopy every 3 months, or open lung biopsy if required for troublesome diagnoses, is relied upon. Patients are also provided with a hand-held peak flow meter, which measures peak expiratory flow (PEF) in a very reproducible manner. Even small decreases in PEF have proven to be reliable predictors of a problem in most patients and may prove to be a sensitive way of suspecting early rejection. It is important at this point to differentiate between rejection and infection. Occasionally, the distinction is very difficult and open lung biopsy may be required. Table 6-6 summarizes the signs and symptoms of rejection.

Rejection can be reversed with intravenous administration of steroids. The frequency and severity of rejection episodes usually decrease after the first 3 months. In a major program, the incidence of lung rejection with or without heart rejection is 0.42 episodes per patient/month in the first 3 months and 0.07 episodes per patient/month after 3 months. Particularly severe rejection may also be treated with equine antithymocyte globulin (ATGAM), Upjohn Company, or OKT3 (murine monoclonal antibody), Ortho Pharmaceuticals. Maintenance immunosuppression, similar to that of heart transplant patients, consists of cyclosporine (Sandimmune) and azathioprine (Imuran) initially with steroids added after approximately 2 weeks. Steroids are delayed in order to maximize healing of the tracheal anastomosis.

PLANNING/REHABILITATION

Discharge Planning

Postoperative teaching is begun as soon as the patient's anxieties are reduced sufficiently for adequate concentration. Areas to be covered by the nurse include medications, observation, reporting of signs and symp-

Table 6-7. **Nursing Priorities for the Heart-Lung and Single Lung Transplant***

- Maintain patent airway
- Promote effective gas exchange
- Maximize activity tolerance
- Promote independence in activities of daily living
- Prevent infection

---

* See also nursing priorities for heart transplantation in Chapter 5.

toms of infection or rejection, and progression of physical activities after discharge. Families as well as patients often will be enthusiastic but fearful of the time of discharge from the hospital when they are no longer under the supervision of the professional staff. An important nursing charge is ensuring that all patients are confident and competent to regain total responsibility for themselves. Although there is no single approach that will ensure smooth transition from hospital to home, a gradual progression favors independence. Gradual permission and expectation for the patient to manage medication and daily routines foster confidence. Nurses may not recognize the power and control they have assumed in a patient's life. The nurse's ability to show regard for the patient's non-illness roles and competence can significantly affect the patient's self-confidence regarding discharge (Christopherson, 1987). The goals of nursing care are found in Table 6-7.

Rehabilitation

Rehabilitation is considered in terms of physical, nutritional, and psychosocial needs. Although all three of these issues need prompt attention in the early postoperative period, patients do not usually benefit from instruction until some amount of physical strength has returned. Physical therapy usually begins on the second or third postoperative day with range-of-motion and bed exercises. Patients are assisted out of bed to a chair as soon as possible and are usually riding a stationary bicycle by postoperative day 5.

Compromised nutritional status is often a problem in patients who have had chronic illnesses. Because of a debilitated preoperative state, heart-lung transplant patients may experience fatigue and loss of appetite. Nutritional counseling with experienced dietitians is important but is supplemented and supported by the nursing staff. Postoperatively, the patient needs protein and calories to heal; therefore, restrictions at this time are usually unwarranted. Family members are encouraged to bring the patient's favorite foods from home to augment the hospital diet. Hyperalimentation has not been encouraged routinely for heart-lung transplant recipients. Risks of fluid overload and infection tend to outweigh the advantages of intravenous alimentation in most cases (Covner and Shinn, 1983).

The psychosocial considerations in heart-lung recipients' recovery and discharge preparations are numerous. Patients undergoing any cardiac operation tend to be somewhat fearful and anxious regarding their rehabilitation and future. Patients recovering from heart-lung transplantation have several additional anxieties. Although success in heart-lung transplantation has improved markedly since 1981, survival rates have still not equaled that of heart transplantation alone. Heart-lung transplantation is associated with longer initial hospitalization, higher morbidity, and more complications.

Even the act of breathing can be stressful. Furthermore, during the reimplantation response when pulmonary compliance is actually decreased, breathing becomes more difficult and exhausting. A vicious cycle is often initiated as the patient feels the need to concentrate on breathing. Due to fear of apnea, patients often avoid sleep, which increases fatigue and exhaustion, contributing to further anxiety. Knowledgeable nursing interventions are crucial to break this cycle (Covner and Shinn, 1983). As patients become more confident in themselves, their caregivers, and their surroundings, anxieties decrease and the work of breathing becomes easier. Patients can then relax and begin concentrating on other postoperative management. Nursing interventions include emotional support, factual information, and frequent rest periods. A visit or phone call from another heart-lung transplant recipient who has recovered is often very helpful.

POST DISCHARGE

After hospital discharge, the patient is followed at weekly to biweekly intervals. Patients record PEF measurements daily and are instructed to report even small decreases in function. In addition to the common post-transplant complications of rejection and infection, heart-lung transplant patients are also at risk for long-term complications. The major long-term complication of heart-lung transplantation has been a progressive and relentless pulmonary disease resulting in obstruction and restriction, described histologically as obliterative bronchiolitis (Burke, et al., 1985). This occlusion of the terminal bronchioles is a result of proliferating granulation tissue infiltrating the small conducting airways as a response to injury (Epler, et al., 1985). This disease process usually occurs after about 9 months and can progress rapidly. A chest x-ray of a heart-lung recipient with a histologic diagnosis of obliterative bronchiolitis is shown in Figure 6-3. Bronchitic signs and symptoms such as cough and mucopurulent

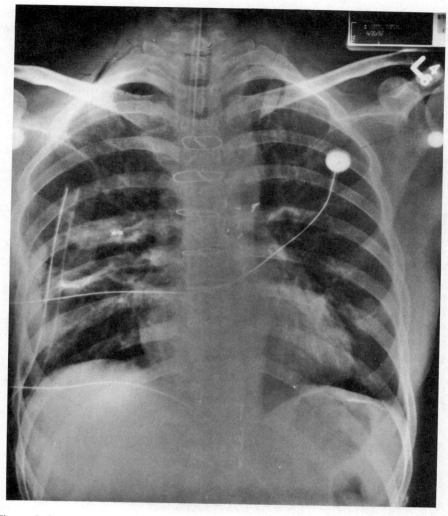

Figure 6-3

Chest x-ray of a heart-lung recipient with a histologic diagnosis of obliterative bronchiolitis.

sputum may precede dyspnea. The chest x-ray shows an interstitial infiltrate described by some as a ground-glass appearance. Obliterative bronchiolitis (also called bronchiolitis obliterans) is characterized by a progressive obstructive and restrictive lung disease with a decrease in total lung capacity. It is largely irreversible with bronchodilators and although it has been reversed in the very early stages with steroids, the obscure and subtle presenting symptoms usually impede early diagnosis (Burke, et al.,

1984; Epler, et al., 1985; Allen, et al., 1986). Although the definitive mechanism of obliterative bronchiolitis in heart-lung transplant recipients is currently still unclear, and may have several contributory components, chronic pulmonary rejection is the most likely cause. The immunogenicity of lung tissue (the expression of class II major histocompatibility antigens, specifically HLA-DR antigens on bronchiolar epithelium) may promote this bronchial disease (Burke, et al., 1987). Measurements of FEV_1 can detect mild changes in pulmonary function. Miniature hand-held spirometry units are inexpensive and easy for patients to use on a daily basis at home. A drop in PEF of as little as 25 to 50 liters per minute, although not specific for etiology, can predict early problems.

SUMMARY

Heart-lung transplantation imposes many risks on the patient who is willing to accept the potential future problems in exchange for the opportunity for a second chance at life. The heart-lung transplant patient imposes a unique challenge to the nurse who has the willingness to invest the time to become knowledgeable about transplantation and the commitment to apply the skills previously learned in caring for postoperative patients, as well as patients with cardiac, pulmonary, and infectious diseases. Combining the skills and principles needed to care for these patients with newly acquired knowledge regarding immunosuppressed patients will provide both patient and nurse with an intimate and rewarding experience.

Bibliography

Adachi, H, et al: Autoperfused working heart-lung preparation versus hypothermic cardiopulmonary preservation for transplantation. J Heart Transplant 6:253, 1987.

Allen, MD, et al: Steroid-responsive bronchiolitis after human heart-lung transplantation. J Thorac Cardiovasc Surg 92:449, 1986.

Augustine, SM: Nursing care of the heart and heart-lung transplant patient. In Baumgartner, WA, Reitz, BA, and Achuff, SC (eds): Heart and Heart-Lung Transplantation. WB Saunders, Philadelphia, 1990.

Balchum, OJ: Pulmonary hypertension. In Sharma, OP and Balchum, OJ (eds): Key Facts in Pulmonary Disease. Churchill Livingstone, New York, 1983, p 385.

Baumgartner, WA and Reitz, BA: Heart-lung transplantation. The SEOPF Newsletter 7(3):14, 1982.

Betts, RF, et al: Clinical manifestations of renal allograft derived primary cytomegalovirus infection. Am J Dis Child 131:759, 1977.

Borkon, AM and Reitz, BA: Heart-lung transplantation. In Konstam, MA and Isner, JM (eds): The Right Ventricle. Martinus Nijhoff Publishing, Boston, 1988, p 321.

Burke, CM, et al: Post-transplant obliterative bronchiolitis and other late lung sequelae in human heart-lung transplantation. Chest 86:824, 1984.

Burke, CM, et al: Late airflow obstruction in heart-lung transplantation recipients. J Heart Transplant 4:437, 1985.

Burke, CM, et al: Lung immunogenicity, rejection, and obliterative bronchiolitis. Chest 92:547, 1987.

Castaneda, AR, et al: Cardiopulmonary autotransplantation in primates. J Cardiovasc Surg 37:523, 1972.

Christopherson, LK, et al: Cardiac transplantation: A psychological perspective. Circulation 75:57, 1987.

Cooper, DK, et al: Acute pulmonary rejection precedes cardiac rejection following heart-lung transplantation in a primate model. J Heart Transplant 5:29, 1986.

Cooper, JD, et al: Technique of successful lung transplantation in humans. J Thorac Cardiovasc Surg 93:173, 1987.

Corris, PA, et al: Reimplantation injury after lung transplantation in a rat model. J Heart Transplant 6:234, 1987.

Covner, AL, and Shinn, JA: Cardiopulmonary transplantation: Initial experience. Heart Lung 12:131, 1983.

Dark, JH, et al: Experimental en bloc double-lung transplantation. Ann Thorac Surg 42:394, 1986.

Epler, GR, et al: Bronchiolitis obliterans organizing pneumonia. N Engl J Med 312:152, 1985.

Eraslan, S, Turner, MD, and Hardy, JD: Lymphatic regeneration following lung reimplantation in dogs. Surgery 56:970, 1964.

Fishman, AP: Update: Pulmonary Diseases and Disorders. McGraw-Hill, New York, 1982.

Fragomeni, LS and Kaye, MP: The registry of the International Society for Heart Transplantation: Fifth official report. J Heart Transplant 7:249, 1988.

Garibaldi, R: Infections in organ transplant recipients. Infect Control 4:460, 1983.

Glanville, AR, et al: Primary pulmonary hypertension: Length of survival in patients referred for heart-lung transplantation. Chest 91:675, 1987.

Goldsmith, J, et al: Clinical and experimental aspects of single-lung transplantation. Heart Lung 16:231, 1987.

Griffith, BP, et al: Asynchronous rejection of heart and lungs following cardiopulmonary transplantation. Ann Thorac Surg 40:488, 1985.

Gurevich, I: The cardiothoracic patient with infection: Effective collection of specimens. Cardiothoracic Nurse 5:5, 1987.

Hardesty, RL and Griffith, BP: Procurement for combined heart-lung transplantation. J Thorac Cardiovasc Surg 89:795, 1985.

Hardesty, RL and Griffith, BP: Autoperfusion of the heart and lungs for preservation during distant procurement. J Thorac Cardiovasc Surg 93:11, 1987.

Hardy, JD, et al: Lung homotransplantation in man. JAMA 186:1065, 1963.

Harvey, P, et al (eds): The Principles and Practice of Medicine, ed 22. Appleton & Lange, Norwalk, CT, 1988.

Jamieson, SW and Oguannaike, HO: Cardiopulmonary transplantation. Surg Clin North Am 66:491, 1986.

Jamieson, SW, et al: Heart and lung transplantation for pulmonary hypertension. Am J Surg 147:740, 1984.

Kontos, GJ, et al: A no-flush, core-cooling technique for successful cardiopulmonary preservation in heart-lung transplantation. J Thorac Cardiovasc Surg 94:836, 1987.

Ladowski, JS, Hardesty, RL, and Griffith, BP: Protection of the heart-lung allograft during procurement: Cooling of the lungs with extracorporeal circulation or pulmonary artery flush. J Heart Transplant 3:351, 1984.

Ladowski, JS, et al: Use of autoperfusion for distant procurement of heart-lung allografts. J Heart Transplant 4:330, 1985.

McGregor, CG, et al: Isolated pulmonary rejection after combined heart-lung transplantation. J Thorac Cardiovasc Surg 90:623, 1985.

McGregor, CG, et al: Combined heart-lung transplantation for end-stage Eisenmenger's syndrome. J Thorac Cardiovasc Surg 91:443, 1986.

Mersch, J: End-stage cardiopulmonary disease: Pulmonary hypertension. In Douglas, MK and Shinn, JA (eds): Advances in Cardiovascular Nursing. Aspen Publishers, Rockville, MD, 1985, p 141.

Michalisko, HO: Psychosocial aspects of recipients undergoing heart transplantation. In Baumgartner, WA, Reitz, BA, and Achuff, SC (eds): Heart and Heart-Lung Transplantation. WB Saunders, Philadelphia, 1990.

Newmark, JH: Eisenmenger's syndrome. Focus on Critical Care 10:34, 1983.

Peterson, PK, et al: Cytomegalovirus disease in renal allograft recipients: A prospective study of the clinical features, risk factors and impact on renal transplantation. Medicine 59:283, 1980.

Preiksaitis, JK, et al: Cytomegalovirus infection in heart transplant recipients: Preliminary results of a controlled trial of intravenous gamma globulin. J Clin Immunol 2(April Suppl):365, 1982.

Prop, J, et al: Why are lung allografts more vigorously rejected than hearts? J Heart Transplant 4:433, 1985.

Reitz, BA, et al: Heart and lung transplantation: Autotransplantation and allotransplantation in primates with extended survival. J Thorac Cardiovasc Surg 80:360, 1980.

Reitz, BA, et al: Heart-lung transplantation: Successful therapy for patients with pulmonary vascular disease. N Engl J Med 306:557, 1982.

Reitz, BA, et al: Diagnosis and treatment of allograft rejection in heart-lung transplant recipients. J Thorac Cardiovasc Surg 85:354, 1983.

Reitz, BA, Pennock, JL, and Shumway, NE: Simplified operative method for heart and lung transplantation. J Surg Res 31:1, 1985.

Robicsek, F, et al: An autoperfused heart-lung-preparation: Metabolism and function. J Heart Transplant 4:334, 1985.

Scanlin, TF: Cystic fibrosis. In Fishman, AP (ed): Pulmonary Diseases and Disorders. McGraw-Hill, New York, 1988, p 1273.

Shinn, JA: New issues in cardiac transplantation. In Douglas, MK and Shinn, JA (eds): Advances in Cardiovascular Nursing. Aspen Publishers, Rockville, MD, 1985, p 185.

Siegelman, SS, Sinha, SB, and Veith, FJ: Pulmonary reimplantation response. Ann Surg 177:30, 1973.

Stevens, PM, et al: Regional ventilation and perfusion after lung transplantation in patients with emphysema. N Engl J Med 282:245, 1970.

Toronto Lung Transplantation Group: Unilateral lung transplantation for pulmonary fibrosis. N Engl J Med 314:1140, 1986.

Traill, TA and Michael, JR: Pulmonary hypertension. In Harvey, P, et al (eds): The Principles and Practice of Medicine, ed 22. Appleton & Lange, Norwalk, CT, 1988, p 85.

Trummer, MJ and Christiansen, KH: Radiographic and functional changes following auto-transplantation of the lung. J Thorac Cardiovasc Surg 49:1006, 1965.

Vander, AJ, Sherman, JH, and Luciano, DS: Human Physiology: The Mechanisms of Body Function. McGraw-Hill, New York, 1980.

Veith, FJ, et al: Lung transplantation. Transplantation 35:271, 1983.

Wahlers, T, et al: Flush perfusion using Euro-Collins solution vs. cooling by means of extra-corporeal circulation in heart-lung preservation. J Heart Transplant 5:89, 1986.

West, JB: Pulmonary Pathophysiology — the Essentials. Williams & Wilkins, Baltimore, 1977.

Whitcomb, ME: The Lung: Normal and Diseased. CV Mosby, St Louis, 1982.

Wilson, RW, Cockerill, FR III, and Rosenow, EC III: Pulmonary disease in the immunocompromised host (second of two parts). Mayo Clinic Proc 60:610, 1985.

Liver
Transplantation

Laurel Williams, RN, MSN

The first human liver transplantation was performed in 1963 by Dr. Thomas Starzl. Over the next 17 years, the one-year survival rate for people undergoing liver transplantation in the United States was approximately 28% (Starzl, et al., 1982a). In the early years of transplantation, candidates for orthotopic liver transplantation were frequently near death from end-stage liver disease due to the experimental nature of the procedure. These early candidates were often in intensive care units, intubated on a ventilator, in deep hepatic coma with kidney failure, and suffering from moderate to severe degrees of malnutrition. The premorbid state of the patient, nonstandardization of the surgical techniques, and problems secondary to the immunosuppressive therapy added to the morbidity and mortality of patients both during and after the operation.

With the introduction of cyclosporine, a more effective immunosuppressive medication, into clinical liver transplantation in 1981, the one-year survival rates increased dramatically to approximately 65% (Wood, et al., 1987). In addition to better immunosuppressive therapy, other improvements were made in the 1980s that helped increase patient survival rates. These included standardization of the surgical procedure, improved anesthesia management, better patient selection due to earlier referral patterns, improved donor management, the introduction of the Wisconsin preservation solution (ViaSpan), and advances in nurses' knowledge of the care and management of patients and their families.

With improved patient survival, the indications for liver transplantation expanded and more patients sought transplantation (Shaw, et al.,

1989d). As more healthcare professionals were needed to manage these complex patients, the multidisciplinary team approach to patient care became an essential part of liver transplantation (Fig. 7–1).

In June 1983, the National Institutes of Health Consensus Conference declared that liver transplantation was an accepted therapeutic modality for a variety of patients with end-stage liver disease (NIH, 1984). Con-

LIVER TRANSPLANTATION TEAM APPROACH

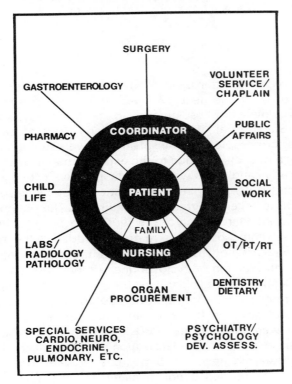

Figure 7–1

The team approach to liver transplantation. (OT = occupational therapy; PT = physical therapy; RT = respiratory therapy.)

comitantly, there was growth in the number of centers initiating liver transplantation programs. In 1988, the United Network for Organ Sharing (UNOS) estimated that there were 1680 transplants performed at 54 institutions in the United States. One center recently reported one-year survival rates as high as 90.4% in low-risk patients and 45% in those with high-risk factors (Shaw, et al., 1989c). The American Council on Transplantation reports an overall patient survival rate of 77% (American Council on Transplantation, 1988). Survival rates following liver transplantation have been shown to exceed survival rates following other forms of therapy for all causes of liver failure (Shaw, et al., 1989d).

The persistent high mortality for high-risk patients underscores the need for earlier referral for transplantation. Patients should be evaluated and activated on transplant lists before advancing liver disease leads to other complications which severely diminish the probability of survival after transplantation.

The goal of liver transplantation is to return patients to activities of daily living. The majority of deaths that occur after transplantation occur in the first year, generally within the first 3 to 6 months. Of those patients who are alive 1 to 5 years after transplantation, 85% to 90% can be considered fully rehabilitated (Shaw, et al., 1989c). The quality of life has been excellent, with most patients returning to a productive life-style (Shaw, et al., 1989a; Shaw, et al., 1985). However, liver transplant recipients still have a lifetime need to take medications and adhere to prescribed medical regimens. Ongoing medical and nursing research may alter these requirements in years to come.

PATHOPHYSIOLOGY OF LIVER DISEASE

The largest organ in the body, the liver performs numerous functions, some of which have not been well-defined by medical science. The basic functions of the liver will be reviewed in this chapter in relation to the pathophysiology of liver disease. These functions of the liver include metabolism of proteins, carbohydrates, and fats; storage of vitamins; waste removal; and secretion of bile (Guyton, 1982).

The liver synthesizes many different proteins, including the three major plasma proteins — albumin, globulin, and fibrinogen. Albumin provides colloid osmotic pressure, which prevents plasma loss from capillaries. Patients with liver disease often have low serum albumin levels, which may contribute to findings of peripheral edema, ascites, and pleural effusions during the nurse's assessment (the last finding more common on the right side).

Globulins perform a number of enzymatic functions and contribute to the integrity of the immune system. Patients with liver disease may suffer from an impaired immune system and are identified by the nurse as being at an increased risk for infections. In addition, the protein-rich ascites provides a culture medium for bacteria. Spontaneous bacterial peritonitis (SBP) is a well-known complication of liver disease.

The protein fibrinogen aids in blood coagulation. Low plasma levels of fibrinogen may result in easy bruisability and impaired clot formation following injury. In addition to low fibrinogen levels, synthesis of other clotting factors may be altered with severe liver dysfunction. Cholestatic liver disease such as primary biliary cirrhosis and sclerosing cholangitis may be associated with decreased vitamin K absorption and decreased levels of coagulation factors II, V, VI, and IX. Safety is therefore a major focus of the nursing care plan.

The liver is a major site of gluconeogenesis, synthesizing amino acids, carbohydrates, and fats to glucose and glycogen to be used for energy. By the same token, the liver's role is essential in maintaining normal blood glucose. Glycogen is stored in the liver when excess glucose is present in the blood stream, and glucose is released from the liver when blood sugar falls (Guyton, 1986). Severe hypoglycemia may complicate end-stage liver disease.

The liver is one of the body's sites of fat metabolism, synthesizing fats from carbohydrates and proteins. Cholesterol and phospholipid produced in the liver are important in the synthesis of hormones and cell membranes. Fat is the body's most important source of fuel in the fasting state (Corliss and Middleton, 1983). Problems with metabolism and malnutrition secondary to liver disease may contribute to the muscle wasting and weight loss seen in patients with liver disease. Malnutrition in women may cause amenorrhea and in men may be associated with gynecomastia and testicular atrophy. The distribution of body hair may be abnormal in patients with liver disease. Patients may also complain of dry, scaly skin. The nurse addresses the psychosocial as well as physical needs related to these manifestations.

Vitamins, particularly the fat-soluble vitamins A, D, E, and K are stored in the liver as well as large quantities of vitamin B_{12} and iron. Vitamin K plays an essential role in blood coagulation and a deficiency may lead to abnormal bleeding. The interrelationship between vitamin D and calcium absorption likewise may result in bone problems in these patients.

The liver is responsible for metabolizing the end-product of protein metabolism, ammonia. Ammonia is converted by the liver into its water-soluble form, urea, and excreted by the kidneys. Patients with liver disease may have elevated serum ammonia. Elevated serum ammonia levels have been associated in some patients with the development of hepatic encephalopathy (Kirk, 1936; McDermott and Adams, 1954; Rikkers, et al., 1978). Encephalopathy is manifested by varying degrees of mental confusion. However, other studies have revealed poor correlation between ammonia levels and encephalopathy (Zakim and Boyer, 1982). If serum ammonia levels are elevated, measures that decrease blood ammonia levels may be beneficial to patients who have encephalopathy. Encephalopathy is usually precipitated by a secondary event such as sedative medications, hypokalemia, infection, or gastrointestinal hemorrhage (Zakim and Boyer, 1982). Since blood is a protein, blood in the gastrointestinal tract from bleeding ulcers or varices increases the protein load in the gut and may result in worsening of encephalopathy. Another finding associated with hepatic encephalopathy is fetor hepaticus, a characteristic offensive odor to the breath, often described as a fruity smell.

One of the most important functions of the liver is detoxification of drugs and other toxins such as alcohol. The liver also detoxifies certain fat-soluble products of metabolism. For example, bilirubin, a fat-soluble substance formed from the breakdown of red blood cells, is converted (conjugated) in the liver to a water-soluble form that is excreted in the bile. Elevation of the serum bilirubin (hyperbilirubinemia) results in jaundice. Hyperbilirubinemia can be the result of hemolysis, a reduction in the liver's ability to conjugate bilirubin, or a reduction in the liver's ability to excrete bilirubin into the bile. Bile, comprised of bile salts, bilirubin, cholesterol, phospholipids, and plasma electrolytes, is excreted in the intestine. The bile salts in bile are responsible for the breakdown of fats and absorption of cholesterol and other lipids in the intestinal tract. Fat malabsorption aggravates the nutritional problems seen in patients with liver disease. The accumulation of bile salts in the skin is in part responsible for the pruritus associated with hyperbilirubinemia. Absence of bile in the gastrointestinal tract results in clay-colored stools. Excretion of conjugated bilirubin by the kidney results in tea-colored urine. The nurse assesses for each of these manifestations in evaluating the patient's condition and response to therapy.

The liver is unique in its dual blood supply. In addition to the arterial blood supply, the liver also receives about 70% of its blood flow from the portal venous system. When the liver is scarred, or cirrhotic, there is increased resistance to flow through the portal venous system. The resistance to portal blood flow results in increased blood pressure in the mesenteric venous system (portal hypertension). This in turn leads to shunting of blood away from the liver through natural collateral channels. The mesenteric blood, in effect, bypasses the liver and returns directly to the heart through the collateral routes. The most common sites in which these collaterals form are the abdominal wall around the umbilicus (caput medusa), through hemorrhoidal veins, and through cross-over connections between gastric and esophageal veins. The latter form dilated veins called varices and peptic erosion of the overlying esophageal mucosa, which can lead to massive hemorrhage. Portal hypertension can also be associated with splenomegaly and hypersplenism. Hypersplenism may be associated with increased consumption and destruction of white blood cells and platelets, leading to leukopenia and thrombocytopenia (Rikkers and Edney, 1986). Constant monitoring of the complete blood count is therefore part of nursing management.

Acute fulminant hepatic failure (AFHF), one of the most severe forms of liver disease, demonstrates the multisystem effect of liver failure. Acute hepatic failure is severe failure of the liver occurring within 6 weeks of the onset of the symptoms of liver disease in an otherwise healthy individual. Causes include infection, chemicals, ischemia, or metabolic abnormalities (Zakim and Boyer, 1982). A patient with AFHF, by definition, will have some degree of hepatic encephalopathy, which may advance to coma, cerebral edema, and death if the process is not interrupted. Acute hepatic failure is also accompanied by coagulopathy. In addition, it may present with hypoglycemia and jaundice. Hypotension may occur secondary to hemorrhage, sepsis, or cardiac or respiratory abnormalities (Zakim and Boyer, 1983). The heart rate, peripheral vascular resistance, and cardiac output tend to be decreased in patients with AFHF. Dysrhythmias are common, especially in patients who are in deep hepatic coma. Hypoxia is often a severe problem, not readily associated with overt pulmonary complications such as pneumonia or adult respiratory distress syndrome (ARDS). Electrolyte imbalance with disturbances in acid-base balance is common. Renal failure is a late manifestation as is portal hypertension. Patients with AFHF have a high incidence of infection and gastrointestinal bleeding (Zakim and Boyer, 1983).

A patient presenting with end-stage liver disease such as AFHF requires a thorough nursing assessment in a head-to-toe systems approach. A baseline assessment using inspection, palpation, percussion, and auscultation is performed and recorded. Alterations in any of the systems are documented.

Appropriate nursing interventions are applied to minimize the patient's risk of complications secondary to the above findings while maximizing the patient's potential for wellness. Early referral to a transplant center should be a consideration in the overall patient care plan. Table 7–1 highlights common nursing diagnoses for the pre-transplant liver patient.

EVALUATION FOR TRANSPLANTATION

The evaluation process of potential candidates for liver transplantation is dependent on each transplant center's unique protocols, but similarities exist. When a patient is referred for transplantation evaluation, the transplant nurse coordinator may provide much information regarding the center's requirements for candidacy, information about the program, and

Table 7-1. Common Nursing Diagnoses for the Pre-Transplant Liver Patient

Health Perception — Health Management
- Health maintenance, altererd
- Health seeking behaviors
- Infection, potential for
- Injury, potential for
- Noncompliance

Nutritional — Metabolic
- Fluid volume, altered: excess
- Nutrition, altered: less than body requirements
- Oral mucous membranes, altered

Elimination
- Constipation
- Urinary elimination, altered patterns

Activity — Exercise
- Activity intolerance
- Cardiac output, decreased
- Diversional activity deficit
- Fatigue
- Home maintenance management, impaired

Sleep — Rest
- Sleep pattern disturbance

Cognitive — Perceptual
- Comfort, altered
  - Pain
  - Pruritus
  - Nausea
  - Vomiting
- Decisional conflict
- Knowledge deficit
- Thought processes, altered

Self-Perception
- Anxiety
- Fear
- Hopelessness
- Powerlessness
- Self-concept, disturbance in: body image; personal identity; self-esteem

Role — Relationship
- Family process, altered
- Self-concept, disturbance in: role performance
- Social interaction, impaired
- Social isolation

Sexuality — Reproductive
- Sexual dysfunction
- Sexuality patterns, altered

Coping — Stress Tolerance
- Adjustment, impaired
- Coping, ineffective individual
- Coping, ineffective family: compromised

Value-Belief Pattern
- Spiritual distress

the process of evaluation. Some centers require physician-to-physician referral for transplantation evaluation. Many centers accept self-referrals of patients or family members. Evaluations may be performed on an inpatient or outpatient basis and the extent and type of evaluation will vary from center to center. An example of one center's evaluation protocol is given in Table 7–2.

Table 7–2. Liver Transplant Evaluation Protocol

1. History and physical as usual

2. Consults
- Liver transplant group
- Liver study group
- Social service
- Psychiatry
- Patient business office

3. Tests
- ECG
- Chest x-ray
- Ultrasound of portal vein
- Urinalysis
- Pulmonary function test

4. Studies if clinically indicated
- Computerized tomographic (CT) bone analysis
- Upper endoscopy
- CT scan of abdomen
- Hand or wrist tray
- Endoscopic retrograde cholangiopancreatography (ENCP)
- Liver biopsy
- Cardiac catheterization

5. Research studies

6. Lab work — minimal blood draw
- Complete blood count (CBC) with differential and platelet count
- Renal panel
    - electrolytes, BUN, creatinine
- Liver function profile
    - bilirubin (treatment discontinued), aspartate aminotransferase (AST), alanine aminotransferase (ALT), gamma-glutamyl transpeptidase (GGTP), alkaline, phosphate, cholesterol
- Nutritional panel
    - total protein, albumin, ionized calcium, magnesium, phosphorus
- Prothrombin time/partial thromboplastin time (PT/PTT)
- Epstein-Barr virus (EBV), cytomegalovirus (CMV) (immune)
- Viral syndrome III (AIDS) and hepatitis B surface antigen
- Chronic hepatitis screen
- Alpha-fetoprotein
- Vitamin levels

The period of evaluation allows nursing and other healthcare professionals the time to assess the patient's and family's knowledge about liver disease and transplantation as well as their response to prior medical treatment. This initial relationship formed with the nursing personnel facilitates the educative and supportive interventions nurses will apply in caring for patients and their families throughout the transplantation process.

An integral part of any evaluation is educating patients and their families about the risks and benefits of transplantation so that they are able to make an informed decision about pursuing transplantation. The transplantation evaluation period is a time to review the risks and benefits of transplantation as well as its phases, including the waiting period, the operative procedure, postoperative routines, and long-term followup care. Patients are given this information during evaluation to allow them time to assimilate the information and ask questions before they are faced with the additional stress of the actual surgery.

Each transplant center has its own criteria for accepting patients as candidates for their active waiting list. The acceptance or denial of patients for transplantation is usually determined by a multidisciplinary team. Table 7 – 3 lists the usual diseases that may require transplantation. With the overall success of the procedure, the indications for transplantation are broadening.

Currently, patients are listed on the United Network for Organ Sharing (UNOS) system by blood type, size, and medical need. Any change in a candidate's medical stability is reported to the transplant center as it may alter the patient's priority status.

WAITING PERIOD

Once a patient is accepted as a transplant candidate, most centers encourage the patient to return home to await a suitable donor organ. Some centers may require their patient to relocate closer to the transplant center. An integral part of the pre-transplantation evaluation is informing the patient and family about the variable length of the waiting period prior to transplantation. Waiting has been described as one of the most difficult times of the transplantation process (Gold, et al., 1986). It is a time that requires close followup by the transplant center staff to monitor changes in the physical as well as the emotional well-being of the candidate. Waiting for a donor organ produces strong emotional feelings in patients and their family members. Some of the most prevalent feelings are hopelessness as the liver disease worsens, guilt in knowing that someone must die to allow them a chance to live, anger at the lack of suitable donor organs, and depression as the wait extends from days to months and even

Table 7–3. Disease States for Which Liver Transplantation Has Been Effective

ADULTS

- Post-necrotic cirrhosis
- Primary biliary cirrhosis
- Primary sclerosing cholangitis
- Fulminant hepatic failure
- Primary liver malignancy
- Laennec's cirrhosis
- Budd-Chiari syndrome

CHILDREN

- Biliary atresia
- Post-necrotic cirrhosis
- Fulminant hepatic failure
- Biliary hypoplasia
- Familial cholestasis

METABOLIC DISORDERS

- Alpha$_1$ antitrypsin deficiency
- Hereditary tyrosinemia
- Wilson's disease
- Crigler-Najjar syndrome type I
- Glycogen storage disease types I and IV
- Oxalosis
- Familial hypercholesterolemia (homozygous) type II
- Gaucher's disease
- Urea cycle deficiencies
- Hemophilia

years (Gold, et al., 1986). Medical followup as well as psychological support is essential during the waiting period.

Each center has its own methods for following and supporting patients during the waiting period. Methods may include periodic letters or postcards to the patients and their local doctors inquiring about recent laboratory work, medical or personal changes, or phone calls to the patients and their family by the nurse coordinators, social workers or other transplant team members. During the waiting period, periodic return visits to the transplant center may be indicated. In addition, referring physicians, patients, or their family members are encouraged to contact the center if the candidate either experiences changes in physical health or needs more emotional support. Families are encouraged to participate in local transplant center or community support group meetings. With the increasing number of transplant patients across the country, more communities are establishing local support groups. National liver organizations such as the American Liver Foundation, Children's Transplant Association, Children's Liver Foundation, Canadian Liver Foundation, and others are also active in providing support to families awaiting transplantation.

DONOR CRITERIA

The criteria for matching donors and recipients for liver transplantation include compatible blood type and liver size. Crossing of blood groups has been done successfully in emergency situations (Gordon, et al., 1986b). The degree of tissue type matching has been investigated retrospectively at some centers but does not appear to be correlated with outcome (Gordon, et al., 1986a). Size matching is usually done by height and weight though some centers rely on ultrasound or other radiologic tests to determine compatible size between the donor and the recipient. In addition to blood type and size, the suitability of donor organs is determined by the donor history, physical exam, and pertinent laboratory studies. These criteria are listed in Table 7-4.

Prior to the 1988 introduction of ViaSpan, the acceptable maximum time that a liver could be maintained outside the body was 8 hours (Shaw, et al., 1989d). This often necessitated the start of the recipient operation prior to the arrival of the donor organ at the recipient hospital. Occasionally, if the donor organ was deemed unsuitable for transplantation, the recipient had already been subjected to anesthesia, the insertion of the major intravenous catheters, a skin incision and the initial dissection of the liver. With the introduction of ViaSpan, preservation time of liver grafts was extended to 30 hours (Shaw, et al., 1989d). The increased preservation time allows centers to perform transplants on a semi-elective basis,

---

Table 7-4. **Donor Criteria for Liver Transplantation**

- Age (newborn to 50+ years)
- Size (compatible with recipient)
- Blood type compatible with recipient
- No history of pre-existing liver disease
- No active sepsis
- Human immunodeficiency virus (HIV) and hepatitis screen negative
- No history of prolonged ethanol alcohol abuse or intravenous drug abuse
- No evidence of ongoing disseminated intravascular coagulation (DIC)
- Coagulation profile normal
- Serial liver function tests — normal or improving
- No prolonged hypoxic episodes
- No prolonged hypotension
- Ideally — dopamine <10 mg/kg/minute

often as part of the routine operating room schedule. The added time factor also decreases the possibility of patients undergoing the initial steps of the operation prior to inspection of the donor liver. In addition, the increased preservation time has allowed for the development of techniques to perform reduced-size transplantation or split-liver transplants, which are now being performed in small adults and children. In reduced-size transplants, the right or left lobe of a larger liver is used for a small patient. In a split-liver transplant, the right lobe and left lateral segment of the liver are used for two different patients (Stratta, et al., 1990). When a donor organ becomes available to a transplant center, it is often the responsibility of the nurse coordinator to contact the potential recipient. In the past, due to the time constraints of the short preservation time, patients had to be able to return to the transplant center within 4 hours, usually necessitating private jet transportation. With the use of ViaSpan and extended preservation times, the patient may be allowed more flexibility in travel time to the transplant center. The patient may be able to drive or travel by commercial airline, which helps defray costs. However, many patients, due to distance from the transplant center or time constraints, still require the use of private planes for expeditious transportation to the transplant center.

Recently, living-related donors have been utilized in limited numbers. A segment of the liver from a living-related adult has been successfully procured and transplanted to children in several cases. The practice is new, evolving, and not without controversy related to the risks to the donor.

After the patient arrives and is admitted to the transplant center, the usual preoperative routines are followed. These routines include history and physical examination; blood work; chest x-ray; urinalysis; the insertion of an intravenous catheter; consultation by the anesthesiologist, surgeon, and clinical nurse specialist; and the signing of a consent form.

As noted above, the operation may begin immediately or be done semi-electively the next day. The time prior to the operation may be stressful to the patient and family. The time immediately pre-transplantation is reserved for answering questions, providing support, and allowing patients to spend time with their families. Thus, preoperative teaching may be more effective if done at the time of evaluation, prior to the arrival at the hospital for surgery.

OPERATIVE NURSING PROCEDURES

The surgical procedure of liver transplantation requires approximately 7 hours with a range of 4 to 24 hours. One to two hours of anesthesia preparation time is needed prior to the skin incision. The anesthesia time includes the time it takes to position the patient on the table, insert catheters and monitoring equipment, and perform skin cleansing prior to the skin incision.

Due to the nature of the operation, special nursing measures are required to assure patient safety throughout the operation. To protect the patient from pressure sores and tissue damage during the lengthy case, the operating room table is padded with an eggcrate mattress covering the patient's body length. A warming blanket is placed under the patient to prevent excessive heat loss. The arms are positioned to eliminate the possibility of brachial plexus injury secondary to hyperextension and the elbows are padded to guard against ulnar nerve injury. A pillow or blanket is placed lengthwise under the thighs to prevent knee hyperextension. The legs are loosely wrapped together to prevent external hip rotation, which can lead to sciatic or peroneal nerve injury; padding placed between the legs prevents pressure sores. The feet are also placed on heel pads.

The long surgical hours involved in liver transplantation may tax the attention span of the operating room personnel; however, the constant anticipation of the needs of staff and concern for patient safety is essential to a successful operation. The procedure itself has been well described in various articles (Shaw and Wood, 1988; Staschak, 1984), as has the use of specialized equipment such as the veno-venous bypass system, and rapid blood transfuser (Winters and Kang, 1986).

OPERATIVE PROCEDURE

A bilateral subcostal incision with possible midline-extension is made and the major structures of the liver (supra- and infrahepatic inferior vena cava, hepatic artery, portal vein, and bile ducts) are visualized and skeletonized prior to removal of the native liver (Shaw, 1984). This part of the procedure is termed the recipient hepatectomy. The recipient hepatectomy is more complicated in patients with severe coagulopathy or in patients with adhesions from previous surgery of the liver or biliary system.

Before the native liver is removed in adult patients, the patient is placed on a venous bypass system. Cannulas are inserted in the femoral, portal, and axillary veins (see Fig. 7-2). The femoral and portal vein cannulas are attached by a Y-connector, removing blood from the portal and systemic venous system, and returning the blood via a nonheparinized pump to the axillary vein and thus back to the heart during the anhepatic phase of the operation. The venous bypass system helps to minimize venous hypertension and maintain normal cardiac hemodynamics (Shaw, 1984). Once satisfactory bypass flow has been established, the vascular structures to the liver are clamped and the liver is removed.

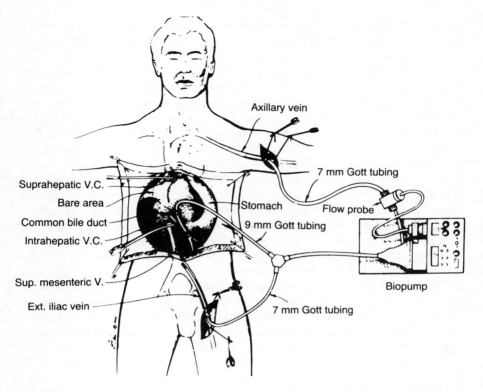

Figure 7–2

Before the native liver is removed in adult patients, the patient is placed on a venous bypass system. Cannulas are inserted in the femoral, portal, and axillary veins. (VC = venous cannula.)

After hemostasis is obtained in the retrohepatic area, the donor liver is sewn into place. First the supra- and then the infrahepatic vena caval anastomoses are completed. Prior to completion of the infrahepatic vena cava anastomosis, the liver is flushed via a cannula in the donor portal vein to remove the preservation solution from the liver and to prevent air embolism. The portal vein limb of the bypass system is clamped, the tubing removed from the recipient portal vein, and the portal vein anastomosis completed. The vascular clamps are released and blood flow is restored to the liver. This is a critical point of the operation and the patient may become unstable when the liver is revascularized. Hemostasis is obtained and the hepatic artery anastomosis is completed.

After the vascular anastomoses are completed and adequate hemostasis is obtained, the bile duct is reconstructed either by duct-to-duct

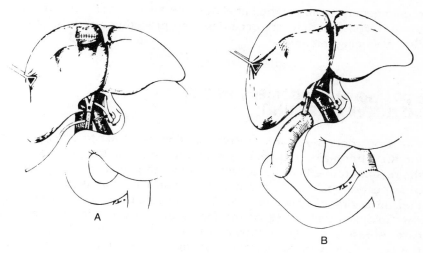

Figure 7 – 3

Completed orthotopic liver transplantation. (A) Biliary tract reconstruction with choledo-chostomy. (B) Biliary reconstruction with choledochojejunostomy, using a Roux limb.

anastomosis, choledochocholedochostomy, over a T-tube (using the pa-tient's native bile duct and sewing it to the donor bile duct) or a choledo-chojejunostomy over an internal stent, (using the donor bile duct and attaching it to a Roux-en-Y limb of the jejunum). A Roux-en-Y intestinal limb is performed in cases when the patient's native bile duct is absent, diseased, or too small to allow the insertion of a T-tube (Fig. 7 – 3). During the biliary tract reconstruction, the patient is usually stable and remains stable through the remainder of the case. After completion of the biliary tract reconstruction, the gallbladder is removed. Finally, closed-suction drains (such as Jackson-Pratt drains) are put in place, and the abdomen is closed. Once the operation is completed, patients are usually taken di-rectly to the intensive care unit for recovery.

RECOVERY FROM ANESTHESIA

After surgery, the anesthetic agents used during the operation are not usually reversed. Initially, in the intensive care unit (ICU), patients are usually hemodynamically stable on full life support and do not typically require the use of pressor agents. In managing these patients, the nurse considers that their sense of hearing may return before other signs of reversal of anesthesia are noted. It is important that nurses bear this phenomenon in mind in the initial postoperative period when the family is present, conversations are occurring, and procedures and routine nursing care are being initiated.

NURSING MANAGEMENT IN THE INTENSIVE CARE UNIT

A postoperative liver transplant patient is similar to other patients in the ICU after major abdominal surgery. In assessing the physical status of the postoperative liver transplant recipient the nurse uses the same skills of inspection, palpation, percussion, and auscultation as pre-transplantation. In addition, effective communication skills and assessment of the psychological well-being of the family are an essential part of nursing care. A baseline body systems assessment is made as a change in any of the systems may be significant. Nursing interventions are geared to the outcome of optimal patient and family well-being.

The patient is intubated on a ventilator, and has a Swan-Ganz or central venous catheter, cardiac monitor, nasogastric tube, arterial catheter, pulse oximeter, multiple intravenous catheters, a large abdominal incision, Jackson-Pratt drains, and a Foley catheter. The more unique aspects of managing liver transplant patients involve the assessment and management of hypertension, rejection, and infection. These problems present themselves throughout the patient's hospitalization and long-term followup. A systemic review of potential problems experienced by liver transplant patients follows. This review is inclusive of most potential problems but is not all-inclusive. The problems seen in patients with liver failure may recur after liver transplantation if the graft does not function.

Neurologic

Generally, anesthetic agents are not reversed in patients following liver transplantation. Patients may show signs of awakening from minutes to hours after the operation. One of the first indications that the liver is functioning adequately is the speed and degree to which the patient awakens. Consistent evaluation of the patient's neurologic system is crucial and is performed on an hourly basis or whenever changes occur.

Pain management may present a problem because analgesics alter the neurologic status and are metabolized in the liver. Any depression of the detoxifying ability of the liver may result in prolonged effects of analgesics (Williams and Rzucedlo, 1985). Small doses of analgesics may however be administered safely. Therefore the level of pain experienced by patients needs to be continually assessed by the nurse. Intervention may require routine comfort measures and strong patient advocacy skills in requesting the physician to order analgesic medications. Care must be given not to over-sedate patients if standing orders for analgesia exist. Surprisingly, many patients do not complain of incisional pain despite the large incision. Pain may be experienced in the rib cage secondary to the use of retractors in the operating room, and in the back, secondary to the length of the operation. Pain from the operation itself is usually limited to the first week. Any prolonged complaints of pain, unrelieved pain, or pain in a new location warrant nursing assessment and intervention.

Another neurologic problem experienced by transplant patients is psychosis, often related to stress, depression, prolonged stays in the intensive care unit, or to a combination of factors, including high doses of steroids or other medications. Usually psychosis or depression is self-limited, but may require assessment and coordination of interventions by the various members of the healthcare team. Assessment and intervention address both patient and family needs.

Seizures may be experienced as sequelae to drugs, electrolyte imbalance, medications, or intracranial bleeds. Damage to the brachial plexus may be experienced secondary to injury occurring during insertion of the axillary limb of the venous bypass system (Shaw, 1984). The diaphragm may be temporarily paralyzed by trauma to the phrenic nerve during the clamping of the suprahepatic inferior vena cava (Carithers, et al., 1988).

Cardiovascular

In assessment of the cardiovascular system, the nursing goal is adequate perfusion of all body organs. The patient's electrocardiogram (ECG) is continuously monitored during the intensive care unit stay. Generally patients are in normal sinus rhythm postoperatively and remain in normal sinus rhythm throughout their hospital stay. Transient episodes of sinus bradycardia have been noted as have episodes of sinus tachycardia, the latter mostly in conjunction with fever. Premature ventricular contractions (PVCs) may be associated with placement of pulmonary artery or central venous pressure catheters, electrolyte imbalance, or intrinsic cardiac disease. The presence of PVCs warrants close assessment and immediate consultation with a physician.

Hypertension is an almost universal phenomenon in liver transplantation patients. The cause of the hypertension is unknown; however, possible etiologies include alterations in the renin-angiotensin system, faulty tyramine metabolism, and side effects of steroid therapy or cyclosporine (Starzl, et al., 1982). Radial or femoral arterial blood pressures are monitored continuously in the intensive care unit. Hypertension is managed by the use of intravenous antihypertensive agents such as nitroprusside, nitroglycerine, and hydralazine.

Hypotension is rare following liver transplantation. Dehydration may alter blood pressure, but hypotension is most commonly a side effect of antihypertensive medications. Hypotension may indicate more serious problems, the two most serious of which are bleeding and sepsis. Bleeding and sepsis are complications that may be related to any of the four vascular anastomoses. Other problems involving the vascular anastomoses include thrombosis and stenosis.

Swan-Ganz catheter readings are routinely monitored in the intensive care unit. The usual hemodynamics following liver transplantation include a high cardiac output with a low systemic vascular resistance (Shaw, et al., 1989b).

Pulmonary

The goal in management of the pulmonary system is maintenance of adequate oxygenation of all tissues. Liver transplant patients are susceptible to pulmonary problems secondary to the long operative procedure and anesthesia time and large abdominal incision. Initially, patients return from the operating room intubated on a ventilator. Usually, if allograft function is adequate, patients are extubated within 24 to 48 hours after surgery. Right pleural effusion in adult patients is common (Wood and Shaw, 1985). Most pleural effusions resolve spontaneously or with diuretic therapy, although some respond only to thoracentesis or placement of a chest tube (Wood and Shaw, 1985). Paralysis of the diaphragm may be caused by injury to the phrenic nerve during clamping of the upper vena cava. Vocal cord paralysis may result from trauma secondary to the endotracheal tube (Wood and Shaw, 1985).

Atelectasis and pneumonia are problematic after any major surgical procedure. Aggressive nursing intervention such as suctioning, chest physiotherapy, coughing and deep breathing, change of position, and use of an incentive spirometer are undertaken throughout the hospital stay.

Gastrointestinal

Technical complications related to the gastrointestinal tract usually occur in the early postoperative period but may occur at any time. Complications of the biliary tract reconstruction include strictures, obstruction, perforations, infarction, infection, and bleeding.

Diarrhea is a complication following liver transplantation that affects the absorption of cyclosporine as well as the nutritional status of the patient. One of the causes of diarrhea in transplant patients is cytomegaloviral (CMV) enteritis, which may be associated with gastrointestinal bleeding, nausea, and vomiting (Shaw, et al., 1989b). Hyperalimenation is instituted early in the postoperative course if patients have complications of diarrhea or anorexia resulting from chronic illness and extensive surgery. Nutritional assessments by the nurse aid are continuous in monitoring the patient's status as well as response to therapy.

Upper and lower gastrointestinal bleeding may occur, often the result of stress-related ulcers, viral enteritis, or infectious colitis. Most cases of gastrointestinal bleeding after transplantation can be treated medically (Shaw, et al., 1989b). Nursing assessment of the gastrointestinal tract includes inspection of the abdomen, assessing for occult blood in drainage fluids, as well as assessment of bowel patterns and nutritional intake.

Renal

Renal dysfunction is not uncommon following liver transplantation, especially if renal function was impaired prior to surgery (Wood, 1987). Intraoperative hypotension will adversely affect renal function, and the use of diuretic and nephrotoxic drugs, including cyclosporine, may also potentiate renal dysfunction. Occasionally, patients will require dialysis in the postoperative period for hyperkalemia or fluid overload. The use of dialysis is usually temporary. Most patients recover adequate renal function prior to discharge from the hospital (Wood, 1987).

Fluid and Electrolytes

The most common abnormalities of serum electrolytes following liver transplantation involve sodium, potassium, and calcium. Frequently, patients have an excess of total body water despite low or normal intravascular volume. Therefore, patients requiring volume replacement receive colloid solution rather than crystalloid solution to replete the intravascular volume. One cause of hypocalcemia may be the citrates used in banked red blood cells.

Metabolic alkalosis, a common occurrence after liver transplantation, is not clearly understood. However, sodium bicarbonate administration in the operating room and prolonged nasogastric suctioning may be predisposing factors.

Extreme sodium shifts intraoperatively have been linked to central pontine myelinolysis, a process of demyelination of central nerve fibers. A patient with central pontine myelinolysis may initially wake up, but over a period of a few days may slip into a deep, irreversible coma and eventually die (Zbigniew, et al., in press). Assessments by nurses caring for liver transplant patients include following up laboratory studies and consultation with a physician when deviations from normal occur. Nursing care includes maintaining accurate intake and output records, obtaining daily weights, and observing for signs of fluid retention.

Hematologic

A properly functioning liver graft dramatically improves the patient's prothrombin time (PT) during the operative procedure. Coagulation studies should normalize in the immediate postoperative period. Abnormal or prolonged clotting times are often signs of a poorly functioning liver graft and, when present, prompt the nurse to closely monitor the patient for signs of bleeding. Anemia may be a problem throughout the hospitalization. Anemia may result from bleeding due to ulcers or gastroenteritis, or from excessive amounts of blood taken for laboratory tests. The nurse functions as the primary patient advocate in assuring that minimum amounts of blood are obtained for all laboratory studies and that repeat or superfluous tests are not ordered.

Hypersplenism secondary to portal hypertension generally resolves slowly over time. Hypersplenism may cause neutropenia and thrombocytopenia. Medications such as azathioprine and antithymocyte globulin, used for the treatment of rejection, and ganciclovir, used for the treatment of cytomegalovirus, may also result in bone marrow suppression and a low white blood count.

Musculoskeletal/Integument

Maintenance of an intact musculoskeletal system and intact integument is essential in nursing management of transplant patients. The skin is the body's first line of defense against infection. In the initial postoperative period and throughout hospitalization, meticulous care of all intravenous lines and careful wound management is needed to prevent infection. Routine turning of patients until they are able to be out of bed (which usually occurs within the first 24 to 36 hours) prevents decubitus ulcers.

Other integument problems are secondary to the use of cyclosporine and include gum hyperplasia and hirsutism or hypertrichosis; these potential problems are discussed before they become problematic and are included as part of discharge teaching. Careful oral care including brushing and flossing of the teeth is initiated early in the postoperative period to minimize chances of gum hyperplasia and oral infections. Hirsutism may be controlled with depilatories, bleaching, or shaving.

Infection/Rejection

Infection and rejection are the most difficult medical problems to manage in all transplant patients. The management of immunosuppressive therapy is intimately linked with both of these problems and may vary from center to center. Nursing management of these complications is geared toward prevention, patient and family education, and support.

Infectious complications may occur in any or all body systems post transplantation. Bacterial, fungal, and viral infections are common following liver transplantation. Bacteria may be the cause of wound infections, intravenous catheter sepsis, urinary tract infections, pneumonia, or intra-abdominal abscesses. Fungal infections, most commonly candidal infections, are usually secondary infections and frequently occur in patients with multiple organ failure. Cytomegalovirus (CMV), Epstein-Barr virus (EBV), and herpes viruses are the most common viral infections seen in transplant patients. Viral infections are either primary infections or reactivation of a latent infection. Liver transplant patients are not routinely placed in isolation following transplantation because the problematic bacteria, fungi, and viruses are usually part of the patient's own body flora. Although certain infections are more common among transplant patients, any type of infection is possible and potentially life threatening. Poor liver function, malnutrition, or multi-organ systems failure increases the risk for infectious complications.

Because liver transplant patients are at risk for infectious complications, nursing care focuses on prevention, including careful hand washing, meticulous intravenous line care, and sterile dressing changes. Hand washing remains one of the simplest, yet most effective ways to prevent infection. Families and the patients themselves are taught the importance of this. Careful assessment of all body systems for signs and symptoms of infection is also important.

Rejection is not usually a problem during the ICU stay following transplantation. However, primary graft nonfunction presents within the first 24 to 48 hours post transplantation and requires immediate retransplantation. Signs and symptoms of primary graft nonfunction include markedly elevated liver function tests, failure of the patient to awaken after surgery or changes in level of consciousness, acute renal failure and marked abnormalities of the clotting studies. Nursing care includes continued monitoring of vital signs with frequent neurologic checks, protection of the patient's airway, and family support.

NURSING MANAGEMENT ON THE SURGICAL/TRANSPLANT UNIT

Patients generally remain in the ICU for 3 to 5 days postoperatively. They are then transferred to a surgical or transplant unit for the remainder of their hospital stay (which averages from 3 to 6 weeks). A wide range of physical as well as psychosocial problems may be encountered during this time.

Neurologic

By the time patients leave the ICU, they are usually alert and fully oriented. Any change in the level of consciousness requires immediate attention. Situational or acute depression requires the nurse's support and consultation with psychologic services or social work staff. Sleep deprivation is a frequent complication that may contribute to feelings of depression. Nursing activities, including administration of medications, are grouped wherever possible and patients are assured blocked periods of time to promote sleep.

Cardiovascular

Cuff blood pressures are followed once patients are transferred from the ICU, and a combination of oral antihypertensive and diuretic medications is used to control hypertension. Careful nursing assessment of blood pressure and the therapeutic as well as side effects of the medications on the patient is necessary. The assessment involves evaluation of patient's blood pressure trends throughout the day. Orders for blood pressure medications include parameters for high and low blood pressure and guidelines for the administration of antihypertensive medication. In addition, the side effects of blood pressure medications are reviewed with patients to promote safety related to side effects such as orthostatic hypotension. Patients receiving antihypertensive medications are routinely instructed to get out of bed slowly, to go from bending/sitting to standing slowly, and to limit the amount of time spent in temperature extremes such as showers.

Headaches are not uncommon after transplantation. Headaches have been noted as a side effect of cyclosporine and stress. The potential for infectious complications causing headaches, however, should be of concern until proven otherwise. Persistent headaches are evaluated, documented, and appropriate physician consultation initiated.

Pulmonary

Patients continue to be at risk for atelectasis and pneumonia after leaving the ICU. Ambulation, coughing and deep breathing, and the use of incentive spirometers is continued. Assessment and documentation of the pulmonary system are performed routinely. Any changes including persistent cough, wheezing, increased respiratory rate, or cyanosis are pursued.

Gastrointestinal

Anorexia secondary to surgery, drugs, and chronic illness puts the patient at risk for inadequate caloric intake, which may predispose the patient to infection. Increased caloric requirements exist after transplantation. It is important to establish positive nitrogen balance to promote healing. Persistent anorexia or inability to meet the caloric demands of the body may be addressed with enteral or parenteral supplementation. Patients are usually encouraged to eat a balanced diet; however, problems secondary to electrolyte imbalance or fluid overload occasionally require special diets or dietary restriction for a short period of time. A registered dietician is consulted on a routine basis for dietary management. Diarrhea may be seen anytime during the postoperative course, and predisposes to the problems already discussed. Patients may also have problems with constipation.

Patients who have undergone previous sclerotherapy may suffer from esophageal strictures. Strictures may result in feelings of dysphagia, further affecting nutritional status.

Musculoskeletal

Ambulation benefits not only the musculoskeletal system but gastrointestinal and pulmonary systems as well. Early and frequent ambulation is included in nursing care plans. Consultation with physical therapy is routine. Consultation with occupational and recreational therapy may be ordered on a case-by-case basis as needed.

Aseptic necrosis, especially of the head of the femur secondary to steroid therapy, is a late complication of the musculoskeletal system seen in transplant patients. Persistent complaints of joint pain unrelieved by comfort measures warrant assessment and consultation with orthopedic physicians.

Infection and Rejection

Infection and rejection continue to be problematic throughout the patient's hospital stay. Infectious complications may require a return to the ICU. Hand washing remains crucial as does meticulous intravenous catheter and wound care.

Rejection is usually diagnosed through laboratory studies and liver biopsy. The first signs of graft rejection may occur as early as 5 to 7 days post transplantation but may occur at any time (Shaw, et al., 1989b). While some patients may not have any symptoms with rejection, other patients may develop fever and flu-like symptoms. Nursing intervention includes administration of prescribed immunosuppressive drugs, and management of symptomatology, education, and support.

The problems associated with infection/rejection and management of the immunosuppressive drugs are often the cause of the prolonged hospital stay. Patients have referred to the ups and downs following surgery as a roller-coaster ride, and not being able to see the light at the end of the tunnel (Gold, et al., 1986). These emotional ups and downs present the nurse with a challenging problem. Time must be devoted to families so they may vent their frustrations. Primary nursing is helpful in dealing with families' feelings of frustration. The transplant clinical nurse specialist, social worker, and other healthcare professionals may provide additional support during these times. Families may also gain support from other patients and their family members who have experienced similar medical problems and feelings. Attendance at patient and family support groups may be helpful during these times.

Retransplantation

Despite the use of cyclosporine and other immunosuppressive medications, rejection is still the most common indication for retransplantation (Shaw, et al., 1989b). Other reasons for retransplantation include graft nonfunction and hepatic artery thrombosis. Usually the need for more than one liver transplant occurs within the first few months after transplantation and usually while the patient remains at the transplant center. A small number of patients who develop rejection have also required retransplantation more than 1 year after the original surgery (Shaw, et al., 1985a). The success of one retransplant is generally quite good, but diminishes with each successive retransplantation.

Discharge Planning

Discharge planning needs to be addressed at an early point in the hospitalization. It is initiated after the patient has left the ICU, has no major complications, and has stable liver function studies. The focus of discharge planning includes medications, diet, activity, wound care, or care of any tubes, such as a T-tube. Followup laboratory studies and instructions on when to call the local physician or transplant center are also included.

If patients are leaving the hospital on blood pressure medications, most centers request that patients not add salt to their food at the table. In returning patients to a so-called normal environment, common sense versus rigid adherence to a strict diet is encouraged. Once the healing process is complete, patients are advised against eating high-calorie foods with little nutritional value. Steroids may stimulate the appetite, and patients who continue on a high-calorie diet once healing is complete will obviously gain weight.

The patient's level of activity will be based on his or her physical abilities upon leaving the hospital. Some patients may require physical therapy for a period of time if they were debilitated prior to surgery or have had a prolonged hospitalization. Most patients will experience fatigue following liver transplantation and are instructed to gear their activity accordingly. After a specific period of time, usually 3 months, patients are able to resume unrestricted activity. Some centers will restrict patients from playing contact sports such as tackle football. Patients are also counseled in the resumption of sexual activity, the risks of pregnancy, and the use of birth control methods (Shaw, et al., 1989d).

The prescribed use, side effects, dose, and timing of medications are reviewed with patients. Medications are scheduled according to the patient's individual routine. Medications are grouped to minimize the number of times per day patients need to take medications, and to aid in patient compliance. Suggestions for managing the side effects of drugs, such as the hirsutism caused by cyclosporine, are discussed. Some centers require patients to routinely check their weight and blood pressure (Overman, et al., 1989). Other centers require patients to check vital signs only if problems occur.

Patients are instructed to avoid the use of over-the-counter medications or medications that have not been prescribed by a physician as such medications may affect liver function or adversely interact with prescribed medications. Patients are also advised to avoid attenuated virus immunizations because of the potential risks that the virus will cause disease in the patient (Shaw, et al., 1989b).

Care of the abdominal incision usually involves checking for redness, pain, or drainage and notifying the appropriate person if problems or changes occur. Patients with open wounds are instructed in the techniques of packing the wound and/or changing the dressing. Care of indwelling catheters (such as a T-tube or central line) is based on transplant center protocols but generally includes keeping the site clean and checking for redness, pain, drainage, or change in the length of the tube outside the body; or loosening or absence of sutures.

The nursing staff begins preliminary teaching early with patients in self-care areas as concerns and questions arise. These concerns may appear during the day-to-day assessment and care of the patient and family members. Transplant clinical nurse specialists and coordinators are involved in reinforcement of patient teaching in conjunction with the staff nurse. They also coordinate outpatient followup care. Transplant center protocols vary in regard to outpatient followup. Usually the initial follow-up is done while the patient remains in the area of the transplant center, with visits to the outpatient clinic and frequent laboratory studies. Once patients return home, both the number of return visits to the transplant center and frequency of laboratory studies will vary dependent on the center's protocol.

Patients are instructed on whom to call if problems arise. Patient problems that warrant a phone call to the physician or clinical nurse specialist include fever of greater than 38°C, abdominal pain, diarrhea, persistent vomiting, persistent headache, persistent cough, jaundice, swelling, or weight gain. In addition, patients are encouraged to call if they have any questions or concerns about their physical or mental well-being.

While at the transplant center as outpatients, the contact person is generally the transplant clinical nurse specialist or coordinator. Once the patient has returned home, the local physician may become the first contact person. Most transplant centers continue to take an active role in caring for patients once they return home and continue to manage the immunosuppressive medications. Local physicians and patients are encouraged to call the transplant physician, clinical nurse specialist, or coordinator when problems or questions arise so a continued team approach can be utilized in dealing with problems. Table 7–5 summarizes nursing diagnoses throughout the post-transplant period. Table 7–6 highlights nursing goals for care.

PSYCHOLOGICAL ASPECTS OF NURSING CARE

Emotional and psychological support are of prime importance to patients and their families after transplantation. The hospital stay can be fraught with ups and downs secondary to any of the problems already discussed. In dealing with the continual unpredictability of the transplantation process, family members develop new attitudes and beliefs to help them cope (Mishel and Murdach, 1987). Educating patients and families about what to expect and the process of rejection and infection, as well as reinforcing treatment plans, becomes an integral part of nursing intervention. Allowing patients and families to ventilate fears and concerns is crucial to their well-being. Consultation and referral to the transplant coordinators, social worker, psychiatric services, and support group are freely initiated. The team approach among the various healthcare members provides a supportive structure for transplant patients, families, and team members. Effective and therapeutic communication among all participants is maintained. The nurse is the primary patient advocate and facilitator of the communication process.

Table 7–5. **Common Nursing Diagnoses for the Post-Transplant Liver Patient**

Health Perception — Health Management
- Health maintenance, altered
- Health seeking behaviors
- Infection, potential for
- Injury, potential for
- Noncompliance

Activity — Exercise
- Activity intolerance
- Diversional activity deficit
- Fatigue
- Home maintenance management, impaired

Nutritional-Metabolic Pattern
- Fluid volume deficit, potential
- Nutrition, altered: potential for more than body requirements
- Nutrition, altered: less than body requirements
- Hyperthermia (potential)
- Oral mucous membranes, altered
- Skin integrity, impaired: potential

Sleep — Rest
- Sleep pattern disturbance

Cognitive — Perceptual
- Knowledge deficit
- Decisional conflict
- Thought processes, altered

Self-Perception
- Anxiety
- Fear
- Hopelessness
- Powerlessness
- Self-concept, disturbance in: body image
- Self-esteem, chronic low

Role — Relationship
- Family process, altered
- Self-concept, disturbance in: role performance
- Social interaction, impaired
- Social isolation

Sexuality — Reproductive
- Sexuality patterns, altered

Coping — Stress Tolerance
- Adjustment, impaired
- Coping, ineffective individual
- Coping, ineffective family: compromised

Value-Belief Pattern
- Spiritual distress

Table 7-6. Nursing Priorities for the Liver Transplant Recipient

- Monitor hepatic function
- Assess for rejection
- Prevent infection
- Promote maximum independence and restoration of activities of daily living
- Foster return to normal sexual functioning

Emotional and psychological support from the transplant center is an ongoing process as late problems with infection and rejection may occur. These usually become less severe after the first post-transplant year (Shaw, et al., 1989b). It should be noted that the perceived quality of life in patients prior to transplantation and 3 months after transplantation is significantly improved (Lobiondo-Wood, et al., unpublished research).

Readmission to the hospital increases tension and anxiety in patients and their families. Primary nursing and consistency among team members provides a familiar base for patients and families during stressful times. In addition, contact with the transplant center and other transplant patients may help patients reintegrate with their home environments. Appropriate referrals are made to local counselors, social workers, public health nurses, and psychiatric services if problems occur concerning transition back into the family and community.

FINANCING TRANSPLANTATION

Although most third-party payers and state Medicaid programs cover the cost of transplantation, some do not. The costs for liver transplantation vary per center, and may be quite high. The American Council on Transplantation estimates the cost range for liver transplantation to be $135,000 to $338,000 (American Council on Transplantation, 1988). Many centers require cash deposits if no insurance support is available. Therefore payment for transplantation may become both a practical and ethical problem for the patient, family, and healthcare professionals.

Hospitals usually have in place a financial adviser or social worker to help patients with financial problems. Some centers have been quite aggressive in helping people pursue legal action against states or third-party payers that have denied transplant benefits. Usually individuals or organizations such as national transplant groups provide the impetus for such legal proceedings. Nurses may play a role as an advocate for patients having financial problems.

The transplant nurse coordinator, clinical nurse specialist, or primary nurse may be placed in the role of intermediary between patient and third-party payers. Involvement in local and national awareness of funding problems and political issues involving transplantation allows nurses a prime opportunity to become more knowledgeable about and contribute to the solution of the funding problem.

FUTURE ISSUES

The future issues of liver transplantation continue to revolve around increasing the supply of donor organs — including living-related — finding more effective methods of immunosuppression, and improving medical and nursing care of transplant patients. A new immunosuppressive drug, FK506, is currently being used in clinical trials; "cluster" organ transplants are being performed for patients with certain cancers; livers are being divided so that two patients benefit from one liver; and trials of total lymphoid irradiation, to prevent or treat rejection, have been initiated. All of the new medical techniques will affect nursing; however, nursing research and nursing publications are needed to document and support the work of nurses who care for patients undergoing transplantation. The nursing literature in this area is sparse, mostly descriptive and anecdotal in nature, and often center-specific. There is a need to address the issues of transplantation such as its effects on quality of life, effects on the family, effects on long-term survival, reintegration into activities of daily living, and the similarities and differences among transplant patients in general. Future issues in transplantation will include medical research with implications for nursing. The future of transplantation, however, is nonexistent without nursing care. Nursing care based on quality research is essential in promoting patient care and the science of nursing.

Acknowledgments

The author wishes to acknowledge the editorial assistance of Dr. R. P. Wood, Dr. G. Lobiondo-Wood, Dr. J. Donovan, Dr. B. W. Shaw, Jr., and Dr. R. J. Stratta and to thank Beth Blackburn, Elvira Keller, and Arleen Kottich for their secretarial assistance.

Bibliography

American Council on Transplantation, Statistics Sheet, 1988.
Carpentino, LJ: Handbook for Nursing Diagnosis. JB Lippincott, New York, 1989.
Carithers, RL, et al: Postoperative care. In Maddrey, WC (ed): Transplantation of the Liver. Elsevier Science Publishers, New York, 1988.
Cerilli, GJ (ed): Organ Transplantation and Replacement. JB Lippincott, New York, 1988.

Corliss, JK and Middleton, HM: Normal liver function: A basis for understanding hepatic disease. Arch Intern Med 143:2291–2294, 1983.

Gold, LM, et al: Psychosocial issues in pediatric organ transplantation: The parents' perspective. Pediatrics 77:5, 1986.

Gordon, RD, et al: The antibody crossmatch in liver transplantation. Surgery 11(4):705, 1986a.

Gordon, RD, et al: Liver transplantation across ABO blood groups. Surgery 11:342, 1986b.

Guyton, AL: Basic Human Physiology: Normal Function and Mechanism of Disease, ed 3. WB Saunders, Philadelphia, 1982.

Guyton, AL: Textbook of Medical Physiology, ed 6. WB Saunders, Philadelphia, 1986.

Kirk, E: Amino acid and ammonia metabolism in liver disease. Acta Med Search 77(Suppl):1, 1936.

Lobiondo-Wood, G, et al: Perceived quality of life in adult liver transplant recipients. Unpublished research, 1987.

McDermott, WV, Jr and Adams, RD: Episodic stupor associated with ECK fistula in the human with particular reference to metabolism of ammonia. J Clin Invest 33:1, 1954.

Mishel, NH and Murdach, CL: Family adjustment to heart transplantation: Redesigning the dream. Nursing Research 36:332, 1987.

National Institutes of Health Consensus Development Conference Statement: Liver transplantation; June 20–23, 1983. Hepatology 4:1078–1108, 1984.

Overman, JA, et al: Role of the nurse in the multidisciplinary team approach to care of liver transplant patients. Mayo Clin Proc 64:690–698, 1989.

Rikkers, LF and Edney, JA: Portal hypertension. General Surgery 3:4, 1986.

Rikkers, L, et al: Subclinical hepatic encephalopathy: Detection, prevalence and relationship to nitrogen metabolism. Gastroenterology 75:462, 1978.

St Joseph's Hospital Standards of Care. Marshfield, Wisconsin, 1988.

Schanwell, A, et al: Hemolysis in ABO-compatible liver transplantation—only after O grafts? Transplant Proc 21(3):352, 1989.

Shaw, BW, Jr: Venous bypass in clinical liver transplantation. Ann Surg 4:524–534, 1984.

Shaw, BW, Jr, et al: Hepatic retransplantation. Transplant Proc 5(1):264–271, 1985a.

Shaw, BW, Jr, et al: Transplantation of the liver. In Moody, F (ed): Surgical Treatment of Digestive Disease. Year Book Medical Publishers, Chicago, 1985b.

Shaw, BW, Jr, et al: Postoperative care. Seminars for Liver Disease, 1989b.

Shaw, BW, Jr, et al: Stratifying the causes of death in liver transplant recipients. Arch Surg 124(8):895–900, 1989c.

Shaw, BW, Jr, et al: Transplantation of the liver. In Moody, F, et al (eds): Surgical Treatment of Digestive Disease, ed 2. Year Book Medical Publishers, Chicago, 1989d.

Shaw, BW, Jr, et al: in press.

Shaw, BW, Jr, Starzl, TE, and Iwatsuki, S: An overview of orthotopic transplantation of the liver. In Flye, MW (ed): Principles of Organ Transplantation. WB Saunders, Philadelphia, 1989a, pp 347–364.

Shaw, BW, Jr and Wood, RP: The operative procedure. In Madry, CW (ed): Transplantation of the Liver. Elsevier, New York, 1988.

Starzl, TE, et al: Evolution of liver transplantation. Hepatology 2:614–636, 1982a.

Starzl, TE, Putnam, CW, and Corman, JL: Transplantation of the liver. In Schiff, L (ed): Diseases of the Liver, ed 4. JB Lippincott, Philadelphia, 1982b.

Staschak, S: Orthotopic liver transplantation: The surgical procedure. AORN 35(1):34–39, 1984.

Stratta, RJ, et al: The impact of extended preservation on clinical liver transplantation. Transplantation 50:438–443, September 3, 1990.

Williams, L and Rzucedlo, SE: Care of the pediatric liver transplant patient in the ICU. Critical Care Quarterly 8(1):13–25, 1985.

Williams, L, Wood, RP, and Shaw, BW, Jr: Role of nursing in the establishment of a liver transplantation program: Impact on nursing or nursing's impact? Transplant Proc 19:4, 1987.

Winters, PM and Kang, YS (eds): Hepatic Transplantation: Anesthetic and Perioperative Management. Progress Publication, New York, 1986.

Wood, RP: The reversal of hepatorenal syndrome following successful orthotopic liver transplantation. Ann Surg 205:415–417, 1987.

Wood, RP and Shaw, BW, Jr: Extra hepatic complications of the liver. Semin Liver Dis 5:377–384, 1985.

Wood, RP, et al: A review of liver transplantation for gastroenterologists. Am J Gastroenter 82:593–606, 1987.

Wood, RP, et al: Optimal therapy for patients with biliary atresia: Porto-enterostomy ("Kasai" procedure) vs primary transplantation? Pediatric Surgical Association (Abstract), May, 1989.

Zakim, D and Boyer, TD (eds): Hepatology: A Textbook of Liver Disease. WB Saunders, Philadelphia, 1982.

Zbigniew, KW, et al: Pontine and extrapontine myelinolyses following liver transplantation: Relationship to serum sodium. Transplantation, in press, 1989.

Pancreas Transplantation

Marilyn Groshek, RN, BSN
Victoria L. Smith, RN, MSN

Diabetes mellitus is a chronic disease indicated by hyperglycemia. It affects more than 12 million Americans, about 1 in every 20 people. As the third leading cause of death in the United States, it is also the leading cause of new blindness and a major cause of heart disease. Although insulin helps to control the manifestations of diabetes, it is not a cure. People with diabetes are at risk for major health complications including cerebral vascular accidents, renal failure, neuropathy, blindness, coronary artery disease, and infection severe enough to result in amputation (ADA, 1985). Classic symptoms of diabetes include polyuria, polydipsia, polyphagia, and weight loss following a rise in serum glucose levels.

Decreased utilization of glucose by the cells results in increased serum glucose levels. Increased mobilization of fat from storage areas in turn causes abnormal fat metabolism and lipid deposits in vascular walls. This results in atherosclerosis. Depletion of protein in body tissues occurs since glucose is not being utilized efficiently and the body must derive its nutritional source from the breakdown of protein. Due to the lack of insulin action, protein anabolism is prevented (Macleod, 1977). The nurse will see a patient with decreased muscle mass upon examination.

Diabetes is a chronic disease that affects the metabolism of carbohydrate, protein, fat, water, and electrolytes. It is associated with permanent and irreversible functional and structural changes in body cells (Guyton, 1977).

The financial impact of this disease is staggering to both the patient and the healthcare system. Governmental statistics indicate this disease represents an $18 billion-a-year drain on the U.S. economy. For the patient, insurance may be very expensive or even difficult to obtain. The available insurance may provide limited or inadequate coverage to meet the financial needs of medical treatment (Polin, 1985).

The goals of pancreas transplantation are to restore glucose control (euglycemia), remain independent from insulin, and halt the progression of long-term diabetic complications. Most important is the goal of restoration of a homeostatic environment that will halt the progression of complications resulting from altered carbohydrate, protein, and fat metabolism. This concept is not new. An unsuccessful attempt to transplant sheep pancreas extract into the abdominal wall of a diabetic comatose patient occurred in 1891. This was 30 years before the discovery of insulin by an English surgeon named Williams.

Currently, most pancreas transplants are performed in uremic patients either simultaneously with (synchronously) or 6 months to 1 year following renal transplantation (dysynchronously). The rationale is that a functioning endocrine pancreas will protect the renal graft and stabilize diabetic complications. (Pancreatic Transplantation in Diabetes, 1987). It also assists in monitoring pancreatic rejection. Renal biopsies can be done to monitor rejection but pancreatic biopsies are not indicated because the pancreas is so vascular.

From December 1966 until June 1988, over 1400 pancreas transplants have been reported to the world registry, half performed in North America and the other half in Europe (Sutherland and Moudry, 1989). The majority of pancreas transplants have been done within the last 5 years. The first pancreas transplant in the world was performed in 1966 by Kelly and Lillehei in Minneapolis, Minnesota. Since then, transplant centers have increasingly added this procedure to their program. The current worldwide graft survival rate at 1 year is 55%. (Table 8–1 reports numbers of transplants performed and graft survival statistics.) This survival rate represents an increase in graft survival from 25% prior to 1982 (Sutherland and Moudry, 1989). These data include all types of pancreas transplants, alone or with a kidney, from all centers reporting. During this early era, transplants were performed on uremic patients with advanced complications. Failures were frequent due to vascular thrombosis and difficulty disposing of the exocrine secretions. These problems resulted in new knowledge, research, and application. Major advances in surgical technique, improvement in immunosuppression, and better management of rejection have provided an impetus for further expansion and research in this area.

Table 8-1. **Pancreas Transplant Graft Survival Worldwide**

| Number of Transplants | | | | Graft Survival % |

* Percentage: Graft Survival Worldwide
Adapted from Pancreas Registry Report Data.

APPLYING PATHOPHYSIOLOGY

The cause of diabetes is still being researched. One or more of the following factors may contribute to this disease: genetic, environmental, viral, autoimmunity, inflammatory disease, metabolic disorders, insulin insufficiency secondary to pancreatic lesions, and abnormal glucagon secretion.

Diabetes is the result of abnormalities in the endocrine and vascular systems. A lack of insulin action alters carbohydrate, protein, and fat metabolism. This disease affects both the macrovascular and microvascular vessels in the body. As a result of macrovascular changes, the risk of myocardial infarctions, cerebral vascular accidents, and peripheral vascular disease is increased. Diabetics also develop retinopathy, nephropathy, and neuropathy due to microvascular changes (Davidson, 1986).

Following the discovery and use of insulin by Banting and Best in 1922 as a treatment modality for diabetes, life expectancy has significantly increased for the diabetic patient. However, with this increase in longevity has come a rise in deaths from renal disease. End-stage renal failure accounts for about half of the morality in young insulin-dependent diabetics diagnosed prior to age 40. On the average, renal failure second-ary to insulin-dependent diabetes mellitus (IDDM) occurs after 20 years (Orie, 1986). It is important to emphasize that rehabilitation following transplantation is superior to dialysis. A transplant is more cost effective, since the cost of transplantation is comparable to the cost of just 1 year of dialysis. Following a transplant, improvements in diabetic gastroenterop-athy and neuropathy are documented to enhance quality of life (Olefsky, 1985). Although no improvement in retinopathy has been documented, pancreas transplant recipients have less frequent and less severe vitreous hemorrhages and decreased need for further laser surgeries.

Assessing for Clinical Signs and Symptoms

INTEGUMENTARY MANIFESTATIONS

The nurse assesses the diabetic patient to be at high risk for skin infections. Elevated glucose concentrations in the skin due to hypergly-cemia and decreased leukocyte function place the patient at risk for moni-liasis and vulvovaginitis. Providing patient education regarding hygiene is a critical nursing intervention. Nystatin is effective in treating these fungal infections when they occur. The nurse also assesses for furuncles, boils, and infected skin ulcers, which may appear. So-called shin spots, which may be found on the extensor surfaces of the lower extremities, are painless lesions. Once healed, they are covered with atrophic scar tissue. Necrobiosis lipoidica diabeticorum is a more extensive lesion that causes ulceration and necrosis of tissue (Skilnan and Tzagournis, 1985).

Preservation of skin integrity of the feet is a priority for patient care in the nursing care plan, considering the high rate of amputation in diabetics. Two common changes that occur in the feet and legs of many diabetics are diabetic neuropathy and decreased circulation. Neuropathy occurs when the nerve's ability to transmit messages of pain from the feet and legs to the brain is impaired. A minor lesion may not be felt and may progress to serious infection. The nurse instructs the patient of the need to check the feet for redness or lesions daily and teaches the visually impaired patient ways to do this. Wearing proper – fitting shoes and keeping skin soft with an emollient are part of the teaching plan. The patient is cautioned that due to the changes in nerves affecting the sweat glands, the skin may become dry, cracked, and later infected. Toenails which are thickened in the diabetic patient, are cut straight across with a nail clipper or file in order to prevent tissue injury caused by scissors. The patient is instructed to always seek assistance in treating corns and calluses, the leading causes of ulcerations and infections. The nurse cautions that over-the-counter medications for ingrown toenails may contain acid and instructs the patient that these can cause severe damage. If precautions are taken and trouble areas are discovered early, amputations can be prevented.

METABOLIC MANIFESTATIONS

When insufficient insulin is produced, glucose cannot be properly utilized, causing serum glucose levels to rise. The renal tubules exceed their capacity to reabsorb glucose from the glomerular filtrate, resulting in glycosuria. In most people this occurs with a glucose exceeding 180 mg/100 mL. The nurse monitors both urine and serum glucose levels as needed. Diuresis occurs due to the excess serum glucose exerting an osmotic effect. This osmotic effect prevents the reabsorption of water, manifested by polyuria and nocturia. The nurse constantly assesses for dehydration of both intracellular and extracellular fluids. This sequela develops due to loss of water and minerals, resulting in polydipsia (Macleod, 1977).

Abnormal carbohydrate metabolism causes the body to shift to another source for fuel, depleting stores of protein and fat. The nurse observes a patient with fatigue and tissue wasting despite increased food intake (polyphagia). As fat metabolism increases, excess ketone bodies are produced by the liver for cellular catabolism. Metabolic acidosis occurs when both the pH and the CO_2 combining power of the blood fall below normal levels. Diabetic ketoacidosis signifies an emergency situation. The primary goal in treatment is to shift fat metabolism to carbohydrate utilization. This is done by an intravenous insulin drip (Luckmann and Sorenson, 1989). The second goal is to treat shock and fluid and electrolyte imbalances. Diabetic management has become easier because of the important role nurses play in patient teaching. The educational content includes improved methods for home glucose monitoring, adequate insulin intake, validating understanding of the dietary regimen, and emphasizing the benefits of exercise.

CARDIOVASCULAR MANIFESTATIONS

Atherosclerosis is more prevalent and occurs at an earlier age in the diabetic than in the nondiabetic. Studies indicate diabetics have higher plasma concentrations of low-density lipoproteins (LDL) and lower than normal concentrations of high-density lipoproteins (HDL). Calcification of the atherosclerotic plaques occurs, and results in hypertension (Skilnan and Tzagournis, 1985). These plaques are related to high glucose and lipid levels common in diabetes. Due to the coronary artery disease that develops in diabetics, a decreased cardiac output reduces blood supply to nerves, eyes, kidneys, and lower extremities. The nursing history and exam reveal intermittent claudication, cold feet, paresthesias, foot infections, inadequate wound healing, ulceration of extremities, and gangrene. All are a result of decreased blood supply (Luckmann and Sorenson, 1989).

Diabetic nephropathy occurs as a result of the changes in the basement membrane of the glomerular capillaries; these changes are termed diabetic glomerulosclerosis. The nurse monitors for symptoms including proteinuria, edema, and hypertension, as well as renal failure and uremia. In addition to the other multifaceted problems associated with diabetes mellitus, the entire clinical syndrome of renal failure, seen in 50% of diabetics into their fifteenth year of the disease, makes this a complex case for nursing management.

Diabetic retinopathy is the most common cause of blindness. Microangiopathy is a thickening of the basement membrane of the capillaries. Along with vascular degeneration, these can cause microaneurysms, retinal hemorrhages, and retinal detachment. The nurse emphasizes routine eye exams to detect early signs of retinopathy. Early diagnosis and destruction of new vessels by photocoagulation before hemorrhage, macular damage, and retinal detachment occur are recommended.

NEUROLOGICAL MANIFESTATIONS

Major causes of diabetic neuropathy are vascular insufficiency, vitamin B deficiency, and elevated serum glucose levels. These lead to metabolic disturbances in the neuron itself. Involvement of changes in the autonomic nervous system may cause diarrhea, neurogenic bladder, impotence, postural hypotension, and an impaired response to hypoglycemia (Macleod, 1977). The nurse assesses for peripheral neuropathy, which presents first as pain in the lower extremities and later as numbness. Because of the loss of sensation, pain, temperature, and position, preventive measures against injury are emphasized with the patient. Assessing for other signs of degenerative motor disease such as muscle atrophy, gross weakness, and footdrop complete the examination (Skilnan and Tzagournis, 1985).

Neuropathy affects the gastrointestinal tract by the delay of gastric emptying and/or diarrhea, which may alternate with constipation. Because bladder dysfunction may occur due to neural impairment, the nurse assesses for infection, interference with urination, and painless retention of urine. Ascending urinary tract infections are also common in patients with neurogenic bladders. A complete nursing history may reveal sexual dysfunction in either sex. About 50% of diabetic males have impotence related to nerve impairment, hindering the dilatation of penile arteries to engorge with blood necessary for an erection. Retrograde ejaculation can also occur from an incompetent bladder neck which allows seminal fluid to flow back into the bladder. Phenylpropanolamine can be prescribed for this problem, resulting in an increase in semen volume, assisting in effective ejaculation. The female diabetic also may encounter orgasmic difficulties.

The diagnosis of diabetes mellitus results not only in physical but also in emotional difficulties to be overcome. The interruption of and change in life-style this diagnosis requires of the patient, coupled with the long-term implications and complications, can be overwhelming. This is a chronic disease with a very uncertain future. Medical management can attempt to control, but does not cure, diabetes. Nursing care and patient education can make the difference in how the patient responds to this condition, and how each will respond to changes in activities of daily living. These include compliance with diet, and monitoring glucose and insulin levels to provide optimum health and function.

Potential nursing diagnoses for the pre-transplant pancreas patient can be found in Table 8–2.

SELECTING THE RECIPIENT

Patient criteria for selection as a candidate for pancreas transplantation are often based on age, stage of renal failure, ophthalmic exam, electromyography (EMG), cardiac workup, ability to withstand surgery, noninvasive vascular studies, and emotional and psychological stability. The age of this population ranges from 22 to 44 years. Since there is an increased incidence of cardiac disease in diabetics, a thallium stress test is indicated for all candidates over the age of 30. About 20% of all diabetics screened prior to transplant exhibit a positive stress test and require further cardiac evaluation, including cardiac catheterization. Of these patients, some can be treated with either medications, balloon angioplasty, or coronary artery bypass grafts (Orie, et al., 1986). If there is a question of cardiac dysfunction, transplantation is usually delayed. Vascular studies of extremities (EMG, noninvasive studies) determine the severity of neuropathy. Ophthalmic exams assess and provide a baseline of retinopathy.

Cadaveric pancreas transplantation is suitable for two subpopulations. One is the patient who has had a previous renal transplant and is already taking the immunosuppressive medications required for a pancreas transplant. The other is the patient who exhibits renal failure and is a qualified candidate for renal transplantation. An isolated pancreas transplant may be indicated for the first, while the latter may be qualified for a simultaneous pancreas and renal graft. Pancreas transplantation in nonuremic diabetics who have not had a renal transplant and would be

Health Perception — Health Management
- Health maintenance, altered
- Health seeking behaviors
- Noncompliance

Nutritional — Metabolic
- Infection, potential for
- Nutrition, altered: more than body requirements
- Oral mucous membranes, altered

Elimination
- Constipation
- Diarrhea
- Urinary elimination, altered patterns

Activity — Exercise
- Activity intolerance
- Cardiac output, altered: decreased
- Diversional activity deficit
- Fatigue
- Home maintenance management, impaired
- Tissue perfusion, altered: peripheral

Sleep — Rest
- Sleep pattern disturbance

Cognitive — Perceptual
- Comfort, altered
  - Chronic pain
  - Pruritus
  - Nausea
  - Vomiting
- Decisional conflict
- Knowledge deficit
- Sensory-perceptual alteration: tactile
- Thought processes, altered

Self-Perception
- Anxiety
- Fear
- Hopelessness
- Powerlessness
- Self-concept, disturbance in: body image; personal identity; self-esteem

Role — Relationship
- Family process, altered
- Self-concept, disturbance in: role performance
- Social interaction, impaired
- Social isolation

Sexuality — Reproductive
- Sexual dysfunction
- Sexuality patterns, altered

Coping — Stress Tolerance
- Adjustment, impaired
- Coping, ineffective individual
- Coping, ineffective family: compromised

subjected first to the side effects of immunosuppressants has been tried. It is being debated whether the risks outweigh the benefits (Sutherland, 1988). The use of living-related donors for segmental donation has also been tried and is another area under discussion.

Providing Patient Education

Nursing care begins with the initial contact with the patient during an interview, and may include a tour of the transplant unit. At this time, the nurse also shares information regarding transplantation with the patient. An assessment is made of the amount of knowledge the patient has regarding diabetes, management of the disease, transplantation, and expectations. Information is shared with the patient regarding admission, length of hospital stay, procedures, unit policies, and followup care. The opportunity to speak to several pancreas transplant patients is made available when possible.

MANAGING THE PATIENT PREOPERATIVELY

Nursing care and education of the patient begin with the initial visit to the transplant center. A potential candidate for either isolated or simultaneous pancreas and renal transplantation must meet the criteria of the center. Initial evaluation will be followed by an interview with the transplant coordinator for any additional workup. Tissue typing, ABO screening, cytomegalovirus (CMV) and human immunodeficiency virus (HIV) titers, hepatitis reactivity, blood urea nitrogen (BUN), and creatinine levels are assessed. Table 8–3 provides a more complete list of evaluation criteria.

When the patient is contacted about the availability of a pancreatic donor, he or she is instructed not to eat, drink, or take any insulin at this point. Insulin is generally given to achieve a serum glucose level of 200 mg/100 mL at the time surgery begins (Vernon and Sollinger, 1989). After the pancreas is placed, glucose levels will begin to equilibrate to a normal level without exogenous intervention.

Psychologically, patients may be difficult to evaluate preoperatively due to uremia dulling mental acuity, depression from ineffective coping, and recognition that the pancreas or pancreas-renal transplant is finally becoming a reality. The combination of fear of the unknown and optimism results in a great deal of anxiety.

Weight and vital signs (orthostatic) are documented. A bed-scale weight and standing weight are recorded by the nurse as a baseline.

Table 8–3. Evaluative Criteria for Pancreas Transplant

- Insulin-dependent diabetes mellitus
- Renal failure
- Negative thallium stress test for coronary artery disease
- Documented medical history
  1. Referral letter from local medical doctor
  2. Hospital discharge summaries
- Nonreactive human immunodeficiency virus (HIV) result
- Laboratory tests: Tissue typing, ABO typing, blood urea nitrogen (BUN), creatinine, hepatitis B profile, herpes simplex virus (HSV) titer, cytomegalovirus (CMV) titer, Epstein-Barr virus (EBV) titer
- Meet with:
  1. Transplant coordinator
  2. Transplant unit nurse
  3. Financial advisor
- Risk factors for pancreas transplant:
  1. Complete loss of eyesight
  2. Major amputations
  3. Cardiovascular disease
  4. Inability to understand procedure
  5. Inability to obtain financial approval
  6. Active infection

Considering postoperative bedrest is 24 to 48 hours, both of these preoperative measurements are necessary for accurate and comparative evaluation. Table 8–4 lists the elements of the nursing admission history.

The nurse has begun teaching at the initial contact. To reduce anxiety and promote cooperation, a brief review of unit policies and orientation to the environment are shared with the patient and family. Preoperative teaching and information regarding the immediate procedures are kept to a minimum. Since the level of anxiety is very high preoperatively, the nurse recognizes that teaching at this point is not well retained. Table 8–5 represents an example of a teaching flow sheet for pancreas transplantation.

Preoperative preparation begins with tap water enemas until clear results are obtained. Since the organs are being placed in an intra-abdominal technique, the nurse explains to the patient that thorough evacuation of stool allows for comfort postoperatively and minimizes the risk of perforation. A steroid ileus may occur preoperatively.

The nurse then instructs the patient on the need for an antibacterial shower. Laboratory reports of serum results are reviewed by the nurse. Also included may be the final crossmatch, ABO typing, chest x-ray report, ECG report, and cold agglutins. Cold agglutins are circulating antibodies that sludge in a cold environment. If this test is positive, the

Table 8-4. **Nursing Admission History**

1. Previous transplants and amount of immunosuppression
2. Genitourinary: Amount of urine in 24 hours as baseline, history of urinary tract infections or retention
3. Years on dialysis
4. Access site
5. Vision
6. Extent of neuropathy
7. Insulin type and amount
8. Number of years with IDDM
9. Subjective recognition of hypoglycemia
10. Monitoring system used for glucose control
11. Type of diet
12. Skin integrity: Lesions, ulcerations, toenails
13. Mobility
14. Cardiovascular: Edema, strength, rhythm and rate of pulses, color, and skin temperature
15. Respiratory: Respiration quality
16. Gastrointestinal: Pain or distension, nausea, emesis, peritoneal dialysis catheter, scars
17. Support systems
18. Initial instructional plan: Literacy, vision, glucose monitoring, taking own vital signs, medications, and activity

surgeon needs to warm the kidney prior to transplantation or blood will clump. Hyperkalemia, if presents, is treated preoperatively. Instruction and a return demonstration of the use of the incentive spirometer are completed before surgery. Instructions to cough and deep breathe using a pillow for splinting of the abdomen are done at this time. The arteriovenous fistula access, if present, is wrapped gently with Kerlix gauze and labeled.

MANAGING THE PATIENT INTRAOPERATIVELY

Surgery for an isolated pancreas transplant takes approximately 3-4 hours and a simultaneous pancreas and renal transplant about 4-6 hours. Patients are sent to the recovery room postoperatively and are returned to the transplant unit when awake and in stable condition. An intensive care unit is not routinely utilized unless indicated. The surgeons and transplant coordinator will report the patient's condition to family members immediately after surgery.

Variations in surgical technique and transplantation of whole or segmental pancreas are left to the individual transplant center's preference and experience. The type of surgical technique is based solely on how the

Table 8-5. Pancreas Transplantation Teaching Flow Sheet

Preoperative
- Inspirometer, coughing and deep breathing practiced with incision splinting
- Explanation of diagnostic tests: chest x-ray, ECG, laboratory values, physical exam
- Surgical prep: Enemas, skin prep and shave, anesthesia consult, IV placement, and medications

Postoperative
- Suture line care and assessment
- Foley catheter care and monitoring of urine output
- Pancreas rejection: Glucoses, urine amylases, and perfusion scan
- Review signs of infection
- Medications: Discuss rationale and side effects
- Keotoconazole, azathioprine or cyclophosphamide, prednisone, cyclosporine, antibiotics, antiviral agents, and antacids
- Practice drawing up cyclosporine
- Discharge planning: Telephone followup, clinic appointments, glucose monitoring, transplant labs, orthostatic vital signs, dehydration and adequate hydration, electrolytes, bicarbonate loss

exocrine secretions are to be directed. Although the pancreas has a dual function, exocrine and endocrine, in which the exocrine portion excretes enzymes that aid in digestion, and the endocrine portion secretes insulin, only the endocrine function is needed. Exocrine function in the native pancreas remains intact despite diabetes mellitus. The three most common techniques to occlude duct drainage of exocrine secretions are: (1) polymer injection (Figure 8-1); (2) intestinal drainage (Figure 8-2); and (3) bladder drainage (Figure 8-3).

The first technique, polymer injection into the pancreatic duct, produces total duct occlusion of the graft, which is used to suppress exocrine secretions. An agent such as Neoprene, a liquid synthetic rubber, is easily injectable and solidifies on contact with pancreatic juices. Other agents may also be used for duct occlusion. The pancreatic graft is placed intraperitoneally and anastomosed to the common iliac vessels with the tail of the graft lying downward with the omentum. A renal graft can be placed using the opposite common iliac vessels in all three techniques. Early graft failure of the pancreas may occur from pancreatitis, which can result immediately postoperatively. Progression of fibrosis can lead to late graft failure but generally the exocrine parenchyma is replaced by loose fibrous tissue surrounding well preserved islets (Dubernard and Monti, 1985).

The second technique is the enteric or intestinal drainage of a pancreatic graft. The anastomosis is similar to the above technique, using the common iliac vessels or distal vena cava. Anastomosis of the pancreatic

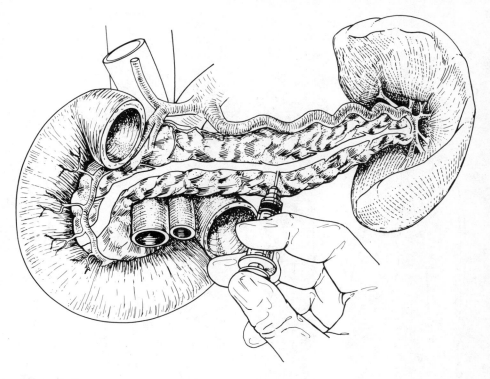

Figure 8–1

Duct injection.

graft to either duodenum or jejunum with a temporary pancreatic duct tube draining to the exterior is known as pancreaticoenterostomy or pancreaticojejunostomy (Corry and Nghiem, 1986). Wound sepsis is a potential disadvantage for this technique if the bowel anastomosis should leak. The nurse assesses for signs of infection to detect this complication.

The third technique is bladder drainage, in which pancreatic vessels are anastomosed to iliac vessels as in the above techniques. Both pancreas and a portion of duodenum containing the pancreatic duct are anastomosed to the bladder, a technique known as pancreaticoduodenocystostomy (Sollinger, 1988). Pancreatic enzymes are secreted in an inactive form and do not cause any damage to the bladder or ureter. Since one of the secretions of the pancreas with a segment of duodenum is bicarbonate, the nurse assesses for metabolic acidosis, observing for hypotension and dehydration. The advantage of this technique is that the nurse can monitor the amylase in urine as a aid in diagnosing rejection of the pancreatic graft if simultaneous pancreas and renal grafts are not used.

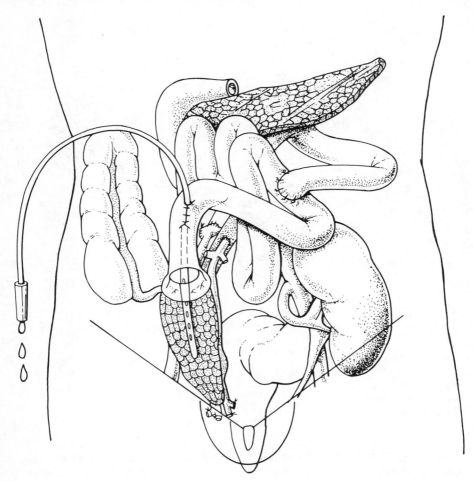

Figure 8-2

Pancreaticoenterostomy.

The Pancreas Transplant Registry reports that no major differences have been shown with one-year graft survival between whole organ versus segmental transplantation. There is also no difference in graft survival related to selected exocrine drainage technique. Differences do occur, however, in graft survival statistics between centers. The treatment of rejection based upon renal dysfunction in simultaneous pancreas and renal grafts has allowed for the successful treatment of pancreatic rejection. Graft survival statistics for simultaneous transplants are much higher than those for a pancreas transplanted alone.

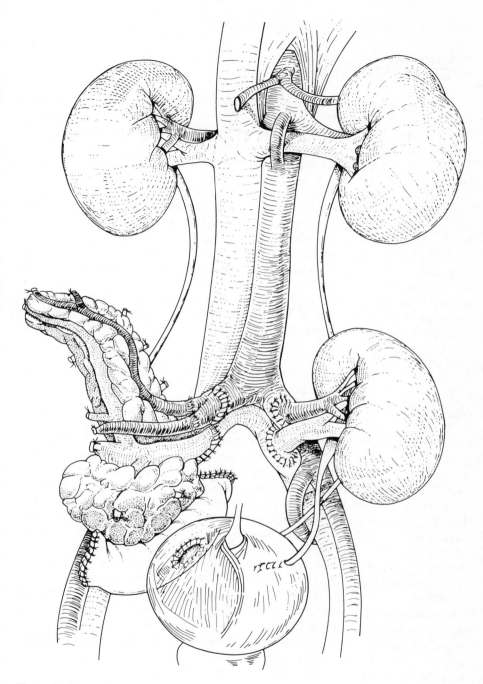

Figure 8-3

Pancreaticoduodenocystostomy.

MANAGING THE PATIENT POSTOPERATIVELY

Changes in the recipient's condition may be rapid, and nursing care postoperatively focuses on changes related to potential complications. (See Table 8–6 for nursing diagnoses for the pancreas recipient.) Fluid balance, respiratory care, and potential for bleeding are primary focal points. The nurse can expect parenteral fluid orders to be titrated to urine output plus 30 cc/hour for a pancreas-renal combination to promote renal function. For isolated pancreas transplant, a set rate of 125–150 cc/hour may be ordered. The nurse recognizes that an osmotic diuresis may occur after surgery in a patient who is uremic and fluid overloaded. However, a patient with a previous kidney transplant may not experience this diuresis due to the already functioning renal graft. To reduce graft edema and promote diuresis, the physician may order albumin and mannitol. For the first 72 hours postoperatively, the nurse measures the patient's abdominal girth every shift, or more frequently if indicted. A central line is utilized to facilitate blood sampling, to provide access as a medication port, and to monitor central venous pressure.

Assessing for Anastomosis Leakage

A Foley catheter is placed during surgery, and remains for approximately 10 to 14 days. The indwelling catheter provides constant decompression of the bladder to minimize pressure on the anastomosis site. Before the catheter is removed, a cystogram is obtained to assure that the anastomosis of the pancreas and duodenal segment is well healed to the bladder without leakage. The Foley catheter is then removed if no extravasation occurred. If a small leak is noted on cystogram, the Foley catheter remains in place for 4 to 6 weeks until the anastomosis has healed. Frequent cultures are obtained and pathogens are aggressively treated. In the case of a large leak at the anastomosis site, the Foley catheter may be attached to Pleurovac suction. The site may need further surgery. Allowing for accurate measurement of urine output, the catheter also serves as a means to irrigate clots and prevent overextension of the bladder at the anastomosis sites (ureter and/or pancreas). Urine retention increases pressure at these sites and can lead to a bladder leak. The nurse measures and assesses urine output. Fluid balance is assessed frequently. Urine is often bloody due to the anastomosis and vascularity of the bladder and clears within a week postoperatively. The nurse assesses for hematuria after clearing, recognizing that it may indicate a complication.

Table 8–6. Common Nursing Diagnoses for the Post-Transplant Pancreas Patient

Health Perception — Health Management
- Health maintenance, altered
- Health seeking behaviors
- Noncompliance

Nutritional — Metabolic
- Fluid volume deficit
- Infection, potential for
- Nutrition, altered: less than body requirements
- Oral mucous membranes, altered

Elimination
- Constipation
- Diarrhea
- Urinary elimination, altered patterns

Activity — Exercise
- Activity intolerance
- Airway clearance, ineffective
- Cardiac output, altered: decreased
- Diversional activity deficit
- Fatigue
- Home maintenance management, impaired
- Tissue perfusion, altered: peripheral

Sleep — Rest
- Sleep pattern disturbance

Cognitive — Perceptual
- Comfort, altered: pain
- Decisional conflict
- Knowledge deficit
- Sensory-perceptual alteration: visual
- Thought processes, altered

Self-Perception
- Anxiety
- Fear
- Hopelessness
- Powerlessness
- Self-concept, disturbance in: body image; personal identity; self-esteem

Role — Relationship
- Family process, altered
- Self-concept, disturbance in: role performance
- Social interaction, impaired
- Social isolation

Sexuality — Reproductive
- Sexual dysfunction
- Sexuality patterns, altered

Coping — Stress Tolerance
- Adjustment, impaired
- Coping, ineffective individual
- Coping, ineffective family: compromised

Promoting Fluid and Electrolyte Balance

Volume depletion is corrected with administration of albumin, Plasmanate, or a fluid challenge. Knowing that hypovolemic shock can cause decreased perfusion to transplanted organs, the nurse assesses for adequate hydration. Vital signs are also parameters that help the nurse assess fluid status. Daily weights are compared, and serial central venous pressure (CVP) readings are evaluated to further assess hydration. The nurse assures that intake and output are accurately monitored.

Metabolic acidosis can occur in pancreas transplants with bicarbonate levels well below normal. Loss of bicarbonate in the urine from the duodenal transplanted segment may be excessive, necessitating replacement. Sodium bicarbonate is administered intravenously while the patient is NPO. Oral supplements may be needed long term. Electrolyte imbalances may occur from fluid replacement, diuresis, or diuretic therapy. The nurse also assesses for hypokalemia and administers potassium supplements when ordered.

Hyponatremia may occur with osmotic diuresis and is usually treated by changing the parenteral solution administered. Frequent monitoring of serum electrolytes is indicated.

Daily serum laboratory values are assessed to monitor for signs of rejection, infection, bleeding, and electrolyte imbalance. Blood glucose, serum amylase, and urinary amylase levels are obtained frequently for the first 48 hours as spot measurements. Frequency is then tapered with the patient's progress. A variety of daily laboratory studies is ordered depending upon the center's postoperative protocol.

Beta-2-microglobulin (B2M) is associated with histocompatibility antigens and is utilized as an immunologic monitor of renal transplant function. Rejection in simultaneous pancreas and renal transplants can be diagnosed earlier because B2M precedes the rise and fall of creatinine by 1 to 2 days. This is not useful in an isolated pancreas transplant, since B2M is catabolized and excreted solely by the kidney.

Monitoring for Pancreatitis

Elevation of serum amylase occurred frequently postoperatively prior to the use of UW preservation solution (from the University of Wisconsin —Madison) (D'Allesandro, 1989). This rise was self-limited and did not require treatment. The use of this solution has eliminated the initial pancreatitis seen postoperatively at some centers. Reflux pancreatitis can occur later in the postoperative course from bladder overdistension and reflux into the pancreatic duct. The nurse carefully assesses for bladder distension regularly. Voiding patterns, including frequency and volume, are recorded. As previously noted, a Foley catheter is initially placed. After the Foley catheter is removed, post-void residuals will be monitored. If a neurogenic bladder is the cause of distension, the patient will be taught intermittent self-catheterization. Urinary tract infections are common. Patient education is a nursing priority to decrease the incidence of these complications. A persistent pancreatitis may indicate infected ascites, necessitating surgical intervention. Elevation of serum amylase is a marker to predict pancreas rejection, but has not consistently been a reliable indicator (Stratta, et al., 1988).

Promoting Normal Serum Glucose Levels

The nurse monitors serum glucose levels every 2 hours postoperatively. Euglycemia usually occurs within 6 hours after transplant without the administration of insulin. Hyperglycemia occurs only late in the immunological rejection process. Glucose intolerance is not manifested until most of the pancreas is destroyed. Only 10% of islet cells are needed for glycemia control. Therefore, reversal of rejection after the onset of hyperglycemia has a low success rate. The nurse assesses for earlier manifestations of a rejection episode by noting slight changes in normal patterns of glucose levels for that patient at comparable times of the day. An elevation of 30–40 mg/100 mL is reported and other variables are assessed.

Monitoring for Rejection

A major problem in pancreatic transplantation is the lack of an early reliable indicator for rejection. (See Table 8–7 for the signs and symptoms of rejection.) Studies have demonstrated that the exocrine pancreas is subject to rejection earlier than the endocrine pancreas and a reduction in exocrine function precedes hyperglycemia (Prieto, et al., 1987). While important, glucose monitoring alone is insufficient to predict rejection

---

Table 8–7. Signs and Symptoms of Pancreas Rejection

- Decrease in urinary amylase without diuresis
- Elevation in creatinine in simultaneous transplant with decrease in renal perfusion
- Decrease in perfusion of pancreas on technetium scan
- Elevation in temperature
- Hematuria
- Elevation in glucose patterns
- Pancreatitis

early enough to permit reversal. At home, pH is measured daily. A lower amylase excretion is reflected in an increased acidity in the urine (Groth and Tyden, 1988).

A major advantage of monitoring urinary amylase is that it represents a direct measure of exocrine function. In pancreaticoduodenocystostomy, the pancreas with the duodenal segment is anastomosed to the bladder. Urine amylase levels are used as an early marker for rejection. Urinary amylase can only be measured by the surgical technique that drains exocrine secretions into the bladder. It can continue to be measured for the life of the organ. In pancreaticoenterostomy, temporary measurement of exocrine secretion is accomplished with a pancreatic duct tube (Groth and Tyden, 1985).

Spot urinary amylase levels increase dramatically in the hours after pancreas transplant. The nurse assesses for an immediate postoperative value of below 100 units/liter, but a steady rise greater than 3000 units/liter or more within 2 days. The level continues to rise during the course of hospitalization. Graft survival is best predicted with concentrations greater than 10,000 units/liter (Stratta, et al., 1988). Urinary amylase levels consistently decrease from the patient's normal pattern before hyperglycemia occurs. Normal ratings for a functioning graft can be widespread, from 10,000 to 200,000 units/liter. Usually the individual's pattern remains in a range within 40,000 units/liter. An example of this type of range may be where one patient's levels vary from 40,000 units/liter to 80,000 units/liter, while another's vary from 60,000 units/liter to 100,000 units/liter. The nurse recognizes that a decline in the range normal for an individual patient is significant and that further assessment will be necessary for diagnosis of rejection. The nurse also assesses for factors such as diuresis, which can cause a precipitous decline in urinary amylase concentrations simply from dilution. Another method of monitoring urinary amylase is the 24-hour collection with ranges usually below 14,000 units/hour.

In isolated pancreas transplants, an additional indicator being used is a decrease in perfusion on a technetium scan. Blood pooling in the transplanted pancreas is measured (the technetium index), with a decrease occurring during rejection episodes (Perlman, et al., 1986). Typically, a baseline scan is done on the first postoperative day. Scans are repeated to diagnose rejection when other parameters have been assessed such as a decrease in urinary amylase levels, a dysfunction in glucose levels, or an elevated temperature. Urine amylase levels and the technetium index consistently decrease prior to the onset of hyperglycemia in pancreas rejection.

In simultaneous pancreas-renal transplants, a major advantage is the use of renal function as an indicator for rejection. The rise in creatinine and decreased perfusion of the renal transplant on a renal scan with no significant change in urinary amylase or decrease in the technetium scan for the pancreas is an important development in identifying pancreas rejection. Anti-rejection therapy used on these grafts often results in continuance of euglycemia, normal urine amylases, and no change in the technetium index. Successful treatment of renal rejection with creatinine returning to normal range signifies that renal rejection in a combined graft is the forerunner of pancreas rejection and is a valid indicator (Sollinger, 1988).

SUMMARY

Pancreatic transplantation offers a valid treatment for those in the IDDM population with severe complications from their disease. Improvement in neuropathy (Solders, et al., 1987) and a protective effect against diabetic microangiopathy (Boham, et al., 1986) in the kidney are now documented. The transplant nurse is a vital member of the transplant team and exhibits assessment skills, acts as educator, and assesses patient and family needs. The nurse is a patient advocate and coordinator during the entire hospitalization and after discharge. The spouse or significant other may stay overnight in the room with the patient. A lounge chair or cot can be provided and is especially appreciated by financially burdened families. The nurse assesses the family's ability to pay for local low-cost housing without straining the family's resources. Added costs of food, transportation, loss of work time, and child care during the time of hospitalization are all factors that can add to patient and family anxiety.

Nurses play an active role in transplant management. Overall nursing priorities are found in Table 8-8. Education, assessment, and advocacy of the patient facilitate the rehabilitation to a normal life-style. The basic philosophy a transplant nurse upholds is to make the hospital experience a beginning of a new life, both mentally and physically. The nurse sets obtainable goals with the patient to make this a time of learning new things and restoring independence. Social interaction with other staff and patients is promoted to provide easier adaptation to health. A patient who is withdrawn and feeling beaten by the disease process can blossom

Table 8-8. **Nursing Priorities for the Pancreatic Transplant Recipient**

- Promote normal serum glucose levels
- Assess for rejection
- Prevent infection
- Monitor renal function in combined renal-pancreas transplants
- Promote maximum independence and restoration of activities of daily living

into a new personality because of nursing support and the hope of a more normal life. At present, financial coverage may be provided by a private insurance company, personal funds, or some type of aid based on the individual's circumstances. Approval of funds is generally completed before transplantation. It is hoped that in the future more insurance companies will recognize the value of pancreatic transplantation and allow available coverage to more patients. The option of pancreas transplantation is available only to those diabetic patients whose complications are, or predictably will be, greater than those of the immunosuppressive regimen required to prevent rejection. The benefits of the combination transplant (pancreas-kidney) include euglycemia and possible stabilization of diabetic complications to prevent future deterioration. At this time it is the preferred treatment for insulin-dependent (type I) diabetics with end-stage renal disease. While rejection is now the leading cause of graft loss, it is readily reversible when diagnosed early.

Bibliography

American Diabetes Association, Inc: Who We Are, What We Do. ADA, New York, 1985.

Bohman, S, et al: Diabetic nephropathy in kidney transplants of diabetic patients, with a note on the protective effect of concomitant pancreas transplantation. Diabetic Nephropathy 5:55, 1986.

Corry, R and Nghiem, D: Transplantation and immunology letter. National Transplantation Immunology Information Network, 3:1, 1986.

Davidson, M: Diabetes Mellitus Diagnosis and Treatment. John Wiley & Sons, New York, 1986.

D'Allesandro, A: Use of UW solution in pancreas transplantation. Diabetes 38:7, 1989.

Dubernard, J and Monti, L: Transplantation and Immunology Letter. National Transplantation Information Network, New Jersey 2:1, 1985.

Groth, C and Tyden G: Transplantation and Immunology Letter. National Transplantation Information Network, New Jersey 2:1, 1985.

Groth, C: Pancreatic Transplantation. WB Saunders, Philadelphia, 1988, p 181.

Guyton, A: Basic Human Physiology: Normal Function and Mechanisms of Disease. WB Saunders, Philadelphia, 1977.

Luckmann, J and Sorenson, K: Medical Surgical Nursing: A Psychophysiological Approach. WB Saunders, Philadelphia, 1989.

Macleod, J: Davidson's Principles and Practice of Medicine. Churchill Livingstone, New York, 1977.

Olefsky, J and DeFronzo, R: Diabetes Mellitus: Management and Complications. Churchill Livingstone, New York, 1985.

Orie JE, et al: Thallium-201 myocardial perfusion imaging and coronary arteriography in asymptomatic patients with end-stage renal disease secondary to juvenile onset diabetes mellitus, Transplant Proc 18:1709, 1986.

Pancreatic Transplantation in Diabetes. Lancet 5:1015, 1987.

Perlman, S, et al: Noninvasive evaluation of pancreas allografts. J Nucl Med 27:909, 1986.

Polin, S: Paying for health care: The high cost of diabetes. Clinical Diabetes 9/10:108, 1985.

Prieto, M, et al: Pancreas transplant results according to the technique of duct management: Bladder versus enteric drainage. Surgery 10:680, 1987.

Skilnan, T and Tzagournis, M: Diabetes Mellitus. Ohio State University and The Upjohn Company, 1985.

Solders, G, et al: Effects of combined pancreas and renal transplantation on diabetic neuropathy: A two-year follow-up study. Lancet 2:1232, 1987.

Sollinger, H, et al: Combined kidney-pancreas transplantation with pancreaticocystostomy. Transplant Proc 21:2837, 1988.

Sollinger, H, et al: Experience with simultaneous pancreas-kidney transplantation. Ann Surg 208:475, 1988.

Stratta, R, et al: Early diagnosis and treatment of pancreas allograft rejection. Transplant International 1:6, 1988.

Sutherland, D: Pancreas transplantation in nonuremic, type I diabetic recipients. Surgery 8:453, 1988.

Sutherland, D and Moudry, K: Pancreas transplant registry report. Transplant Proc 21:2845, 1989.

Toledo-Pereyra, LH: Pancreas Transplantation. Kluwer Academic Pubs, Norwell, MA, 1988.

Vernon, WB and Sollinger, HW: Management of combined pancreatico-renal allograft recipients. Transplantation Management 1:565, 1989.

CHAPTER

The Pediatric Transplant Patient: Donor and Recipient

Laurel Williams, RN, MSN
Mary Anne House, RN, MSN
Carol Hill, RN, BSN, CCRN

Whether dealing with a potential pediatric donor or a pediatric recipient, the situation presents a special challenge to the nurse. Both scenarios involve special management problems not necessarily encountered in the adult population. Regardless of whether you are the nurse caring for the donor or the recipient, there is one rule that *must* be remembered: the pediatric patient is not just a little adult. Children have distinctly different laboratory values and drug dosages, as well as management problems that require the nurse to deal with the pediatric transplant patient in a different manner from the adult patient. The psychological and emotional impact of transplantation on the pediatric patient, the family, and the staff differs from that of the adult patient.

THE DONOR

This section explains the psychological and qualitative variables of the pediatric organ donor and outlines specific medical interventions designed to maximize pediatric organ viability prior to transplantation.

169

Psychological Variables

There are three main psychological variables that the nurse must be aware of in dealing with the child as an organ or tissue donor. It is imperative for the nurse to understand the interrelatedness of these variables in order to effectively support the donor family, referring physicians, and nursing staff. These psychological variables include:

1. the different facets of the pediatric donor family
2. the hesitation of the physician or other healthcare providers to refer potential pediatric donors
3. the difference between the nursing staff interactions with the pediatric donor family and the adult donor family.

There are often more individuals actively involved in the family dynamics of the pediatric donor. Prior to discussing donation, it is imperative to identify the key support person(s) upon whom the parents rely. Many times, significant others actually make, or control, decisions. Although every donor scenario has some element of tragedy, the death of a child is usually devastating and unexpected, and it often appears to be illogical. The level of guilt, justified or unjustified, borne by the parents is usually extremely high. It is vital for the nurse to understand as much as possible about the dynamics of the situation in order to provide proper support. Intervention by a chaplain or social worker to provide independent support for the family is important in helping to work through the grieving process, allowing the family members to deal with the death of the child as well as the option of donation.

For many physicians, as well as other healthcare providers, the death of a child is a major defeat. All caregivers need support throughout the process of managing the case. The nurse can sometimes make the situation at least tolerable by discussing feelings common to healthcare providers. It is our obligation as healthcare providers to offer organ and tissue donation as an option, and to provide the family with the necessary information they need to make an informed decision. We must then support the family in that decision.

The nurse takes time to provide support for fellow staff. Nurses play a vital role in the evaluation and management process of a donor. It is critical that the nursing staff recognize the importance of interaction with the organ procurement coordinator. Allowing the coordinator to become a part of the nursing team makes the evaluation and management of the pediatric donor more fluent.

Qualitative Variables

The qualitative variables related to organ donation are divided into brain death determination and laboratory values.

The diagnosis of brain death may differ in children. Clinical observations vary with the age of the child. Use of confirmatory testing, that is, electroencephalograms, arteriography, and radionuclide studies, varies with the child's age and the preference of the physician, but is also influenced by state legislation and hospital policy. In the child, electrolyte imbalances may influence the physical examination. The temperature, as with adults, must be within normal limits for accurate evaluation of brain death to be made. Careful history and drug screening are mandatory parts of the assessment. A careful review of all laboratory studies must be undertaken.

Many laboratory values differ in children from those in adults; the nurse should be familiar with the standards used in each particular setting. The pattern of change over the time since admission is also very important. Observation of trends will have major influence on whether or not the child is accepted for donation. Calculating body surface area assists in using certain laboratory values in evaluation and in determining drug dosages.

Management

Once the child has been pronounced brain dead, physiological management becomes crucial to the successful recovery of viable organs for transplantation. As in adult cases, the main goal of organ donor management is to maintain optimal conditions to promote healthy organ recovery.

Organ viability can be maintained with adequate hydration, adequate urine output, maintenance of serum electrolytes within normal limits, and hemodynamic stability (Table 9–1).

The systolic blood pressure is maintained within normal limits for age and size. Hypotension is the most frequent management problem in the donor. Early correction is essential to minimize organ damage from decreased perfusion. In assessing the blood pressure, the nurse remembers that brain stem herniation, collapse of peripheral vascular resistance, or hypovolemia (secondary to neurologic management, hemorrhage) and excessive urine output all influence vital signs. The blood pressure is monitored accurately by arterial line or with a cuff that is two thirds the size of the upper arm.

Table 9–1. **Parameters for Maintenance of Organ Viability**

• Central venous pressure	8–10 mmHg
• Urine output	2cc/kg/hour
• Serum electrolytes	within normal limits
• Oxygenation	PO_2 >95 mmHg
• Hemodynamics	within normal limits for age/size

The nurse assesses the type and function of intravenous line placement just as would be done in the adult. Patent IV lines, preferrably in the upper extremities, are used. A central venous pressure (CVP) line is an asset, especially in the management of the multiple organ donor. Electrolyte status is monitored regularly. In the volume-depleted pediatric patient, the infusion rate is typically at least 5 cc/kg every 10 minutes until adequate hydration status is restored.

Vasopressor therapy is used if hypotension continues after aggressive hydration. Use of low-dose dopamine is preferable to other agents. The nurse titrates in order to use the lowest dose possible to maintain a normal blood pressure for the child.

Maintenance IV fluids are selected as is appropriate according to the serum electrolyte levels. Maintenance fluids are generally $D_5/0.2NS$, with the addition of potassium as needed. Maintenance rates are 2 cc/kg/hour plus the previous hour's urine output. If the serum sodium is elevated after the donor has been rehydrated, restriction of sodium intake by using D_5W instead of saline-containing solutions is necessary. Utilization of all available resources in those instances where difficult management problems arise helps assure organ viability.

The urine output is maintained at greater than 2 cc/kg/hour. The nurse is cognizant of signs and symptoms of diabetes insipidus (Table 9–2). Treatment includes replacement of urinary losses, and if approved by the organ recovery team, administration of vasopressin. The use of vasopressin may be as a drip, subcutaneously, intramuscularly, or intranasally. Vasopressin should not be administered within 2 hours of organ recovery.

Pediatric donors are especially susceptible to hypothermia due to their small body surface area. Hypothermia often accompanies brain death due to loss of hypothalamic regulation. Body temperature is maintained at greater than 97°F. A significant decrease in core temperature can result in cardiac dysrhythmias or asystole. Due to impaired electrical impulses in the brain, brain death declaration cannot be made if hypothermia exists. The nurse uses warming blankets and heat lamps, in addition to wrapping the head and extremities, to assist in maintaining the child's temperature. Use of humidified, warm oxygen via the ventilator and warmed IV fluids and blood products are frequently administered to prevent temperature loss.

The dosages of drugs routinely given to the pediatric organ donor

---

Table 9–2. **Signs/Symptoms of Diabetes Insipidus**

- Serum sodium > 150 mEq/L
- Serum osmolarity > 310 mOsm/L
- Specific gravity > 1.006
- Urine output > 7cc/kg/hour

Table 9–3. **Common Pediatric Drug Dosages**

Drug Name	Dosage
Calcium chloride	10 mg /kg
Calcium gluconate	100 mg/kg
Methylprednisolone sodium succinate (Solu-Medrol)	30 mg/kg
Furosemide (Lasix)	1.0 mg/kg
Mannitol	0.5 gm/kg
Phenoxybenzamine hydrochloride (Dibenzyline)	2 mg/kg
Chlorpromazine (Thorazine)	1.0 mg/kg
Phentolamine mesylate (Regitine)	1.0 mg/kg
Heparin	300 units/kg

vary according to the weight of the child (Table 9–3). Care should be taken when administering any medications to the pediatric donor. Most of the drugs routinely used in donor management can cause dysrhythmias if administered too rapidly.

Special Considerations in Death and Dying

An important aspect of caring for a pediatric donor patient is caring for the family experiencing the death of a child. Critical to any care plan is the treatment of the family as a whole. The family unit may include siblings, grandparents, significant others, or legal guardians. The nurse recognizes that each family member often has different emotional needs as they individually attempt to grasp the reality of the death of the child. For the pediatric donor, this is almost always a sudden and unexpected death. The family has little time to prepare for the rapid development of events or to deal with their emotions.

As parents struggle with their own pain — and frequently guilt, if the death was due to trauma — siblings of the donor may not receive adequate support. Siblings are also experiencing grief and may find their usual support system, their parent(s), unable to help them. The support of nurses, other healthcare professionals, and friends of the family may provide the necessary resources to comfort siblings who are struggling with feelings of hurt and anger.

There are many ways that nurses can directly help the surviving the siblings. By openly and honestly discussing feelings and the death, the nurse can help to alleviate fears and fantasies. Encouraging the sibling to see and/or touch the deceased child can possibly lead to questions that the nurse may best be prepared to answer. Therefore, the nurse finds it important to assist all family members, including surviving siblings, during this acute phase of the grief process.

Maintaining a pediatric donor patient on support equipment in order to preserve organ function may also provide the family with time to say good-bye. Surviving siblings are included in this time to say good-bye as well. Those who are not included often experience nightmares and fantasies. By including them in this important — and certainly painful — family experience, feelings of isolation may be avoided. The family is encouraged to touch the deceased child, and to support each other during this time.

For some donor families, the final good-bye may need to be after the support machines are removed. Since this will not occur until after the organs are procured in the operating room, the family may insist on seeing the patient again after surgery. This decision is usually supported. The family may need to be assured that the body was not disfigured. They may wish to hold the child again. Providing the family with private time to themselves, both before and after the organs are removed, will allow ventilation of feelings (i.e., love, guilt, and anger). These needs are important and the nurses and other healthcare professionals are crucial to the support of the family.

There are many theories of grief, and often stages of grief are identified. Importantly, healthcare professionals provide the family with the essential information that there is not specific or only way to express grief. While there will be similar emotions experienced such as shock, numbness, pain, anger, and isolation, each individual in the family may experience these at different times, each individual is unique. The nurse also informs the family that there is no time limitation to grieving. They will always experience some sadness because of their loss.

Care of the pediatric donor is twofold. First, the nurse is involved in the crucial tasks related to maintaining organ perfusion. But no less importantly, the nurse cares for all members of the family who are giving generously of their child during their time of great grief and sorrow.

The identification, evaluation, and management of the pediatric organ or tissue donor is a challenge to any healthcare provider. For the nurse caring for the potential donor, it presents a special challenge. Careful management of the donor, as well as support for the family, is vital in allowing a successful organ or tissue recovery. The experience, although very stressful, is ultimately rewarding for all of the healthcare providers involved.

THE RECIPIENT

Children and their families facing the process of transplantation deal with multiple and unique issues. These issues involve the developmental level of the child, the family dynamics, and the fact that many of the children are very young and have little or no participation in or control over their own care. Different healthcare problems and issues are encountered depending on the organ that a child receives. This section reviews the psychosocial issues that are most common for children undergoing the process of transplantation and their families.

End-stage organ failure differs from other life-threatening childhood diseases in that transplantation offers the chance of long-term survival and rehabilitation. However, children with organ failure are at risk for experiencing similar physical and emotional problems as are children with other chronic or life-threatening illnesses. Prior to transplantation, children often incur repeated hospitalizations, which may involve separations from family members, school, friends, and familiar environments. Instead, a new environment, the hospital, with a confusing number of new healthcare professionals and the additional threat of painful medical procedures, becomes necessary (Matteson, 1972). Throughout the process of transplantation, the child is influenced by previous experiences with hospitals and healthcare professionals. The child's perception of these experiences both pre- and post-transplantation will be affected by his or her developmental age.

Pre-Evaluation

Children requiring transplantation and their parents may travel a great distance for transplantation evaluation. Prior to visiting a transplant center, children and their families may have preconceived ideas about evaluation for transplantation, and the risks and benefits of transplantation. The nurse coordinator makes initial phone contact with the family prior to their arrival at the transplant center to establish rapport, clarify misconceptions, and facilitate plans, and to explain the process of the transplantation evaluation. Written material sent out to children and their families, which describes the evaluation process and provides details specific to the transplant center and surrounding community, is often helpful prior to the visit.

Evaluation

During transplantation evaluation, a thorough family history is obtained in an attempt to identify family strengths and weaknesses to better help the family through the stress of hospitalization. (Table 9–4 lists common pre-transplant nursing diagnoses.) Attention is directed to identification of previous exposures to and outcomes at healthcare settings. Individual time is spent with both the child and parents to help them better understand the process of transplantation. Children require age-ap-

Table 9–4. Common Nursing Diagnoses for the Pre-Transplant Pediatric Patient

Health Perception — Health Management
- Health maintenance, altered, possibly related to
  - denial of illness
  - inadequate energy
  - depression
- Health seeking behaviors
- Noncompliance (potential for), possibly related to
  - denial of illness
  - lack of belief that therapies can help
  - developmental needs

Nutritional — Metabolic
- Nutrition, altered: less than body requirement, possibly related to
  - decreased appetite
  - malabsorption
  - fatigue with eating

Activity — Exercise
- Activity intolerance, possibly related to
  - circulatory problems
  - respiratory problems
  - sedentary habits
- Fatigue, possibly related to
  - effects of chronic illness
  - poor rest and sleep
- Self-care deficit: total, possibly related to
  - fatigue
  - musculoskeletal changes
  - developmental delays

Cognitive — Perceptual
- Knowledge deficit, possibly related to
  - possible treatment modalities
  - health-promoting activities

Self-Perception — Self-Concept
- Anxiety, possibly related to
  - unknowns of transplantation
  - uncertainty of transplantation success rates
- Fear, possibly related to
  - inability to receive a graft
  - possibility of death
- Hopelessness, possibly related to
  - low donor supply
  - length of waiting time
  - failing health
  - long-term stress
- Powerlessness, possibly related to
  - inability to receive a graft
  - loss of role functions
  - illness-related regimen

Table 9-4. **Common Nursing Diagnoses for the Pre-Transplant Pediatric Patient (*Continued*)**

- Self-concept, disturbance in: body image, possibly related to
  - chronic illness
  - weight loss
  - hair loss
- Self-concept, disturbance in: self-esteem, possibly related to
  - loss of role functions
  - appearance

Role — Relationship
- Family process, altered, possibly related to
  - change in roles
  - ineffective communication
- Parenting, altered: potential, possibly related to
  - fear for survival of child
  - financial stress
  - inability to adapt to sick child's role
- Self-concept, disturbance in: role performance, possibly related to
  - dependency
  - loss of student role
  - changes in family roles
- Social interaction, impaired
- Social isolation, possibly related to
  - fatigue with activities
  - loss of social and school contacts

Coping — Stress Tolerance
- Coping, ineffective individual, possibly related to
  - inability to use previous coping mechanisms
  - inability to develop new coping mechanisms
  - loss of support systems
- Coping, ineffective family: compromised, possibly related to
  - despair
  - conflict of coping mechanisms
  - ineffective relationships

Sexuality — Reproductive
- Sexual dysfunction, possibly related to
  - endocrine imbalances
  - fear
  - change in relationships
  - transition of roles

propriate assessment and teaching to help them understand transplantation and organ donation. Medical play kits and books about the hospital may be helpful if more specific teaching tools are not available. Children and siblings may benefit from seeing pictures of other children both before and after transplantation to desensitize and support the child or sibling. Also, touring the hospital often alleviates fears that the child may have about a new environment. While visiting the respective units that the child will encounter, for example the intensive care unit and/or post-ICU unit, the rules and expectations, and sights and sounds are discussed to help orient and desensitize both the child and family. Other information that should be discussed includes the visitation hours; types of other patients on the units; tubes, lines, and monitoring equipment; and support systems or group meetings that may be available to help the child and the family.

When talking to parents about the risks of transplantation, care is taken in how the information is presented if children are present. Discussions of complications and the possibility of death may be frightening and misunderstood by children depending on the child's developmental level. Discussions with the family also address the concerns and learning needs of siblings. Siblings, too, require developmentally appropriate educational tools to help them deal with their sibling's illness, parental separation, fears about their own health, and ways to cope with these problems. A qualified healthcare professional should be available to help families plan for the eventual transplant. Child, sibling, and parental needs are also anticipated so they can be addressed prior to and during transplantation.

Physical needs are also addressed during the evaluation for transplantation. In looking at growth and development, the child's immunization status is assessed. Immunizations are administered prior to transplantation when possible. Alterations in the immune system after transplantation may render immunizations ineffective. The use of live-virus vaccination post transplantation is also controversial at present, with many centers discouraging their use.

The assessment of growth and development and feeding patterns in children prior to transplantation is extremely important. Children with failure of any major organ are at risk for problems secondary to malnutrition (Lebenthal, 1989). Malnutrition can result from physical causes such as end-stage organ failure, and is complicated by anorexia secondary to chronic illness. Malnutrition may also result from psychosocial factors due to the lack of emotional and sensory stimulation (Whaley and Wang, 1983). Malnutrition may lead to problems with vitamin deficiencies, rickets, anemia, muscle wasting, and poor physical and mental growth and development. Improvement in nutritional status has been noted to have a direct impact on survival for some solid organ transplant recipients (Kaufman, et al., 1987). The caloric intake required to obtain reasonable growth and development is ascertained during the evaluation period. Nutritional therapies to achieve caloric needs are instituted. Nutritional therapies may include caloric supplementation through continued nasogastric or parenteral feedings, vitamin supplementation, fluid restrictions, or other dietary manipulation. Anthropometric and developmental analysis has been advised to classify and assess growth (Drash, et al., 1968).

Children with body changes secondary to organ failure are encouraged and helped to maintain developmental skills and discuss concerns about self-image and self-concept. Encouragement of normal developmental skills may involve consultation and intervention with physical therapy, early childhood intervention programs, and educational support services.

Children use play and mobility to explore and master the environment as well as cope with stress (Matteson, 1972). Medical procedures performed on the child during evaluation and hospitalization are arranged so that the child has adequate time to recover and regroup emotionally before being subjected to additional stresses. Simple, honest, age-appropriate preparation for procedures will dispel fantasies and build trust with the child and the parent. When possible, parents should be allowed to remain with the child for emotional support during procedures.

Although a health history is obtained and a physical examination is performed during evaluation, all body systems are reviewed and assessed in relation to transplantation. Any therapy that will maximize a child's health prior to surgery should be initiated.

Information given at the transplant center during the evaluation should be reinforced once the child has returned home. The child and siblings are given opportunities to ask questions and voice fears and misinterpretations. The family continues to provide appropriate play materials while awaiting transplantation.

The shortage of pediatric donor organs across the nation makes waiting for transplantation an extremely difficult time for parents. Parents may travel to different centers in an attempt to increase the child's chances of transplantation by being on multiple transplant lists. Families may involve the media in their attempts to increase organ donation or raise funds for transplantation and the subsequent expenses. Families are counseled on the effects that the media may have on the child's and family's privacy, both before and after transplantation. In addition they should be counseled on whom to contact to set up appropriate trust funds.

During the evaluation process, families are given the name of national and local organizations, and contacts in those organizations, for support and possible financial advice. Families may find it helpful to meet with other individuals in their communities who have experienced the process of transplantation, or who are also awaiting transplantation. Families are encouraged to normalize their lives whenever possible. This might include spending holidays with out-of-town relatives; maintaining children in school; and involving local agencies for infant stimulation or respite care for the parents, so they may have some private time.

Followup of the child and family is done on a regular basis by the transplant team throughout the waiting period and includes assessment of the whole family. If stress becomes evident and unmanageable by any family member, referral is made to an appropriate local agency, hospital-

---

Table 9–5. Nursing Priorities for the Pediatric Transplant Recipient

- Monitor organ function
- Assess for rejection
- Prevent infection
- Promote maximum independence and restoration of activities of daily living
- Foster return to normal role functions, particularly student roles
- Facilitate socialization with peers

---

based healthcare professional, or member of the transplant team. Table 9–5 lists nursing priorities for the pediatric recipient, while Table 9–6 lists common post-transplant nursing diagnoses.

The Operative Procedure and Hospitalization

Arrival at the center for transplantation is stressful for all concerned. More fear and anxiety may be created when the child is separated from the parents going into the operating room. Appropriate use of sedation or premedication may be helpful prior to taking the child to the operating room. In addition, depending on the child's developmental level, the nursing staff prepares the child for what will occur in the operating room, the sights, sounds, and smells of the operating room, with reassurance that the child will be safe and comfortable.

The parent(s) should be allowed to remain with the child as long as possible prior to the operation. If medically feasible, sedation is administered to the child in the parents' presence prior to taking the child to the operating room. Another approach that may help the child to deal with separation from the family at the time of operation is to have a primary nurse or the nurse coordinator go into the operating room with the child after rapport has been established.

Offering the child choices during this time is helpful, if developmentally appropriate. For example, the child is offered the choice of flavors to be applied to the oxygen mask that will be used in the operating room in order to make it smell familiar or better. If time is available, the older child might be given the oxygen mask to play with prior to surgery. The child is encouraged to bring a favorite toy or a stuffed animal to the operating room for comfort.

The presence of parents during induction of anesthesia may be beneficial to the physical and emotional well-being of the child. However, in many hospitals, parents are not allowed to be present for the induction of

Health Perception — Health Management
- Health seeking behaviors
- Noncompliance (potential for), possibly related to
  ◦ denial of post-transplant status
  ◦ denial of potential graft loss
  ◦ depression

Nutritional — Metabolic
- Nutrition, altered: less than body requirements, possibly related to
  ◦ steroids
  ◦ anorexia

Activity — Exercise
- Activity intolerance, possibly related to
  ◦ circulatory problems
  ◦ respiratory problems
  ◦ previous low activity level
- Fatigue, possibly related to
  ◦ poor rest and sleep
  ◦ increased activity
- Growth and development, altered, possibly related to
  ◦ steroids
- Self-care deficit: total, possibly related to
  ◦ developmental delays

Cognitive — Perceptual
- Knowledge deficit, possibly related to
  ◦ survival rates
  ◦ functional ability after surgery
  ◦ operative procedure
  ◦ medications and side effects
  ◦ length of recovery time

Self-Perception — Self-Concept
- Anxiety, possibly related to
  ◦ threat of graft rejection
  ◦ return to role functions
  ◦ change in sick role
  ◦ uncertainty of transplantation success rates
  ◦ overload of information regarding transplantation
- Fear, possibly related to
  ◦ potential failure of graft
  ◦ return to roles
- Hopelessness, possibly related to
  ◦ continued changes in activities of daily living
- Powerlessness, possibly related to
  ◦ inability to change appearance
  ◦ illness-related regimen
- Self-concept, disturbance in: body image, possibly related to
  ◦ moon face
  ◦ truncal obesity
  ◦ hirsutism
  ◦ scars and striae
  ◦ acne

(*continued*)

Table 9–6. Common Nursing Diagnoses for the Post-Transplant Pediatric Patient (Continued)

- Self-concept, disturbance in: self-esteem, possibly related to
    - change in role functions
    - new changes in appearance

Role — Relationship
- Family process, altered, possibly related to
    - changes in roles
    - ineffective communication
- Parenting, altered: potential, possibly related to
    - fear for survival of child
    - financial stress
    - inability to adapt to child's change from sick role
- Self-concept, disturbance in: role performance, possibly related to
    - return to student role
- Social interaction, impaired
- Social isolation, possibly related to
    - continued fatigue

Coping — Stress Tolerance
- Coping, ineffective individual, possibly related to
    - ineffective existing mechanisms
    - inability to develop effective mechanisms
    - change of support systems
- Coping, ineffective family: compromised, possibly related to
    - conflict of coping mechanisms
    - ineffective relationships

Sexuality — Reproductive
- Sexual dysfunction, possibly related to
    - endocrine imbalances
    - fear
    - change in relationships
    - transition of roles

---

anesthesia (Berry, 1986). The presence or absence of parents during induction of anesthesia is dependent on several variables. These variables include the training and attitudes of the anesthesiologists, the hospital facilities for induction, and most critically, the medical condition of the child (Berry, 1986). Children undergoing transplantation are usually categorized as high-risk patients by anesthesiologists. The time of induction may be hazardous. It may therefore be safest for the high-risk child to have induction of anesthesia, intubation of the trachea, and ventilation in the operating room, where emergency drugs and equipment are readily available and a parent is not present.

PARENTAL FEELINGS POST TRANSPLANTATION

Parents often experience a sense of exhilaration after the surgery is completed (Gold, et al., 1986). They then can resume the traditional parent role of nurturer and relinquish the healthcare provider role assumed at the time of diagnosis. However, because of their intense requirement to provide medical care pre-transplantation, many parents need to maintain a sense of control over their child's care after transplantation. The initial positive response of parents after the completion of the operation may be mixed with negative responses to postoperative complications. Parents often struggle with feelings of loss of control, powerlessness, fears of death, or guilt (Gold, et al., 1986). Guilt may be associated with seeing their child restrained and attached to many machines. Guilt may also be associated with the knowledge that another child had to die before their child could survive. In addition, parents may feel guilt because their child received an organ when other children are also in desperate need of transplantation (Gold, et al., 1986).

Parents may also experience feelings of depression, anger, and hostility toward staff in dealing with the emotional roller coaster ride of the transplantation aftermath. Feelings of isolation from family and friends may be made worse when, and if, a spouse returns home for financial or personal reasons. These parental feelings may be picked up by the children and influence their sense of security and ability to cope with recuperation from surgery. In addition, the child's immobility and restriction of activity in the immediate postoperative period may increase the child's stress and thus the parents' level of stress. The physical and emotional well-being of the child and family are included in the nursing care plans. The developmental age of the child will determine appropriate nursing intervention.

RESPONSE TO HOSPITALIZATION BASED ON DEVELOPMENTAL STAGE

Children's response to illness and hospitalization depends upon their developmental stage. These stages of development do not necessarily correspond to chronological age. A review of some of the basic principles of child development is outlined in Table 9–7. A brief review of developmental tasks and the possible effects of hospitalization follows.

Infancy. Erik Erikson describes infant development as a time alternating between trust and mistrust (Erikson, 1963). The infant develops trust through the relationships with primary caregivers. The infant begins to respond to and explore the extended environment (James and Mott, 1988). Hospitalized infants are at risk for problems associated with separation from their primary caregivers, loss of function and control, and pain. An infant in the hospital might therefore respond to stress by exhibiting

Table 9–7. Guidelines for Assessing Growth and Development

Skill	Infancy: Neonate
Gross motor	• random kicking of legs and arms • reflex movement
Cognitive	• discriminates color and brightness • discriminates sound, particularly mother's voice • avoids noxious stimuli • sensitivity to tactile stimuli
Language	• cries • body movements
Social	• consoles self or accepts consolation from adults • responds with eye control • displays satisfaction

Skill	Infancy: 1–3 Months
Gross motor	• minimal head lag when pulled to sitting • head bobs in sitting position • lifts head from side to side when prone
Cognitive	• begins to replace reflex behavior with more deliberate behavior • repeats pleasurable chance movements
Language	• attention to voices and noises • patterns of cry vary • responds differently to voice of primary care giver
Social	• watches face intently • engages in eye control • shows consistent social smile • shows predictable behavior and routines • reciprocates in interaction with parent(s)

Skill	Infancy: 3–6 Months
Gross motor	• minimal head lag when pulled to sitting position • head steady when supported • supports weight on arm when prone • rolls intentionally
Cognitive	• recognizes familiar objects, faces • discovers own body parts • interest in repeat behaviors • does not look for objects out of sight
Language	• squeals, coos, vocalizes when spoken to • localizes sound by turning head • laughs, varies tone
Social	• reciprocal interaction between parent-infant • preferential response to care giver • discriminates familiar people from strangers

Table 9–7. Guidelines for Assessing Growth and Development (*Continued*)

Skill	Infancy: 6–9 Months
Gross motor	• bears weight on legs when held • no head lag • sits without support • stands holding on • creeps, crawls, rolls
Cognitive	• initiates simple sounds, gestures • obtains object by pulling on string • uses well-developed behavior for mouthing, shaking, banging, dropping • looks for objects dropped from sight
Language	• laughs and squeals • enjoys listening to own voice • imitates sounds • talks to toys • recognizes familiar words
Social	• wary of strangers • increased interaction and exploration • increased interest in objects • peek-a-boo, looks in mirror • shows joy and anger

Skill	Infancy: 9–12 Months
Gross motor	• sits steadily • rights self if falls • pulls to stand • stands alone briefly • walks holding on or with help
Cognitive	• continued interest in environment • intentional behavior • imitates novel behavior • associates symbols with events • searches for hidden objects
Language	• uses expressive sounds • uses "ma ma," "da da" specifically • understands simple words
Social	• heightened attachment to mother • separation anxiety • protests at bedtime • sensitivity toward approval or disapproval • enjoys simple games

(continued)

Table 9-7.	Guidelines for Assessing Growth and Development *(Continued)*

Skill	Infancy: 12-18 Months
Gross motor	• stands alone • walks well • creeps up stairs • stoops and recovers • drinks from cup • uses spoon • scribbles
Cognitive	• continues curiosity, exploration • interest in books • finds hidden objects • imitates parents' behavior
Language	• uses gestures to ask for objects • shakes head "no" • says several intelligible words
Social	• increased autonomy • ventures briefly from parents, then returns • temper tantrums • less wary of strangers • shows affection • changes mood frequently • purposefully does things that are forbidden and watches response

Skill	Early Childhood: 18-24 Months
Gross motor	• runs clumsily • pushes and pulls toys • seats self in small chair • walks backward • walks up stairs with 1 hand held
Cognitive	• locates hidden objects • deferred imitation • infers a cause while only seeing an effect
Language	• uses several words • combines 2 words in a phrase • points to body parts • names an object • follows simple directions
Social	• increased autonomy but remains dependent on parents • insists in self-feeding • separation anxiety but better coping skills • comfort/security objects • ritualistic • begins to be possessive • understands most limits but does not have self-control

Table 9-7. Guidelines for Assessing Growth and Development (Continued)

Skill	Early Childhood: 2-3 Years
Gross motor	• jumps in place • rides a tricycle • balances briefly on 1 foot • undresses self
Cognitive	• imaginative play/magical thinking • egocentric • states own sex • infers cause from observing effect
Language	• speaks in sentences • follows simple directions • uses plurals
Social	• increased independence but still needs "refueling" • negativism • performs simple tasks • tolerates separation better • actively initiates projects and exploration though doesn't finish

Skill	Early Childhood: 4 Years
Gross motor	• one-sided functioning established • jumps twice on one foot • alternates feet on stairs • catches ball
Cognitive	• understands concept of "long" or "short" • counts 3 objects • imaginative • less egocentric
Language	• uses sentences of 4 or 5 words • recognizes 3 colors • understands analogies
Social	• verbalizes feelings • usually separates easily • increased independence • fears about body integrity • defines acceptable/unacceptable tasks behaviors but does not allow acceptable limits • displays sexual curiosity • possible sibling jealousy, attraction to parent of opposite sex

(continued)

Table 9–7. Guidelines for Assessing Growth and Development (*Continued*)	
Skill	**Middle Childhood: 4.5–8 Years**
Gross motor	• jumps rope • runs on toes • prints numbers, letters
Cognitive	• identifies 4 colors • improved memory • interested in learning facts and solving problems • developing sense of humor • pre-operational to concrete thinking
Language	• uses complete sentences • follows 3 commands • increased vocabulary
Social	• sexual curiosity • awareness of individual attributes • increased sense of self-esteem • becomes self-critical • separates easily from parents • controls behavior • collections and hobbies • engages in cooperative play outside • relates appropriately to adults
Skill	**Late Childhood: 8–12 Years**
Gross motor	• does tricks on bikes • increased skill fluidity, control • improved coordination • increased stamina • increased precision and speed
Cognitive	• major advancement toward complex intellectual tasks • enjoys reading • wants to acquire new facts • concrete operational to formal thinking • understands relationships between time, speed, or distance • trial/error approach to problem solving
Language	• increased vocabulary • speech entirely understandable • oral, written stories (logical)
Social	• obeys rules • better able to take on another perspective • increase in number of authority figures • self-critical, proud of accomplishments • self-concept redefined in terms of peers • understands health concepts

Table 9-7. Guidelines for Assessing Growth and Development (*Continued*)	
Skill	**Adolescent: 12 – 18 Years**
Gross motor	• progresses from awkward to more adult-like motor skills • choice of activity influenced by personal preferences • competitive/organized sports
Cognitive	• concrete to formal thinking • increased ability for abstract reasoning • plans ahead • capability of imaginative, inactive, inventive thinking
Language	• speech, writing totally understandable • reads, writes complex sentences • uses peer dialect
Social	• formulates personal beliefs and values • establishes sense of identity • tries out new roles • introspective, demands privacy • daydreams • emotionally labile • establishes several identity peer groups as predominant orientation • vacillates between independent and dependent

Adapted from James, SR and Mott, SR: Child Health Care Nursing: Essential Care of Children and Families. Addison-Wesley, Redwood City, CA, 1988.

signs of anxiety or despair such as crying, screaming, rejecting strangers, withdrawal, or disinterest in the environment. Emotional distress may increase with immobility from restraints and the infant may exhibit signs of lethargy and increased dependence on caregivers (James and Mott, 1988).

Nursing intervention with the infant includes consistency among caregivers in promoting feelings of trust. This may include assignment of a primary nurse or case manager who formulates a plan of care with the parent and outlines such things as the child's usual schedule, how the child is comforted, and any special needs the child may have. The infant will respond to talking and singing, holding, rocking, and touch during procedures. The nurse provides the infant with a pacifier or allows sucking on fingers or a bottle when appropriate. Parents are encouraged to stay with the child if they are capable of providing nurturance and helping the child cope. Parents are also allowed and encouraged to help with their child's daily care. Security objects, mobiles, and age-appropriate toys are provided. Whenever possible, the child's environment is nonrestrictive. Normalizing the environment by allowing the child to be out of the room in a playroom or nonbedroom helps the child and parent begin to step out of the sick role and move toward transplantation and wellness.

Support of the parents is also crucial to the care of an infant. Anxious and fearful parents may cause the infant to be fretful and irritable. Support for the parent includes adequate, ongoing information and education about the progress of the child, involvement in the daily care of the child, and avenues for expression of their emotions. Parents may need encouragement to take breaks away from their child to meet their needs for rest and recreation. A parent who is unable to be present during any part of the child's hospitalization also is provided with information and support. Parents are viewed as an integral part of the healthcare team and included in the decision-making process whenever possible.

Early Childhood. The developmental years of early childhood are a struggle between autonomy and shame and doubt, and initiative versus guilt (Erikson, 1963). In early childhood, new skills are developed for mobility and communication. Relationships with family members are further developed and the child continues to learn through exploration of the environment. Children hospitalized during early childhood are at risk for separation anxiety, which may be apparent in several ways. Anxiety may cause the child to cry, have angry outbursts such as physical attacks, or cling to the parent.

Regression in self-care and loss of newly learned motor functions may lead to a sense of failure (James and Mott, 1988). In early childhood, the child has little comprehension of the cause of illness or the nature of the treatment. Children may therefore associate pain as the symptom and punishment for some wrongdoing (Matteson, 1972). For example, some heart transplant patients imagined that their heart was damaged by playing too hard (Willis, et al., 1982). During early childhood, children are upset by changes in their body image especially if the changes are associated with bleeding from invasive procedures (James and Mott, 1988). One child believed a blood transfusion was removing blood instead of replacing blood. Such misperceptions heighten the child's sense of vulnerability and may result in nightmares and fears of the dark, strangers, or people in uniform.

Nursing interventions during early childhood include minimal use of restraints. Prolonged physical restraint of a young child may cause temper tantrums, withdrawal, or serious management problems (Matteson, 1972). Therefore, the child is provided as much mobility as possible during and after procedures. The child is given adequate time to play, since play is the medium for children to express their fears and anxieties. Play should include diversional play (for example, sand play, developmental play, using walkers or push toys), and medical play (using bandages or syringes, or reading books about the hospital). The nurse facilitates rooming-in when possible, and is available to parents to explain child behaviors such as regression. As with the infant, a nonrestrictive environment reinforces the patient to crawl, pull-up, cruise, walk, and explore. Children learn a balance between testing and restrictions. Therefore, positive, consistent discipline is paramount to the child's development. Whenever possible the parents' rules and routine are respected. When parents lack appropriate knowledge and skills, healthcare professionals provide education by role modeling and direct teaching of parenting skills. Physical therapists are consulted to promote development of age-appropriate motor skills for all age groups.

Middle and Late Childhood. During middle and late childhood development alternates between industry and inferiority (Erikson, 1963). Middle childhood is a time when children establish peer relationships and develop physical abilities. Children in middle-childhood are better able to understand the reasons for hospitalization but still require the presence of their parents. They are capable of learning based on understanding and reasoning, and not just by modeling or by means of reward and punishment as are younger children (Harris and Liebert, 1984). Middle-childhood children find it easier to consider what may happen in the future based on current events (Harris and Liebert, 1984). They may exhibit concern over separation from their school routines and classmates, and show signs of anger or frustration from fear of dependence, prolonged immobility, and boredom. They may be embarrassed about crying due to fear of losing emotional control, and show signs of hostility or withdrawal. During middle childhood, children have fears about body disfigurement or mutilation and have a particular fear of surgery involving the genital area (James and Mott, 1988). They need to discuss illness and hospitalization, and are concerned about the appropriate expression of feelings or loss of emotional control. Privacy and embarrassment about exposure become important issues at this age (James and Mott, 1988).

The developmental task of late childhood, children ages 8 through 12 years, is an extension of industry versus inferiority that emerged during middle childhood (Erikson, 1963). During late childhood, skills are developed for problem solving, controlling emotional responses, cooperating with peers, and improving social and math skills. A major concern is separation from school peers. Parental presence is important but not needed at all times. Children may be afraid to ask questions about body changes that occur from the disease state, medications, or surgery, causing them more feelings of confusion and uncertainty (Matteson, 1972). Fear of death and long-term disability becomes more prominent during late childhood. There is fear associated with changes in body appearance and whether peers will continue to accept them.

One way children exhibit signs of coping with hospitalization may include direct questions about their disease course. Nurses may find these questions difficult to answer. Simple concrete answers to each question should be given, and referral made to other healthcare professionals if deemed necessary by the clinical nurse (Petersen, 1989). Nurses continue to act as role models for parents in setting and enforcing limits during middle and late childhood. Since middle and late childhood is a period of concrete thinking, procedures and routines are explained in a simple, precise manner. The child is allowed uninterrupted play time with as much freedom of movement as possible and is permitted choices within acceptable limits. Opportunities for expression of fears and misconceptions may be encouraged with medical play, keeping a journal, group discussions, and one-on-one conferences with appropriate healthcare professionals. School activities are provided as are interaction with siblings and peers when feasible. Ways to help the child cope with painful procedures such as counting or relaxation techniques may also be helpful. Privacy is ensured at all times and parents are allowed to be present during procedures if the child requests their presence and their presence does not compromise medical care.

Adolescence. Adolescent development is a time when struggle with identity versus role diffusion occurs (Erikson, 1963). Adolescents have more understanding of illness but are also struggling with physical and emotional changes that are difficult for even a healthy adolescent to understand. During adolescence, the child learns gender-related roles and begins to establish new social roles with friends and peers. Hospitalized adolescents view separation from their friends as more significant than separation from their parents. They may withdraw from their friends especially if they have perceived changes in their physical appearance. Treatments causing fear of body image changes may be met with uncooperative behavior. Adolescents may exhibit fear or anger at loss of independence and may have difficulty in accepting emotional or physical assistance (James and Mott, 1988).

Adolescents require independence in the hospital as well as parental attention. The adolescent who has more adult-like, abstract thinking skills may require detailed explanations about procedures. Nurses actively listen to the adolescent for cues that he or she wants to talk or needs more detailed explanations about treatment plans and outcome. Games and other activities may facilitate discussion. Time is allowed for the adolescent to be with peers. School work is initiated when appropriate. Privacy is also ensured during all procedures. Whenever possible, adolescents are grouped together on inpatient units. Both parents and the adolescent are involved in any decision-making process.

SIBLINGS

The interaction between siblings is important to both patient and sibling; therefore, sibling visits are initiated if possible. Letters, videotapes, tape-recorded messages, and pictures are alternative ways to maintain sibling contact. This makes the hospital experience easier for the child and sibling. Siblings are made to feel a part of the transplantation process, and the child in the hospital is kept informed of events in siblings' lives outside the hospital. Consultation with a child life specialist, social workers, transplant coordinators, psychologists, and other healthcare providers is freely initiated in dealing with any child or sibling experiencing stress.

Death

Despite the advances in transplantation, a percentage of patients still die following surgery or awaiting transplantation. Dealing with death of a family member is difficult at any age. Reactions to death also differ depending upon whether the death is anticipated or sudden in nature (Sahler and Stanford, 1981). Infectious complications are the most common cause of death after transplantation. Many of the children who die after transplantation are often too sick to be counseled about death. The concerns of siblings and peers need to be addressed at the time of death. Children's understanding of and emotional reaction to the death of a sibling is, again, determined by their developmental level, past experiences, family background, and the emotional climate provided to them (Schowalter, 1980). Young children, below the age of 4 years, do not understand that death is an irreversible process. It is not until ages 6 to 10 years that children develop a concept of death as a logical biologic process (Schowalter, 1980). Children learn about the emotions of loss by experiencing loss. Therefore children who are unfamiliar with death may appear to act inappropriately (Sahler and Stanford, 1981). A sibling needs special attention after a death to be protected from feelings of abandonment, guilt, or fear (Bell and Esterling, 1986). Parents should show understanding and care for the sibling, while allowing themselves to appropriately express their own grief. Children should be addressed at eye level. Touch or holding is important during this time. Explanations should be simple and honest. The use of the words *death* and *dying* are less confusing to children than euphemistic terms such as *passed on* or *taken from us* (Bell and Esterling, 1986). The young child should be provided with opportunities to express and work through any emotions through play. Siblings may benefit from being involved in the funeral arrangements if possible. However, taking an infant or a toddler who has not internalized the concept of death to a funeral may cause feelings of fear and confusion. Any child who is firm about not wishing to attend a funeral should not be forced to go; emotionally, the child may not be ready to attend (Schowalter, 1980).

Children of all ages exhibit grief reactions. Their reaction may include denial, panic, fear, sadness, regression, school problems, anger, or guilt —depending on the child's age and level of understanding. As in all new and unfamiliar situations, the sibling needs to be told what has happened and what is expected behavior during the immediate post-death situation (Sahler and Stanford, 1981). Adults need to listen and be observant of the child's behaviors, and be available during stressful times. Extended family members and friends should also be aware that bereaved parents may be emotionally incapable of maximally supporting the child. Involvement of other resources is often mandatory (Sahler and Stanford, 1981). Literature should be made available for children and adults to help them deal with this most difficult time.

Preparations for Discharge

Once the child's medical condition stabilizes and the need for medical procedures lessens, both parent and child typically feel in better emotional balance (Gold, et al., 1986). Discharge teaching is initiated at this point. In addition to diet, activity, and medical followup, limit-setting becomes an important topic during discharge planning. Although appropriate discipline is encouraged and modeled during hospitalization, parents may be reluctant to initiate limit-setting after dealing with a chronically ill child who has undergone an extensive operation. However, limit-setting is crucial to children as they participate in school and other age-appropriate activities. The type of limit-setting used prior to transplantation is discussed, and alternatives suggested if necessary. Matteson (1972) found that families of kidney transplant patients tended to be overprotective, which is particularly difficult for adolescents who are striving for independence and autonomy.

Parents are faced with the transition and adjustment to home care. This may include adaptation to a new parent role, fear of graft rejection, and readjustment of the family structure. Gold and associates (1986) reported that many mothers had trouble in dealing with a well child. The return of the child to school may add stress as parents worry about the risk of infection. The child's self-concept may be altered due to side effects of medication. Programs should be developed to help transplant children successfully re-enter the school system.

The family is encouraged to regroup as a total unit. The patient is not singled out for individual attention as this alienates the child from siblings as well as peers. Parents may need to spend individual time with siblings who were left at home during transplantation. Family activities that help all family members redefine their roles and responsibilities are encouraged.

Growth and development continue to be concerns for children undergoing transplantation and their families. A number of centers have published articles regarding the improved growth patterns and rehabilitation rates for patients undergoing kidney transplantation (Broyer, et al., 1989; Van-Diemen-Steenvoorde, et al, 1987) liver transplantation (Urbach, et al., 1987; Zitelli, et al., 1987); bone marrow transplantation (Kaleetan, et al. 1989); and heart transplantation (Fricker, et al., 1987; Starnes, et al., 1987).

Issues for the Future

Future issues for pediatric transplantation include organ donation, medical management, and facilitation of a return to a more normal life-style by the family. Use of reduced size or split livers, xenografts, anen-cephalic donors, and living-related donors are possibilities to increase the supply of available organs.

Education of primary care physicians is ongoing and stresses the need to refer patients early in the disease course More specific immunosup-pressive drugs are under trial. More studies addressing post-transplanta-tion quality of life and facilitation of normalcy are needed. Extensive longitudinal studies on growth and development, school performance, emotional development of children, and long-term effects on the family are now possible with the number of successful pediatric transplant pa-tients and programs across the country. Future issues of sexual maturation, fertility, and long-term drug effects on the first and second generations will become important in the years to come. Difficulties in obtaining life and health insurance for pediatric transplant patients will need to be addressed. Ways of facilitating treatment compliance and dealing suc-cessfully with changes in body image among adolescent patients will need to be strengthened.

In summary, the child's developmental level is a major consideration in caring for the child throughout the transplantation process. The child's disposition, family milieu, and social support system are also instrumental in predicting the child's vulnerability to stress (Garmezy, 1987). Nurses caring for children undergoing transplantation and their families have the unique challenge of gearing their care to the appropriate developmental age of the child and the specific needs of the whole family. The unique aspects of caring for children, through the implantation process impact the family, the institution, and even the outcome of the transplantation.

Acknowledgments

The author would like to thank Geri Lo-Biondo Wood, Ph.D., R.N., Chair, Maternal Child Nursing; Randy Lagrone, Ph.D., Department of Child Psychology; Jacque Bell, Child Life Specialist; and Myrna Newland,

M.D., Department of Anesthesiology, for their assistance and support in the writing and editing of this chapter, and Elvira Keller and Arleen Kottich for their secretarial assistance.

Bibliography

Bell, J and Esterling, LS. What Will I Tell the Children. Ne: American Cancer Society, University of Nebraska Medical Center, Omaha, NE, 1986.

Berry, FA (ed): Anesthetic Management of Different and Routine Pediatric Patients. Churchill Livingstone, New York, 1986.

Broyer, M, et al: Organ transplantation in children. Intensive Care Med 15 (Suppl 1):576–579, 1989.

Drash, A, Reese, D, and Brasel, TA: Clinical material: Anthropometric and developmental analysis. In Cheek, R (ed); Human Growth. Lea & Febiger, Philadelphia, 1968.

Erikson, EH: Childhood and Society. Norton, New York, 1963.

Fricker, FJ, et al: Experience with heart transplantation in children. Pediatrics 79(1):138–146, 1987.

Garmezy, N: Stress, competence, and development: Continuities in the study of schizophrenic adults, children, vulnerable to psychopathology and the search for stress-resilient children. Am J Orthopsychiatry 57:159, 1987.

Gold, LM, et al: Psychosocial issues in pediatric organ transplantation: The parents' perspective. Pediatrics 77:738–744, 1986.

Harris, JR and Liebert, RM: The Child: Development from Birth through Adolescence. Prentice-Hall, Englewood Cliffs, NJ, 1984.

House, 1983.

James, SR and Mott, SR: Child Health Care Nursing: Essential Care of Children and Families. Addison-Wesley, Redwood City, CA, 1988.

Kalecta, TA, et al: Normal neuro development in four young children treated with bone marrow transplantation for acute leukemia or aplastic anemia. Pediatrics 83(5):753–775, May 1989.

Kaufman, SS, et al: Nutritional support for the infant with extra hepatic biliary atresia. J Pediatr 110:679–686, 1987.

Lebenthal, E (ed): Textbook of Gastroenterology and Nutrition in Infancy, ed 2. Raven Press, New York, 1989.

Lobato, D, Faust, D, and Spirito, A: Examining the effects of chronic disease and disability in children's sibling relationship. J Pediatr Psychol 13(3):389–407, 1988.

Matteson, A: Long-term physical illness in childhood: A challenge to psychosocial adaptation. Pediatrics 50(5):801–809, 1972.

Petersen, L: Coping by children undergoing stressful medical procedures. Some conceptual, methodological, and therapeutic issues. J Consult Clin 57(3):380–387, 1989.

Shaler, OT and Stanford, BF: The dying child. Pediatrics in Review 3(5):159–165, 1981.

Schowalter, TE: Children and funerals, Pediatrics in Review 1(10):337–339, 1980.

Starnes, VA, et al: Cardiovascular Surgery 1986: Part 2: Cardiac transplantation in children and adolescents. American Heart Association Monograph 10 Supplement 76(5):V43–V47, November, 1986.

Shaw, BW, Jr, et al: Liver transplantation therapy for children: Part 1. 7:157–166, 1988.

Shaw, BW, Jr, et al: Liver transplantation therapy for children: Part 2. 7:797–818, 1988.

Urbach, AH, et al: Linear growth following pediatric liver transplantation. Am J Dis Child 141:547–549, 1987.

Van-Diemen-Steenvoorde, R, et al: Growth and sexual maturation in children after kidney transplantation. J Pediatr 110(3):351–356, March, 1987.

Whaley, LF, and Wong, DL: Nursing Care of Infants and Children. CV Mosby, St Louis, 1983.
Willis, DJ, Elliot, CH, and Toy, S: Psychological effects of physical illness and its concomi-
    tants. In Tuma, J (ed): Handbook in the Practice of Pediatric Psychology. John Wiley and
    Sons, New York, 1982.
Zitelli, BJ, et al: Pediatric Liver transplantation: Patient evaluation and selection, infection
    complications, and life-style after transplantation. Transplant Proc 19:3309–3316,
    1987.

CHAPTER

Immunosuppressive Therapy

Patricia D. Weiskittel, RN, MSN, CNN

THE IMMUNE SYSTEM

The success of organ transplantation depends on the effective suppression of the body's rejection response. The rejection response is a natural phenomenon initiated by the immune system. The immune system is the body's sophisticated alarm system responsible for protection against invasion by foreign substances. When invasion occurs, as it does with a transplant, the alarm is sounded and a specialized group of cells is mobilized to attack and destroy the invader. Phagocytes and helper T cells are the first-line defenders. Phagocytes attempt to surround, engulf, and destroy the invader. Helper T cells are messengers that carry the description of the invaders to the spleen and lymph nodes in order to recruit other cells for defense. Killer T cells are recruited and B cells are mobilized to begin antibody production to destroy the invader. Antibodies are chemical weapons used to neutralize invaders. If the invasion is successfully thwarted, suppressor T cells are left to guard against further attempts of invasion by the intruder (Jaret, 1986). Figure 10–1 illustrates this immune response.

Transplantation of any organ triggers the immune system to action. Implantation of the allograft stimulates a cascade of events designed to seek, attack, and destroy the foreign invader, or organ. There are two phases to the rejection response. These phases are activated through the recognition of class I and class II antigens present on the cell surfaces of the allograft.

199

VIRUS

Needing help to spring to life, a virus is little more than a package of genetic information that must commandeer the machinery of a host cell to permit its own replication.

MACROPHAGE

Housekeeper and frontline defender, this cell engulfs and digests debris that washes into the bloodstream. Encountering a foreign organism, it summons helper T cells to the scene.

HELPER T CELL

As a commander in chief of the immune system, it identifies the enemy and rushes to the spleen and lymph nodes, where it stimulates the production of other cells to fight the infection.

KILLER T CELL

Recruited and activated by helper T cells, it specializes in killing cells of the body that have been invaded by foreign organisms, as well as cells that have turned cancerous.

B CELL

Biological arms factory, it resides in the spleen or the lymph nodes, where it is induced to replicate by helper T cells and then to produce potent chemical weapons called antibodies.

ANTIBODY

Engineered to target a specific invader, this Y-shaped protein molecule is rushed to the infection site, where it either neutralizes the enemy or tags it for attack by other cells or chemicals.

SUPPRESSOR T CELL

A third type of T cell, it is able to slow down or stop the activities of B cells and other T cells, playing a vital role in calling off the attack after an infection has been conquered.

MEMORY CELL

Generated during an initial infection, this defense cell may circulate in the blood or lymph for years, enabling the body to respond more quickly to subsequent infections.

Figure 10-1

1) As viruses begin to invade the body, a few are consumed by macrophages, which seize their antigens and display them on their own surfaces. Among millions of helper T cells circulating in the bloodstream, a select few are programmed to "read" that antigen. Binding to the macrophage, the T cell becomes activated. 2) Once activated, helper T cells begin to multiply. They then stimulate the multiplication of those few killer T cells and B cells that are sensitive to the invading viruses. As the number of B cells increases, helper T cells signal them to start producing antibodies. 3) Meanwhile, some of the viruses have entered cells of the body—the only place they are able to replicate. Killer T cells will sacrifice these cells by chemically puncturing their membranes, letting the contents spill out, thus disrupting the viral replication cycle. Antibodies then neutralize the viruses by binding directly to their surfaces, preventing them from attacking other cells. Additionally, they precipitate chemical reactions that actually destroy infected cells. 4) As the infection is contained, suppressor T cells halt the entire range of immune responses, preventing them from spiraling out of control. Memory T and B cells are left in the blood and lymphatic system, ready to move quickly should the same virus once again invade the body. (From diagram by Allen Carroll, National Geographic Art Division, and Dale Glasgow, in National Geographic [Jaret, 1986], borrowed with permission of the National Geographic Society.)

Recognition of Class I antigens (A and B loci on the sixth chromosome) by T lymphocytes triggers the production of cytotoxic or killer T cells, which are stimulated to proliferate by interleukin-2. These killer cells migrate to the "invading" organ and cause cell destruction. This comprises the cytotoxic or cellular phase of the immune response.

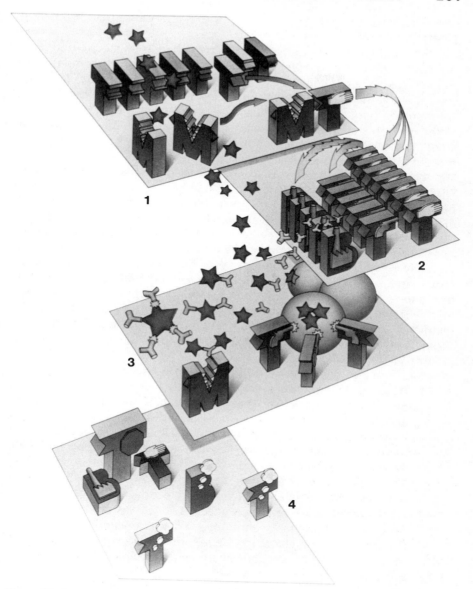

Figure 10–1

(*continued*)

    Recognition of class II antigens (D loci on the sixth chromosome) by helper T lymphocytes stimulates B cell production of antibody and stimulates macrophages to release interleukin-1, which in turn enhances the stimulation and proliferation of antibody-secreting B lymphocytes. Without introduction of suppressant agents to block this cascade, allograft destruction results (Roitt, et al., 1989; Strom and Carpenter, 1983; Ting, 1988).

Immunologic testing performed pre-transplant is utilized to determine the ABO type of the recipient for the purpose of red cell compatibility. Human leukocyte antigen (HLA) typing is performed to identify class I and class II antigens in the recipient. This allows selection of the most tissue-compatible donor. The human leukocyte group A antigens (HLA), known as the major histocompatibility antigens, are located on the sixth chromosome. These antigens are present on most tissues of the body, allowing for tissue typing to be performed simply from a blood sample. Six HLA antigens are identified from A, B, and D loci on the sixth chromosome. These antigens are inherited in pairs, known as haplotypes from each parent. Siblings within a family can therefore be a one-haplotype (half-match), two-haplotype (identical match), or a zero-haplotype match (Kottra-Buck, 1986). A white cell crossmatch is also performed to determine the presence of preformed circulating antibodies against the potential donor. Transplantation is only performed in the presence of a negative crossmatch — validating the absence of preformed antibodies. In the case of related-donor transplantation, a mixed lymphocyte culture is obtained to determine the degree of lymphocytic response of the donor to the recipient. Since this test requires that cells must incubate for 5 days before the response is read, it is impractical for use with cadaver transplantation (Kottra-Buck, 1986).

Four types of rejection response are seen with transplantation:

1. **Hyperacute rejections**, which primarily involve the humoral limb of the immune cascade. The recipient has preformed circulating antibodies sensitized to the transplanted organ. These antibodies have been formed during blood transfusions, pregnancy, or a previous transplant. Immediately upon exposure to the recipient's blood, the organ becomes dark and flabby, and thrombosis occurs. The organ must immediately be removed. A negative crossmatch is necessary to prevent this kind of rejection.

2. **Accelerated acute rejection** occurs 1 to 2 days after transplantation and is a humoral or antibody-mediated rejection response. At the time of transplant, low levels of circulating antibodies are present, and with exposure to antigen, quick proliferation of antibody-secreting cells occurs, with resulting rejection. No successful treatment has been found for this type of rejection.

3. **Acute rejection** occurs within weeks to months following transplantation and is the most common type of rejection seen. It is primarily a cellular response but may have a humoral component. Biopsy of the organ shows lymphocytic infiltration of tissues. Several regimens are utilized to treat this type of rejection. These will be discussed under specific immunosuppressive agents.

4. **Chronic rejection** occurs months to years after transplantation and is a gradual process of deterioration in organ function. Both the cellular and humoral immune response are involved in chronic rejection (Jett and Lancaster, 1983; Kottra-Buck, 1986; Weiskittel, 1988).

Table 10-1 summarizes clinical considerations in rejection of vascular organs. The success of organ transplantation depends upon the ability to block the humoral and cellular immune responses. Several processes have been utilized both historically and currently in an attempt to modify the immune response prior to renal transplantation. These include: total lymphoid irradiation; thoracic duct drainage; splenectomy; third-party transfusions; and donor-specific transfusion.

MODIFICATIONS OF THE IMMUNE RESPONSE

Total Lymphoid Irradiation

Total lymphoid irradiation (TLI) has been used historically in the treatment of Hodgkin's disease. T cell suppression occurs as a result of TLI. TLI has been administered to the mantle field, which includes the lymph nodes of the neck, axilla, and mediastinum, and to the Y field, which includes the aortic, iliac, and pelvic lymph nodes. Wide-field radiation has been employed using low-dose treatment from the base of the skull down to the pelvis (Waer and Strobu, 1988). Studies utilizing TLI have been performed in high-risk patients including diabetics, second transplants, and recipients over 55 years of age. In the four trials described in the literature, only one resulted in better graft survival than control groups treated with cyclosporine (Waer and Strobu, 1988).

More intensive clinical trials are necessary to evaluate cost-benefit, effects with regard to reduction in long-term drug therapy, incidence of rejection episodes, and infectious complications for an optimal TLI treatment regimen.

Thoracic Duct Drainage

Thoracic duct drainage (TDD) has been utilized as an adjunct immunosuppressive therapy pre-transplant and at the time of transplantation. TDD involves cannulating the thoracic duct using a double-lumen catheter. Heparinized saline is infused in one lumen to maintain patency and lymph is collected from the other lumen (Starzl, et al., 1979).

Successful use of TDD has been reported as a pre-treatment for re-transplants, high sensitized patients, and one-haplotype living-related

Table 10–1. Rejection

Organ	Manifestion	Method of Diagnosis	Common Treatment Regimens
Kidney	Elevated BUN and creatinine Decreased creatinine clearance Decreased urine output Graft tenderness Graft enlargement Low-grade temperature Elevated blood pressure	Renal biopsy	Solu-Medrol bolus 250 mg – 1 gm IVP × 3–4 days Antilymphocyte sera 10 – 14 days Monoclonal antibody 10 – 14 days
Heart	Fever, anxiety Low back pain Atrial or ventricular dysrhythmias Gallop, JVD Pericardial rub Hypotension Decreased cardiac output	Cardiac biopsy	Solu-Medrol 250 mg – 1 gm IVP × 3–4 days Antilymphocyte sera 10 – 14 days Monoclonal antibody 10 – 14 days Retransplant for intractable rejection
Liver	Malaise, fever Abdominal discomfort Swollen tender graft Tachycardia RUQ or flank pain Cessation of bile flow Change in bile color Jaundice Elevated enzymes	Liver biopsy	Solu-Medrol 250 mg – 1 gm IVP × 3–4 days Antilymphocyte sera 10 – 14 days Monoclonal antibody 10 – 14 days Retransplant for intractable rejection
Pancreas	Hyperglycemia Pancreatitis No clear manifestations	Very difficult to diagnose; when combined with kidney transplant — Kidney is used as the marker for rejection	Solu-Medrol 250 mg – 1 gm IVP × 3–4 days Antilymphocyte sera 10 – 14 days Monoclonal antibody 10 – 14 days

BUN = blood urea nitrogen; IVP = intravenous push; JVD = jugular venous distension; RUQ = right upper quadrant.

transplants (Johnson, et al., 1977; Oshima, et al., 1988; Starzl, et al., 1979).

TDD is not a widely used therapy and has disadvantages that include: duct cannulation, which may be technically difficult; prolonged hospitalization; increased risk of infection; and problems maintaining patency of catheter (Oshima, et al., 1987).

Splenectomy

The spleen is considered a secondary lymphoid organ containing both T and B cells (Roitt, et al., 1989). Splenectomy has been utilized in an attempt to improve graft survival. Significant improvement in graft survival was proven by a Minneapolis group in 1981. However, long-term followup of splenectomized patients has shown an increase in patient mortality from infection negating the benefit of improved early graft survival (Morris, 1988).

Transfusions

It has been determined over the last 15 years that nontransfused cadaver-donated renal allograft recipients were at the highest risk for failure. A 20% improved graft survival in the transfused group has been attributed to the so-called transfusion effect. The mechanism is not clearly understood but has been reproduced in clinical and experimental settings (Opelz, 1988). It has therefore become customary to require pre-transplant transfusions as a mechanism to increase renal allograft survival. Recently, however, the beneficial effect of transfusion with the use of cyclosporine has presented controversy. Collaborative data have shown a decrease in the strength of the transfusion effect. The difference between transfused and nontransfused recipients has narrowed. It is hoped that further data with reproducible results, accounting for center-to-center variability, will serve to validate the importance of the transfusion effect in renal allograft survival (Opelz, 1988).

Donor-Specific Transfusion

Improved renal graft survival with one-haplotype (half-match) related-donor transplants was reported by Cochrum and Salvatieria (in Alexander, et al., 1987) utilizing donor-specific transfusions. The recipient was given small volumes of the donor's blood at frequent intervals prior to transplantation. Crossmatches were performed to detect the appearance of antibodies to donor antigens between transfusions. Graft survival at one year was reported at 94%, compared with previous graft survival of 56% in this population (Alexander, et al., 1987; Kottra-Buck, 1986).

IMMUNOSUPPRESSIVE AGENTS

Azathioprine (Imuran)

Azathioprine was first used in renal transplant recipients to prevent rejection in 1961 at the Peter Bent Brigham Hospital in Boston.

Action. It is one of a group of drugs known as thioprines and is metabolized in the liver to its active form. It inhibits both RNA and DNA synthesis, slowing metabolism and proliferation, including antibody production (DuToit and Heydenrych, 1986; Kottra-Buck, 1986; Strom, 1984; Walker and d'Apice, 1988) (Fig. 10–2).

Dosage. May be given IV or PO 2 – 3 mg/kg/day as a single dose.

Side Effects. The major side effects include: bone marrow suppression (decreased white blood cell count); megaloblastic anemia (long-term); hepatic dysfunction; and hair loss.

Drug Interactions. Metabolism of azathioprine is by direct oxidation by xanthine oxidase. Allopurinol blocks this pathway of oxidation, creating a fourfold increase in immunosuppression and an increase in marrow toxicity. Allopurinol must be used with extreme caution and dose adjustment in the patient receiving azathioprine (Walker and d'Apice, 1988).

Corticosteroids (Prednisone)

Corticosteroids have been used since the early 1960s in combination with azathioprine to prevent renal allograft rejection. They have also been used historically in large doses to reverse rejection episodes.

Action. Steroids have a complex effect on the immune system. These effects include: inhibition of T cell migration to sites of antigen disposition; and blocking lymphocyte proliferation and the interaction between monocytes and lymphocytes (DuToit and Heydenrych, 1986; Walker and d'Apice, 1988) (see Fig. 10–2).

Dosage. May be given IV or PO. Variable from center to center starting at 1 – 5 mg/kg/day or initial high dosages of 100 – 150 mg/day tapering to 10 – 15 mg/day during the first month post transplant (Kottra-Buck, 1986; Walker and d'Apice, 1988).

Side Effects. Most of the early side effects (see table on p. 208) are associated with higher doses of steroids and diminish with tapering doses. Some centers have gone to alternate-day steroids (particularly in children and adolescents) to reduce side effects.

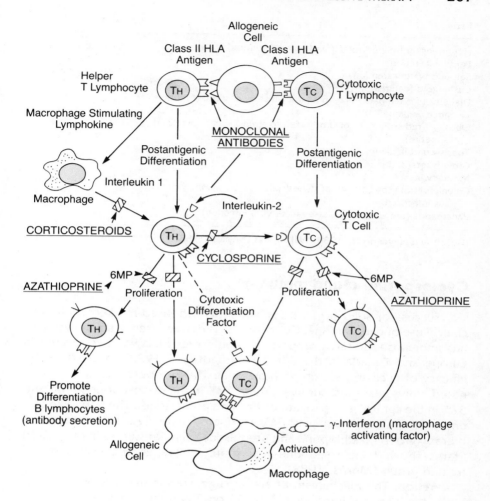

GRAFT REJECTION

Figure 10-2

Schematic representation of sites of action of the commonly used immunosuppressive agents — corticosteroids, azathioprine, cyclosporine, and monoclonal antibodies — in the cellular cascade responsible for graft rejection. (From Flye, MW: Principles of Organ Transplantation. WB Saunders, Philadelphia, 1989, with permission.)

Early	Late
Hypertension (related to salt and water retention)	Cataracts
Peptic ulceration	Osteoporosis
Salt and water retention	Avascular necrosis
Cushingoid features	
Diabetes (seen in patients with a family history of glucose intolerance or diabetes)	
Obesity (redistribution of body fat to trunk area, increased appetite)	
Poor wound healing	
Growth retardation in children	
Mood swings	
Colonic perforation (history of diverticulitis, overt cytomegalovirus infection)	
Pancreatitis (Pre-existing disease, acute viral infection)	

(DuToit and Heydenrych, 1986; Walker and D'Apice, 1988)

Cyclosporine (Sandimmune)

Success of solid organ transplants has increased markedly with the clinical use of cyclosporine. Cyclosporine is derived from a soil fungus and has immunosuppressive properties. Multicenter trials were conducted in Europe and Canada in the late 1970s and early 1980s to evaluate the efficacy of cyclosporine on graft survival. The European multicenter trial noted a one-year graft survival rate of 72% in the cyclosporine group and 52% in the control group (azathioprine and prednisone). The Canadian trial one-year graft survival was 84% compared with 67% in the standard therapy group (azathioprine and prednisone). Similar studies in the United States showed increased one-year graft survival in the cyclosporine-treated group (Morris, 1988).

Action. The mechanism of action suggested is that cyclosporine inhibits the effect of interleukin-2 (IL-2) on T lymphocyte proliferation. It appears to impair IL-2 production, therefore blocking the proliferation of cytotoxic T lymphocytes (Bauman, 1986; Cohen, 1984; Morris, 1988; Wisk, 1986) (see Fig. 10–2).

Dosage. May be given IV or PO. The manufacturer suggests an oral dosage of 15 mg/kg/day initially and tapered to 5–10 mg/kg/day 1 to 2 weeks post transplant. Individualized dosing is recommended based on serum creatinine and cyclosporine drug levels.

Recommended IV dosage is 5–6 mg/kg/day. Clinical experience has shown that doses of 4–5 mg/kg administered by continuous infusion to attain steady-state drug levels can be used effectively (Jensen and Flochmer, 1987; Keown and Stiller, 1987). The cyclosporine molecule is lipid soluble and insoluble in water. Oral cyclosporine and IV cyclosporine are supplied as liquid preparation in an ethanol base. Oral cyclosporine is absorbed from the gastrointestinal (GI) tract with peak concentration occurring in 2 to 4 hours. The absorption in the GI tract is variable and incomplete. Distribution of cyclosporine is higher in the liver, pancreas, and fat; the primary binding site in blood is the erythrocyte. The drug is extensively metabolized via the liver.

Cyclosporine and its metabolites are excreted primarily through the biliary system (Beveridge, 1982; Follath, et al., 1983; Mauer, 1985; Ptachinski, et al., 1985; Van Buren, 1986; Wood, et al., 1983).

Dose adjustments are made depending on drug levels and manifestation of adverse side effects (e.g., nephrotoxicity) in individual patients.

Side Effects. The side effects of cyclosporine vary in severity and can affect the following systems: renal, gastrointestinal, liver, integumentary, cardiovascular, and neurologic.

Nephrotoxicity is the most disturbing and clinically significant side effect of cyclosporine. Manifestations of nephrotoxicity include an elevated serum creatinine and blood urea nitrogen (BUN) with a decreased creatinine clearance, all while maintaining an adequate urine volume.

Nephrotoxicity may occur at different time intervals following renal transplantation. Acute toxicity occurring in the first week post transplant has been associated with ischemic damage to the kidney due to prolonged perfusion and donor hypotension or prolonged anastomotic times.

There is no treatment available for acute toxicity except avoiding the use of cyclosporine preoperatively or intraoperatively in the above mentioned instances. Some centers delay the introduction of cyclosporine until adequate renal function has been established. Cyclosporine has also been associated more frequently with primary nonfunction of grafts leading to failure in 1% to 2% of patients (Kahan, 1986; Morris, 1988).

A less acute form of nephrotoxicity occurs frequently in the first few months after transplantation. This type is associated with deterioration in renal function and may or may not correlate with elevated blood levels of cyclosporine. This type of toxicity usually responds to dose reduction (Kahan, 1986; Morris, 1988).

The third form of nephrotoxicity is chronic toxicity, manifested by an increase in serum creatinine greater than 3 mg/dl that is unresponsive to dose reduction. Renal biopsy findings include vascular changes, interstitial fibrosis, and tubular atrophy (Kahan, 1986; Morris, 1988).

A less common abnormality seen on renal biopsy is acute vasculopathy. This abnormality is seen in patients who have good graft function, which suddenly deteriorates. These patients are found to have features similar to those with hemolytic uremic syndrome. This condition, if detected early, is responsive to discontinuing the cyclosporine (Keown and Stiller, 1987).

GI side effects include nausea, vomiting, anorexia, and diarrhea.

Some patients find cyclosporine unpleasant to take because of its oily consistency even though attempts are made to disguise the taste by mixing it with juices or milk. The GI side effects are usually mild and transient.

Hepatotoxicity manifested by a rise in liver enzymes and bilirubin has been a transient and dose-related phenomenon. Elevation of liver function studies have regressed in most cases with cyclosporine dose reduction. Patients with abnormal liver function studies before transplantation are of concern because of the increased potential for liver injury and altered cyclosporine metabolism (Keown and Stiller, 1987; Morris, 1988).

Two common side effects involving the integumentary system are hypertrichosis and gingival hyperplasia. These side effects generally occur within the first 6 months of cyclosporine therapy, are mild to moderate in severity, and remain for the duration of therapy. Increased hair growth occurs over the face, neck, trunk, and limbs. Gum hypertrophy may be preceded by soreness of the gums and is usually more pronounced in patients with a history of poor dental hygiene. In severe cases of gum hypertrophy, gingival tissue may require surgical resection (Venning, 1988).

Cardiovascular effects include a high incidence of hypertension in cyclosporine-treated patients (Morris, 1988; Steinmuller; 1985) and an increase in LDL cholesterol (Raine, 1988). This is of concern because cardiovascular complications remain a major cause of death following renal transplantation (Raine, 1988).

The metabolic aberrations that may be seen in patients treated with cyclosporine include hyperkalemia, hypermagnesemia, hyperglycemia, and elevated urate levels. Hyperkalemia is the most common metabolic side effect and is easily controlled with dose reduction, dietary restrictions or the use of sodium polystyrene sulfonate (Kayexalate) orally (Morris, 1988).

Neurologic manifestations that have been associated with cyclosporine include paresthesias, tremors, and convulsions. Fine tremors are the most common side effect along with parasthesias, and both do respond to dose reduction. Convulsions have occurred in patients with a previous history and are possibly attributed to both hypomagnesemia and the concomitant therapy with bolus steroids (Kahan, 1986; Morris, 1988).

Drug Interactions. The last major topic of concern related to cyclosporine is drug interactions. Since metabolism occurs almost entirely in the liver, drugs that increase or decrease hepatic enzyme activity may have an effect on cyclosporine metabolism. Drugs that increase hepatic enzyme activity may increase cyclosporine metabolism, resulting in a drop in therapeutic levels of cyclosporine in the blood. Conversely, drugs that decrease hepatic enzyme activity may block the metabolism of cyclosporine and result in markedly increased levels of cyclosporine in the blood.

Table 10-2. Cyclosporine Drug Interactions

Increase Cyclosporine Levels	Decrease Cyclosporine Levels	Possible Added Nephrotoxicity
When taken with:	*When taken with:*	*When taken with:*
Steroids	Phenytoin	Sulfamethoxazole and/or
Erythromycin	Phenobarbital	trimethoprim (oral)
Ketoconazole	Rifampin	cimetidine
Diltiazem	Isoniazid	ranitidine
Nicardipine	Sulfamethoxazole and/or	aminoglycosides
Cimetidine	trimethoprim (IV)	Amphotericin
Ranitidine		Furosemide
Danazol		Mannitol
		Indomethacin

(Adapted from Wadhwa, et al.)

Drugs that are potentially nephrotoxic may result in an additional risk of nephrotoxicity when used concomitantly with cyclosporine (Keown and Stiller, 1987; Morris, 1988; Wadhwa, et al., 1987).

Table 10-2 lists commonly used drugs that increase and decrease cyclosporine levels, and those that may cause additive nephrotoxicity.

Antilymphocyte Sera

Antilymphocyte sera or polyclonal antibody preparations are used both prophylactically to prevent rejection, and in the treatment of acute rejection episodes. Polyclonal preparations are made by injecting human lymphocytes, thymocytes, or cultured lymphoblasts into a horse, goat, or rabbit so the animal will produce antibodies to human antigens. The globulin fraction is separated from sera, purified, and prepared for administration as an intravenous or intramuscular drug (Cosimi, 1988; Kottra-Buck, 1986).

Action. Polyclonal preparations deplete the number of circulating T cells and decrease their proliferative function.

Dosage. Primarily given IV through a central line, 15-30 mg/kg/day for 5 to 14 days prophylactically or as treatment of rejection.

Side Effects. Fever, chills, rash, joint pain, itching, thrombocytopenia. These side effects primarily occur with the first two doses and decrease with subsequent doses (Cosimi, 1988).

Monoclonal Antibody

Orthoclone OKT$_3$ is a murine monoclonal antibody used to treat acute cell-mediated organ rejection. Monoclonal antibody is prepared in four steps:

1. Mice are immunized with antigen.
2. Four to 6 weeks later, spleen cells from the mice are isolated and fused with mycloma cells to increase lifespan.
3. Selection of hybrid (specific antibody-producing cells).
4. Preservation of clones of hybrids.

Monoclonal antibodies have specific advantages over polyclonal preparations; these advantages include homogeneity, specificity, and consistent potency and predictability with regard to efficacy and adverse reactions (Farrell, 1987; Cosimi, 1988).

Action. The mechanism of action includes removal of all T cells, interaction with the T$_3$ antigen recognition complex on late thymocytes and mature T cells, and blocking the immunologic functioning of these cells. OKT$_3$ coats or opsonizes circulating T cells, which are removed by the reticuloedothelial system in the liver and spleen; modulates the T$_3$ antigen structure, rendering it ineffective; and may block later T cell functions (Goldstein, 1987; Moir, 1989).

Dosage. It is administered as a 5-mg IV bolus dose daily for 7 to 14 days.

Side Effects. The majority of side effects or adverse reactions commonly occur after administration of the first dose and to a lesser extent following subsequent doses. These reactions usually occur within 60 minutes of the first dose and may persist for several hours. They are thought to be the result of mediators released during rapid T cell lysis and removal by the reticuloendothelial system.

Common reactions include: fever, chills, tremors, headache, generalized aching, photophobia, dyspnea, chest pain, wheezing, nausea, vomiting, and diarrhea. In the early clinical trials, five cases of pulmonary edema occurred following the first dose. This adverse reaction has been prevented by assuring that there is no evidence of fluid overload, as evidenced by a clear chest x-ray and a weight gain of less than 3% over dry weight before administration of OKT$_3$. If fluid volume excess is present, the patient may be treated with diuretics or ultrafiltration to attain dry weight before OKT$_3$ is administered (Cosimi, 1987; Farrell, 1987; Moir, 1988).

There have been some reports of a syndrome of aseptic meningitis, which is manifested by fever, neck stiffness, and headache. This syndrome has been self-limiting and no infectious agent has been identified (Cosimi, 1988).

Cyclophosphamide

Cyclophosphamide (Cytoxan) is an immunosuppressant agent used in place of azathioprine in patients with liver dysfunction. Its mechanism of action includes destruction of proliferative lymphoid cells and decreasing immunoglobulins. Side effects include: leukopenia, thrombocytopenia, nausea, vomiting, and hemorrhagic cystitis (Bass, 1986; Morris, 1988).

New Drug Trials

FK 506 is a newly introduced immunosuppressive agent. Derived from a soil fungus, this antirejection medication is showing early indications of great success at the University of Pittsburgh (Starzl, et al, 1989a; Starzl, et al, 1989b). Clinical trials at this one center have shown fewer side effects than cyclosporine; specifically less nephrotoxicity has been demonstrated. However, most studies to date have been done on animals. Use in humans for heart, kidney, and renal transplants has been limited. Multicenter studies are needed to confirm early results.

SIDE EFFECTS OF IMMUNOSUPPRESSION

All transplant recipients will be maintained on a combined regimen of immunosuppressive agents for the life of the graft. The short- and long-term side effects of immunosuppression have been documented in the renal transplant population. The early common side effects seen in the first few weeks post transplant are those associated with specific immunosuppressive agents. These have been covered under the specific agents earlier in this chapter.

Brunkwall and his colleagues (1987) have reported a higher incidence of deep-vein thrombosis during the first three weeks post transplant than that of patients in a comparable age group undergoing other types of major surgery. Deep-vein thrombosis occurred in 24.1% of patients receiving azathioprine and high-dose steroids and 9.3% of patients receiving cyclosporine and low-dose steroids. Insulin-dependent diabetes was found to be a risk factor for development of deep-vein thrombosis (Brunkwall, et al., 1987).

The long-term combined effects of immunosuppression include infection, cardiovascular complications, skin disorders, and malignancy.

Infection

Despite the advances in immunosuppression and transplant success, infection continues to remain a major cause of morbidity and mortality following transplantation (Cohen, et al., 1988; Rubin and Tolhoff-Rubin, 1988). Risk factors present in this population include: diabetes, age, nutritional status, neutropenia, potential poor graft function; the experience of a major surgical procedure; and the administration of immunosuppressive agents, which have broad effects on immune competence (Cohen, et al., 1988). The pre-transplant workup is designed to identify pre-existing conditions that may increase risks of infection post transplant.

Post-transplant infection has been well documented in the renal transplant population and occurrences can be divided into three time periods — those that occur within the first 4 weeks, 1 to 6 months, and more than 6 months after transplantation (Rubin and Tolhoff-Rubin, 1988). Table 10–3 lists the common post-transplant infections by time interval and system affected.

Bacterial infections are the most common during the first 4 weeks post transplant. Transplant surgery violates the body's first line of defense including the skin, mucous membranes, and body secretions. Therefore, common early sites of bacterial infection include drains, catheters, intravenous lines, dialysis access sites, chest tubes, urinary tract, and wounds. These infections are usually conventional nosocomial infections seen in surgical patients, but may be more severe in the immunosuppressed population.

In the renal transplant population, wound infection rates vary from 1% to 10% (Cohen, et al., 1988). Wound infections are more common in diabetics and after urine leaks, or hematoma or lymphocele information. The wound is inspected by the nurse each 8 hours for redness, swelling, tenderness, and foul-smelling drainage. All wound drainage is cultured. If infection develops, it may extend down to the graft, increasing morbidity and mortality.

Prevention of infection can be enhanced by adherence to aseptic technique when handling IV lines and catheters, good pulmonary toilet, hand washing, and assessment for signs and symptoms of infection (Chmielewski, 1987).

Herpes simplex virus infection can occur within the first 4 to 6 weeks post transplant and is usually the result of reactivation of latent virus. Lesions may appear in the anogenital area, or on the lips, nose, or mouth, and can extend down into the throat and esophagus. These lesions tend to be painful and localized. Dissemination is uncommon. The treatment of choice is topical and/or oral acyclovir (Cohen, et al., 1988; Levin, 1988; Rubin and Tolhoff-Rubin, 1988). Emphasis on hygiene is of importance in the nursing care plan to prevent spread of the lesions. Painful lesions on

Table 10–3. **Post-Transplant Infections**

1–4 Weeks	1–6 Months		Over 6 Months
Bacterial: Wound	Viral:	CMV	Chronic CMV
Pneumonia		EBV	Non-A, non-B hepatitis
IV lines		VZV	Opportune infections
Urinary tract		Adenovirus	
Access sites			
Hepatitis B	Hepatitis:	Non-A, non-B	
Herpes simplex virus			
	Fungal:	*Cryptococcus*	
		Candida	
		Aspergillus	
	Parasitic:	*Pneumocystis*	
		Strongyloides	
		Toxoplasma	
	Bacterial:	*Mycobacterium tuberculosis*	
		Pneumococcus	
		Staphylococcus	
		Gram negatives	
		Legionella	
		Nocardia	

SYSTEMIC

Pulmonary	*CNS*
Bacteria	*Listeria*
Fungi	*Cryptococcus*
Viruses	*Mycobacteria*
Parasites	

the oral mucosa may prevent adequate intake of nutrients. The use of topical anesthetics may provide palliative relief, allowing for adequate oral intake. The nurse monitors nutritional status and initiates calorie counts and measurement of intake and output as indicated.

Other infections that can be seen in the first month include tuberculosis, strongyloidiasis, and specific mycoses that may be common in particular geographic areas of the country, such as histoplasmosis, coccidiomycosis, and blastomycosis (Rubin and Tolhoff-Rubin, 1988).

One to 6 months post transplant encompasses a critical period of risk from infection. This is the peak period for the cumulative effects of early anti-rejection therapy. The patient is at risk for life-threatening infections. Pulmonary infection can be the result of bacteria, fungi, viruses, or parasites. Patients who present with a fever and infiltrates on chest x-ray frequently undergo bronchiolar lavage for rapid identification of the organism and appropriate therapeutic response (Cohen, et al., 1988). Common bacterial organisms in this population include *Pneumococcus, Staphylococcus, Hemophilus,* gram negatives, *Legionella, Nocardia,* and *Mycobacteria.* There are no specific clinical signs to differentiate *Legionella* from other organisms. Once identified, the treatment of choice is erythromycin. Nocardiosis is usually caused by the acid-fast bacterium *Nocardia asteroides* and can present as a respiratory illness without a productive cough. The patient may complain of malaise and pleuritic chest pain with fever. Chest x-ray may show nodular lesions. Nocardia can spread to the brain, or it can manifest as a skin abscess or joint infection.

Cytomegalovirus (CMV) is potentially the most important and devastating viral infection seen in transplant recipients. Reactivation rather than primary infection is the most common mechanism for this infection. Pretransplant screening has shown that 50% to 60% of patients awaiting transplantation have antibodies to CMV, indicating a previous CMV infection.

CMV typically presents around 40 days post transplant manifested by a spiking temperature that may be accompanied by leukopenia, thrombocytopenia, dyspnea, arthralgia, myalgia, elevated liver enzymes, and renal dysfunction. Severe CMV infections may result in pulmonary, hepatic, and gastrointestinal manifestations.

Gastrointestinal disorders occurring as a result of CMV carry a poor prognosis. Cohen and colleagues (1988) reviewed ulcer specimens from eight renal transplant patients with peptic ulceration and found active CMV in five of the eight patients. Gastrointestinal ulceration and hemorrhage can occur in the presence of severe CMV infection.

CMV is the primary cause of morbidity and mortality during this time interval. It has been estimated that 60% to 96% of patients have laboratory and/or clinical evidence of CMV infection 1 to 6 months post transplant (Garibaldi, 1983). It produces a variety of clinical infectious syndromes and produces an additive immunosuppressed state predisposing the transplant recipient to the potential for other opportunistic infections (Rubin and Tolhoff-Rubin, 1988).

Antiviral agents (gancyclovir) and hyperimmune anti-CMV globulin preparations are being studied and hold some promise for prophylaxis against and treatment of CMV infection. However, at the present time, the clinical management of patients with CMV infection remains difficult and challenging (Cohen, et al., 1988; Rubin and Tolhoff-Rubin, 1988).

Epstein-Barr virus (EBV) infection may occur as a primary infection, may remain asymptomatic, or frequently runs a course of elevated temperature and glandular swelling and tenderness. More commonly, reactivation of seropositive patients occurs with secretion of the virus into the throat. Throat washings of immunosuppressed patients reveal that 50% of the patients have EBV in these washings compared to 10% to 20% in normal seropositive people. The major concern about EBV is the long-term suppression of the T-lymphocyte population, which results in their inability to check the proliferation of EBV-infected B lymphocytes. Proliferation of the EBV-infected B lymphocytes has been implicated as a possible causative factor in the malignant lymphoma frequently seen in transplant recipients (Cohen, et al., 1988; Rubin and Tolhoff-Rubin, 1988).

Varicella zoster virus (VZV) infection occurs in approximately 10% of transplant recipients. The most common presentation is pain and a blistering rash localized over a dermatomal region. Dissemination is uncommon but can occur, leading to pneumonitis, encephalitis, or meningitis. Treatment with oral acyclovir is routine management for dermatomal distribution. If dissemination begins, hospitalization and IV acyclovir are employed (Cohen, et al., 1988; Rubin and Tolhoff-Rubin, 1988).

Pneumocystis carinii is a protozoan infection that produces a diffuse interstitial pneumonia in the transplant recipient. The clinical picture is an acute or subacute onset of dyspnea, fever and a low PO_2. Chest x-ray shows a diffuse interstitial or shadowing pattern. This can be effectively treated with trimethoprim/sulfamethoxazole (TMP-SMX). Patients on triple immunosuppressive therapy are commonly placed on TMP-SMX as prophylaxis against *Pneumocystis* (Cohen, et al., 1988; Rubin and Tolhoff-Rubin, 1988).

The two most common central nervous system (CNS) pathogens occurring during this time period are *Listeria* and *Cryptococcus*. Listeria may present with signs and symptoms of meningoencephalitis. Spinal tap may reveal an increased polymorphonuclear count and reduced glucose, and the organisms may be seen on Gram's stain. Treatment includes ampicillin for 14 days and sometimes the addition of gentamicin.

Cryptococcus infection is probably acquired by inhalation and spread in the blood, causing a subacute meningitis. Presentation includes headache, photophobia, varied symptoms of reduced cerebral function, focal neurological signs, and potential seizures. Rapid diagnosis is made by examination of cerebrospinal fluid, which shows an elevated protein, reduced glucose, lymphocytosis, and positive India ink stain. Initial treatment with amphotericin B and flucytosine for 6 weeks is further followed by a repeat lumbar puncture (Cohen, et al., 1988; Rubin and Tolhoff-Rubin, 1988).

Infections occurring more than six months after transplantation include chronic viral infection progressing to problems such as chorioretinitis due to CMV, liver disease due to hepatitis C (non-A, non-B hepatitis), and EBV-associated lymphoproliferative disease. Patients with good graft function on small maintenance dose immunosuppression have infection problems similar to the general population. Patients with chronic infection, poor graft function and large cumulative doses of immunosuppressive agents are at risk for life-threatening opportunistic infections (Rubin and Tolhoff-Rubin, 1988).

Symptoms of fever, pulmonary changes on x-ray, or CNS abberations require aggressive diagnostic workup to document the pathogen, institute rapid therapy and hopefully prevent life-threatening illness in this population.

Cardiovascular Complications

Vascular events and myocardial infarction are common causes of morbidity and mortality following transplantation. Factors that have been associated with vascular events include hypertension, abnormal calcium metabolism post transplant, accelerated atherosclerosis developing on dialysis, and hyperlipidemia.

Factors that contribute to hypertension following transplant include acute and chronic rejection, steroids, cyclosporine, and the presence of diseased native kidneys that may have increased renin production and fluid overload. Sudden acute onset of hypertension may be the result of acute rejection, renal artery stenosis, or fluid overload. Management of hypertension focuses on drug therapy, followed by native nephrectomy if control is not attained with medications.

Vascular complications occur most frequently in diabetics with evidence of pre-existing vascular disease prior to transplantation. The incidences of occlusive vascular disease and myocardial infarction remain increased in the transplant population.

Persistent lipid abnormalities occur after transplantation with elevation in cholesterol and triglycerides. Lipid abnormalities have been associated with corticosteroid dosing and cyclosporine in some studies. However, no definitive causal relationship has been identified between lipid abnormalities and atherosclerosis in this population.

Current clinical practice is directed at correction of risk factors through early and vigorous treatment of hypertension, dietary modifications to alter lipid abnormalities, and the use of lipid lowering medications (Raine, 1988).

Skin Disorders

Skin disorders are a common complication of immunosuppression. Transplant recipients are susceptible to bacterial, fungal, and viral lesions as well as premalignant and malignant lesions. Bacterial lesions include impetigo, folliculites, abscesses, cellulitis, furuncles, and erysipelas. Superficial skin fungus is very common in this population. *Candida albicans* may occur in sites that are moist: inframammary folds, the groin, and digital web spaces. Predisposing factors include obesity, diabetes, and occlusion. Common warts, flat warts, and plantar warts have been reported in this population. Patients usually have multiple warts that are resistant to treatment and occur commonly on sun-exposed skin (Venning, 1988).

Cancer

Malignancies occurring in transplant recipients have been reported since 1968. Tumors appear on the average of 64 months post transplant in the standard therapy group (azathioprine and prednisone) and 25 months average in the cyclosporine-treated group. Data from the tumor registry shows a higher incidence of lymphomas, Kaposi's sarcoma, and renal carcinoma in the cyclosporine-treated group. The standard therapy group has a higher incidence of skin cancers, uterine cervical cancer, and cancers of the vulva and perineum. The most common malignancies in the standard therapy group were skin and lip cancers, with a predominance being squamous cell in nature. Non-Hodgkin's lymphomas were predominant in the cyclosporine-treated patients, occurring on an average of 12 months after transplant. Data available at this time appear to reveal that the incidence of cancer is not increased with cyclosporine treatment. However, it does appear that the types of malignancies and their behavior are different between the two forms of therapy (Penn, 1988).

SUMMARY

This chapter has outlined the major short- and long-term side effects of immunosuppression. Nursing assessment, nursing diagnosis, care planning, and patient education are major factors that will impact on the recognition and proper treatment of these side effects.

Bibliography

Alexander, JW, et al: The transfusion effect. In Habual, M (ed): Chronic Renal Failure and Transplantation. Semith Offset, Turkey, 1987.

Bass, M: Common complications of immunosuppression in the renal transplant patient. ANNA Journal 13(4):196–199, August, 1986.

Beveridge, T: Pharmacokinetics and metabolism of cyclosporine A. In White, D (ed): Cyclosporine A. Proceedings of an International Conference on Cyclosporine A. Elsevier Biomedical Press, Amsterdam, 1982, pp 35–44.

Brunkwall, J, et al: Postoperative deep vein thrombosis after renal transplantation. Transplantation 43(5):647–649, 1987.

Bauman, WA, et al: Cyclosporine A inhibits IL 2-driven proliferation of human alloactivated T-cell. J Immunol 136:4035–4039, 1986.

Chmielewski, C: Early recognition of infection after renal transplantation. ANNA Journal 14(6):389–391, 408, 1987.

Cohen, DJ, et al: Cyclosporine: A new immunosuppressive agent for organ transplantation. Ann Intern Med 101:667–682, 1984.

Cohen, J, Hopkin, J, and Kurtz, J: Infectious complications after renal transplantation. In Morris, P (ed): Kidney Transplantation Principles and Practice, ed 3. WB Saunders, Philadelphia, 1988, pp 533–573.

Cosimi, AB: OKT₃: First-dose safety and success. Nephron 46(S1):12–18, 1987.

Cosimi, AB: Antilymphocyte globulin and monoclonal antibodies. In Morris, P (ed): Kidney Transplantation Principles and Practice, ed 3. WB Saunders, Philadelphia, 1988, pp 343–369.

DuToit, DF and Heydenrych, JJ: The application/mechanism of action and side effects of immunosuppression agents in clinical transplantation. South African Medical Journal 70:687–691, November 22, 1986.

Farrell, ML: Orthoclone OKT₃: A treatment for acute renal allograft rejection. ANNA Journal 14(6):373–376, December, 1987.

Follath, F, et al: Intravenous cyclosporine kinetics in renal failure. Clin Pharmacol Ther 34:638–643, 1983.

Garibaldi, RA: Infections in organ transplant recipients. Infect Control 4:460, 1983.

Goldstein, G: Monoclonal antibody specificity: Orthoclone OKT₃ T-cell blocker. Nephron 46(S1):5–11, 1987.

Jaret, P: Our immune system—the wars within. National Geographic 169(6):702–734, 1986.

Jett, MF and Lancaster, LE: The inflammatory-immune response: The body's defense against invasion. Critical Care Nurse (September/October, 1983):64–85.

Jenson, C and Flochmer, S: Exacerbation of cyclosporine toxicity by concomitant administration of erythromycin. Transplantation 43:263, 1987.

Johnson, HK, et al: Immunologic preparation for cadaver renal transplant by thoracic duct drainage. Transplant Proc IX(3):1499–1503, September, 1977.

Kahan, BD: Cyclosporine nephrotoxicity: Pathogenesis, prophylaxis, therapy, and prognosis. Am J Kidney Dis VIII(5):323–331, November, 1986.

Keown, PA and Stiller, CR: Cyclosporine: A double-edged sword. Hosp Pract (May 15, 1987):207–220.

Keown, PA, et al: The clinical relevance of cyclosporine blood levels as measured by radioimmunoassay. Transplant Proc 15(4/Suppl 1):2438–2441, 1983.

Kottra-Buck, C: Renal transplantation. In Richard, C (ed): Comprehensive Nephrology Nursing. Little, Brown & Co, Boston, 1986, pp 407–423.

Levin, MJ: Antiviral therapy of herpes virus infections in renal transplant recipients. Transplant Proc XX(6/Suppl 8):19–23, 1988.

Mauer, G: Metabolism of cyclosporine. Transplant Proc 17(4/Suppl 1):19–26, 1985.

Moir, E: Nursing care of patients receiving orthoclone OKT₃. ANNA Journal 16(5):327–328, August, 1989.

Morris, PJ: Cyclosporine. In Morris, P (ed): Kidney Transplantation Principles and Practice, ed 3. WB Saunders, Philadelphia, 1988, pp 285–310.

Oshima, S, et al: The beneficial effect of thoracic duct drainage pretreatment in living related kidney transplantation. Transplant Proc XX(1/Suppl 1):415–417, February, 1988.

Opelz, G: Comparison of immunosuppressive protocols in renal transplantation: Multicenter view. Transplant Proc XX(6/Suppl 8):31–36, December, 1988.

Penn, I: Cancers after cyclosporine therapy. Transplant Proc XX(1/Suppl 1):276–279, 1988.

Ptachinski, RJ, Burchart, GJ, and Venkataramanan, R: Cyclosporine. Drug Intell Clin Pharm 19:90–100, 1985.

Raine, AEG: Cardiovascular complications after renal transplantation. In Morris, P (ed): Kidney Transplantation Principles and Practice, ed 3. WB Saunders, Philadelphia, 1988, pp 575–601.

Roitt, I, Brostoff, J and Male, D: Immunology, ed 2. 1989. Cell cooperation in the antibody response, pp 8.1–8.12; Cell mediated immune responses, pp 9.1–9.14. CV Mosby, St. Louis.

Rubin, RH and Tolhoff-Rubin, NE: Opportunistic infections in renal allograft recipients. Transplant Proc XX(6/Suppl 8):12–18, 1988.

Starzl, TE, et al: Thoracic duct fistula and renal transplantation. Ann Surg 190(4):474–484, October, 1979.

Starzl, TE, et al: Clinical trials of FK 506. IV Congress of the European Society for Organ Transplantation. Barcelona, 1989a.

Starzl, TE, et al: FK 506 for liver, kidney, and pancreas transplantation. Lancet 2:1000, 1989b.

Steinmuller, DR: Cyclosporine and organ transplantation. Cleveland Clinic Q 52(2):263–270, 1985.

Strom, TB and Carpenter, CB: Transplantation: Immunogenetic and clinical aspects — part II. Hosp Pract (January, 1983):135–150.

Strom, TB: Immunosuppressive agents in renal transplantation. Kidney Int 26:353–365, 1984.

Ting, A: HLA matching and crossmatching in renal transplantation. In Morris, P (ed): Kidney Transplantation Principles and Practice, ed 3. WB Saunders, Philadelphia, 1988, pp 183–213.

Van Buren, CT: Cyclosporine: Progress, problems, and perspectives. Surg Clin North Am 66(3):435–447, June, 1986.

Venning, VA: Non-malignant skin lesions in renal transplant patients. In Morris, P (ed): Kidney Transplantation Principles and Practice, ed 3. WB Saunders, Philadelphia, 1988, pp 619–634.

Wadhwa, N, et al: Cyclosporine drug interactions: A review. Ther Drug Monit 9(4):399, 1987.

Waer, M and Strobu, S: Total lymphoid irradiation. In Morris, P (ed): Kidney Transplantation Principles and Practice, ed 3. WB Saunders, Philadelphia, 1988, pp 371–381.

Walker, RG and d'Apice, AJF: Azathioprine and steroids. In Morris, P (ed): Kidney Transplantation Principles and Practice, ed 3. WB Saunders, Philadelphia, 1988, pp 319–341.

Weiskittel, P: Renal transplant. In Swearinger, P, Sommers, M, and Miller, K (eds): Manual of Critical Care Applying Nursing Diagnosis to Adult Critical Illness. CV Mosby, St Louis, 1988, pp 192–198.

Wish, JB: Immunologic effects of cyclosporine. Transplant Proc 18(3/Suppl 2):15–18, 1986.

Wood, AJ, et al: Cyclosporine pharmacokinetics, metabolism and drug interactions. Transplant Proc 15(4/Suppl 1):2409–2412, 1983.

Followup Care of the Transplant Patient

Joan Miller, RNC, MSN

The fragility of health following organ transplantation is well recognized. Recipients must undergo a major adjustment to their altered life-style and require continuous health surveillance. These changes can have a considerable impact on family, friends, and the work setting. The effectiveness of immunosuppression will become the focus of medical followup as will common side effects of the therapy. These side effects can impose problematic physical complications or changes, as well as emotional disturbances. A major focus of nursing intervention is directed at helping these individuals learn to monitor their health status and assisting them with the adjustment period. This period often coincides with a time when the recipient and family are depleted of emotional energy. They will require help to plan for their new life-style, while adjusting to the enormity of what has happened to them.

It is important that nurses who work with these patients be knowledgeable about the myriad of side effects that can occur in long-term immunosuppressed patients. Survival can be dependent on patients' knowledge about their condition, and compliance with therapy. Knowledge of common complications associated with immunosuppressive therapy and key nursing strategies that can be used to assist these patients are critical to successful nursing interventions.

REJECTION

Rejection is a major life-threatening event for the recipients if it progresses undetected and untreated. It can be silent and clinically difficult to detect.

The nurse instructs patients in the importance of adherence to their medical regimen to reduce the risk of a rejection episode. The patient is also taught to be aware of the early and often subtle changes in graft function that may herald the onset of rejection. Some of the signs that may present early in a rejection episode are listed in Table 11 – 1.

The nurse reassures the patient that rejection episodes are not unexpected, and that treatment is usually routine and often without complication. The patient is prepared for emotional and physical changes that may occur. Emotional lability, changes in appetite, and increased cushingoid features are commonly experienced by patients on increased doses of corticosteroids.

INFECTION

Infection is the leading cause of morbidity and mortality in organ transplant patients (Stinson, et al., 1971). The availability of cyclosporine in the early 1980s and the subsequent mushrooming of transplant programs worldwide was a reflection of the major step forward in the management of infection in these groups of patients. Cyclosporine has clearly made infectious complications more manageable by allowing a certain degree of bone marrow activity and immune response to persist. Figure 11 – 1 illustrates the major differences in survival at one center between immunosuppressive regimens before 1980, based on azathioprine, and those after 1980, based on cyclosporine. While the actual number of infectious episodes does not change between the groups, the incidence of death secondary to these infections is clearly improved in the cyclosporine group.

The key to successful outcome, however, is early diagnosis and treatment. Fundamental in this process is a well-educated patient, versed in the signs and symptoms of infection to be alert for and to report. Patients are taught by the nurse to take their own temperature daily following discharge from the hospital. The nurse stresses the importance of establishing a regular midafternoon pattern to increase the possibility of noting a low-grade fever. Patients are instructed to report any temperature elevation associated with additional symptoms and any isolated elevation to 38°C (100.4°F) or higher. Serious signs and symptoms of infection are to be reported immediately. The nurse stresses to the patient that a productive cough, flank pain, painful and/or bloody urination, severe headache

Table 11-1. **Possible Early Clinical Signs of Graft Rejection**

Organ	Fever	Malaise	SOB	Tenderness at Graft Site	Atrial Disrhythmia	Dark Urine, Light Stools	Decreased Urine Output
Heart	±	±	±	−	±	−	−
Kidney	±	+	−	±	−	−	+
Liver	−	+	−	−	−	±	−
Heart/Lung	±	±	±	−	±	−	−

SOB = shortness of breath
± = can be seen
− = not usually seen
+ = usually seen.

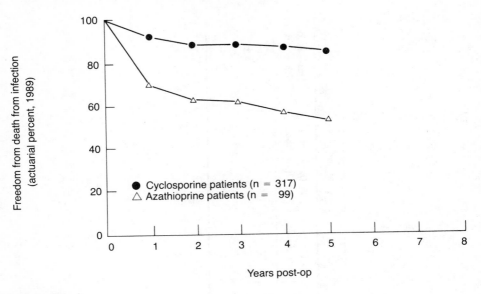

Figure 11–1

Survival rate differences between azathioprine and cyclosporine as immunosuppressive regimens.

associated with emesis, and vesicular rash are all serious occurrences that must be reported immediately.

Patients require a clinical exam at regular intervals. The nurse directs special attention to inquiries relevant to infection. It is recommended that this occur every 6 weeks. Groin and axillary lymph nodes are examined and chest x-rays obtained to screen for silent pulmonary infection.

When infection is suspected, aggressive attempts at diagnosis are undertaken before antibiotic therapy is begun. All culture specimens are processed for Gram's stain, aerobic and anaerobic (where appropriate) culture, acid-fast organisms, and fungus. In addition, all plates are held for *Nocardia* (a genus of gram-positive aerobic bacteria). All specimens obtained from the pulmonary tree are screened with silver staining for fungal and protozoal organisms or malignant processes. Blood is drawn for routine culture, *Legionella*, and for determination of viral titer rise when appropriate.

When infection is suspected, the nurse ascertains that all appropriate cultures have been obtained before antibiotics are administered. As many drugs can alter the metabolism of cyclosporine, the nurse verifies with the physician and pharmacist if any change in dosage is indicated (See also Table 10–2).

Pulmonary infections are the most frequent and potentially serious for the immunosuppressed patient. For these reasons, the nurse instructs the patient to wear protective masks when in the hospital setting to reduce the risk of exposure to airborne organisms. These microbes are often more resistant strains. They are also encouraged to avoid obvious sources of infection in their environment. Visiting between transplant patients who are hospitalized may be discouraged and avoidance of those with obvious infection is necessary. Because cyclosporine does leave a level of immune response intact, these patients usually can weather common colds and influenza. For this reason, the nurse does not recommend any disruption in normal family interactions if family members contract these infections.

The nurse will also encourage the patient to rely on non-aspirin-containing compounds such as acetaminophen for febrile and minor pain relief. Aspirin can temporarily impair blood-clotting time and may increase the risk of complication if invasive techniques are utilized to diagnose infection. The patient will also be reminded to carefully screen over-the-counter remedies, (e.g., antihistamines and cough syrups) for potential interaction with other drugs such as antihypertensives.

The collection of a sputum sample for bacteriologic analysis, while a common intervention, is not always possible and rarely sufficient or rapid enough to be reliable. The nurse anticipates the need for more aggressive methods of specimen retrieval. Transtracheal aspiration, transthoracic needle aspiration, or fiberoptic bronchoscopy is performed when changes on the patient's x-ray are suggestive of a pulmonary infection.

Viral infections, primary or reactivated, are common in organ transplant patients. Since virus can be transmitted from donor to recipient, most centers screen prospective recipients and donors for pre-existing titers to the more common viral agents, such as cytomegalovirus (CMV), varicella zoster (HZ), herpes simplex, hepatitis B, and the human immunodeficiency virus (HIV). While most problems associated with these viruses occur early after surgery, the patients can reactivate or contract them any time. CMV can present as a flu-like syndrome or as a tenacious, often fatal, pneumonia. CMV retinitis can have tragic consequences for the patient because vision can be permanently lost. At this time, there is no reliable treatment for this virus. A newly developed antiviral agent, gancyclovir (DHPG), is currently being evaluated for efficacy. Until appropriate therapies are available, the form of treatment is determined by the severity of the illness. Mild titer rises with accompanying flu-like symptoms require only symptomatic febrile relief and close observation for any acceleration of the disease. CMV retinitis requires the attention of a skilled ophthalmologist to follow its progress carefully. Laser treatment is utilized, when indicated, in an attempt to interrupt the spread of the lesion in the retina.

Patients will be instructed by the nurse that birth defects have been associated with CMV.

They should discuss with their physician the risk, if any, to pregnant women.

Herpes simplex frequently presents in the oropharyngeal mucosa, but can erupt anywhere on the body. Topical or systemic treatment with acyclovir (Zovirax) is usually effective in controlling the lesions. The nurse instructs the patients that the virus can be transmitted sexually.

Varicella zoster (shingles), while not one of the most common of the viruses plaguing these patients, can be one of the more painful. The initial symptom is usually pain, followed a few days later by a red, vesicular rash. Varicella zoster almost always erupts along expected dermatome patterns, but can present atypically. Smears of the vesicular fluid are analyzed to determine a differential diagnosis. Topical treatment with acyclovir is seldom helpful, but systemic treatment is often effective in shortening the course and alleviating pain. Varicella zoster can be associated with serious pain, and patients may require narcotics for relief. Topical applications of agents do not appear to alter the course of the disease, but may encourage drying of lesions and may be therapeutic and soothing. Rarely, a patient will experience long-term herpetic pain as a result of an infection with the varicella zoster virus. Such a patient is referred to a pain clinic for management. Therapy may include temporary or permanent nerve block.

ACCELERATED GRAFT ATHEROSCLEROSIS

Accelerated graft atherosclerosis (AGAS) was first seen in the animal laboratory (Kosek, et al., 1968, 1969). It is a malignant proliferation of the intima of the coronary arteries in transplanted hearts and may be the major limiting factor to long-term survival for recipients. A recent study reported that 37% of patients studied had angiographic evidence of coronary disease. Of these patients, disease was detected in 34.5% the first year, 59.2% the second year, and 91% five years after transplantation (Gao, et al., 1988).

Nerve supply to the heart is severed at the time of transplant, so these patients will not have the typical response of angina to cardiac ischemia. Without this early clinical symptom, evidence of the process may not become apparent until electrocardiographic changes occur or symptoms of heart failure secondary to a myocardial infarction are experienced. For these reasons, annual coronary arteriography is performed to document onset and/or progression of AGAS.

The nurse reinforces the importance of regular periodic arteriography to augment normal followup care. Denervation of the heart eliminates the possibility of angina as a presenting symptom. Electrocardiography may demonstrate changes consistent with myocardial infarction, conduction defects, or ST depression; if these are observed, coronary arteriography would be performed to rule out the onset or progression of disease.

The nurse also encourages the patient to be "heart healthy" by maintaining a regular exercise program, keeping weight within acceptable limits, reducing intake of saturated fats, and avoiding smoking.

When AGAS is observed, the study is repeated in 6 months to ascertain the rate of progression. If a patient demonstrates significant narrowing (greater than 70%) or occlusion of major vessels, elective re-transplantation is recommended. This process presents in a concentric and longitudinal pattern and is not conducive to coronary artery bypass grafting, as there is no patent vessel to receive a graft.

The etiology of this process is not well known, but is assumed to be an immune response to intimal injury associated with rejection. Because platelet aggregation is seen histologically, attempts at interrupting this process with antiplatelet agents (dipyridamole and aspirin) are utilized by many centers.

When AGAS is diagnosed, the nurse allows the patient and family an opportunity to discuss their concerns and anxieties in order to reassure them and to support them with their decision to proceed or not to proceed with elective re-transplantation.

MUSCULOSKELETAL CHANGES

Osteonecrosis

The association between avascular necrosis and corticosteroids was first reported over 30 years ago (Pietrogrande and Mastomarino, 1957). As survival following organ transplantation has increased over the past 25 years, avascular necrosis of joints, or osteonecrosis, has emerged as an increasingly important problem in long-term management of these patients. Some studies have put the average incidence at 16% (Ibels, et al., 1978). Weight-bearing joints are most often affected, with the femoral head the most prevalent. Some patients require bilateral hip replacement. Additional patients can have significant impairment of ankles, knees, and/or elbows.

Avascular necrosis can present as early as 2 months post transplant, with pain the presenting symptom (Bradford, et al., 1984). Early radiographic changes are not always apparent, but eventually verify the diagnosis. As the disease progresses, a subchondral arc in the femoral head or so-called moth-eaten lucencies in the femoral condyles, tali, and humoral head can be visualized (Pietrogrande and Mastomarino, 1957). The roentgenographic changes tend to be uniform in all patients.

Collaborative management of patients with avascular necrosis includes pain relief, anti-inflammatory agents, and the use of crutches or canes to reduce weight bearing. While some patients may respond, the majority will eventually require corrective surgery. Patients who have undergone bilateral hip replacement with insertion of a long-stem endo-prosthesis have experienced rapid return of function, relief of pain, and no serious complications.

The nurse reinforces the need for patients to be systematic in their use of prescribed non-aspirin-based pain relief and anti-inflammatory agents to enable them to be as functional as possible. Also encouraged is care with ambulation to reduce the risk of accidental injury to affected or nonaffected joints. The patient is encouraged to discuss fears and anxieties regarding any possible future surgical interventions.

Osteoporosis

A bigger management problem for an additional number of patients is osteoporosis. Again, corticosteroids appear to be the suspected cause. Glucocorticosteroids are well known to have a direct effect on bone. They can interfere with bone formation and may increase bone resorption (Jowsey, 1970). The onset of back pain can be gradual or sudden and often presents less than 6 months after transplantation. Early management includes analgesia, support (corset/brace), and weight loss where applicable. These are rarely more than temporary measures and often patients will require long periods of total bedrest. Supplemental calcium and calcium infusions have been ineffective in reducing the expected length of disability.

The nurse instructs the patient to lie flat or stand, and to avoid sitting when possible. Again reinforced is the patient's need to be systematic in the use of prescribed non-aspirin-based pain relief and anti-inflammatory agents. The patient is encouraged to assume responsibility for wearing any prescribed supportive device. The patients and their families are allowed the opportunity to discuss the diagnosis and its long- and short-term ramifications.

DERMATOLOGIC CHANGES

While rarely life-threatening, dermatologic changes and complications following organ transplantation can be very distressing and problematic for the patient. Most dermatologic conditions seen in these patients are easily treated with early detection and diagnosis. A recent report categorized the most common disorders into three groups: tumors, infections, and drug-related disorders (O'Connell, et al., 1986).

Tumors of the skin include basal cell and squamous cell carcinomas. Although usually treated easily with surgical removal, there is a low incidence of recurrence. At least two deaths in one group were a result of metastatic squamous cell carcinomas of dermatologic origin. Premalignant lesions, including actinic keratosis, parakeratosis, and keratoacanthoma, are usually also easily controlled and removed.

Not surprisingly, infectious skin complications are common in these patients. Viral lesions seen include verrucae (common warts), herpes simplex (cold sores), condyloma (venereal warts), varicella zoster (shingles), and molluscum contagiosum (firm, round, translucent crateriform papules). Treatment for these disorders is usually routine and effective. The nurse reinforces the importance of regular use of the oral and/or topical agents prescribed to treat these lesions. If the skin lesions are potentially contagious, the patient is instructed to implement isolation precautions to protect persons at risk, such as other compromised hosts, patients with malignancy, children, and pregnant women. Verrucae and molluscum contagiosum respond well to cryotherapy. Condylomata that are resistant to podophyllin therapy may respond to a combination of laser therapy and surgical removal. The viral disorders almost all respond to topical, oral, or intravenous acyclovir (O'Connell, et al., 1986).

Fungal infections, including tinea corporis (body ringworm) and tinea versicolor (multiple macular patches all shapes, sizes, white to brown), are not uncommon. More rarely, nail onychomycosis (dystrophic, discolored, friable) can be a result of *Candida albicans*. The use of topical, broad-spectrum antifungal agents usually controls these infections. Again, the nurse encourages regular use of prescribed antifungal agents and reassures the patient that the infection should be controlled or eliminated.

Many patients have skin complications as a result of immunosuppressive therapy. Dry, irritated, and itchy skin is very prevalent and is normally responsive to keratolytic and emollient therapy. Steroid-induced acne is not uncommon and can be of significant concern among younger patients. Rarely confined to the face, it affects the neck, shoulders, chest, back, and upper arms. Frequently, it is responsive to steroid reduction. It can show significant improvement with topical application of vitamin A gel preparations. Some patients have been treated with isotretinoin (Accutane) for severe steroid-induced acne with good results.

Patients, especially adolescents, need to be encouraged to maintain good skin hygiene: to wash with a pHisoHex-type soap twice a day; to dry the skin carefully; and to be vigilant in the use of prescribed topical and oral agents. If the patient is treated with Accutane, the physician will be monitoring triglyceride levels known to increase with the use of isotretinoin. The nurse arranges a dietary consultation or instructs the patient in a low-triglyceride diet. The need for adequate, reliable birth control to be used during the entire course of therapy, and for a minimum of one month after the drug is stopped, is reviewed with the female patient.

Hypertrichosis (increased hair growth) is seen in almost all patients treated with cyclosporine (O'Connell, et al., 1986). If patients wish, they may shave the extra hair growth or bleach it to reduce the effect. Depilatories are used with caution due to uncertain skin reactions. The nurse cautions the patient against hot wax treatments because of the increased risk of skin injury by burning.

Due to the prevalence and ease of treatment of skin disorders, all patients are encouraged by the nurse to report any changes in their skin early. Regular visits to a reliable dermatologist can not only result in appropriate treatment for the disorder, but can also enhance the patient's feeling of well-being, since so many of these changes can be emotionally distressing.

The incidence of neoplastic (nonmelanotic) disease in the transplant patient is 20 times that of the normal population (Urbach, 1983). Therefore, strict adherence to preventative measures, such as regular use of sun-blocking agents and protective clothing, are stressed in patient teaching plans.

PEDIATRIC CONCERNS

Two situations specific to the younger transplant population are decreased growth rate and changes in facial appearance (Fine, et al., 1977; Reznik, et al., 1987). Since prednisone appears to be the agent responsible for decreased growth (Fine, et al., 1977), many centers with pediatric transplant patients are reserving steroids for treatment of rejection only or placing their patients on steroids every other day in an attempt to improve growth potential.

Changes in facial appearance have been seen in children treated with cyclosporine following transplantation (Reznik, et al., 1987). They report coarsening of features, with thickened nares, lips, and ears, puffiness of cheeks, prominence of supraorbital ridges, and mandibular prognathism (marked protrusion of the jaw).

The implications for nursing care concerning these changes, coupled with expected cushingoid changes common to patients on prednisone, are significant. The major cause of graft failure among young renal transplant patients is immunosuppressant noncompliance. Helping these patients, especially adolescents for whom any changes in their appearance can have significant emotional impact, is of the utmost importance.

COMPLIANCE

Many inherent factors assist in promoting compliance. These include bending to the pressure of one's own desire to survive, the need to reassure family members of improved/continued good health, and maintaining a mutually respectful relationship with one's physician and transplant nurse. These are usually all that is required to guarantee compliance with healthcare management.

Occasionally, however, patients are noncompliant. When this occurs with adults, it is usually the result of misunderstanding or misinterpretation of instructions. Noncompliance may even be the result of a psychosis. The disturbed patient clearly needs professional psychiatric intervention, and the confused or misinformed patient needs the healthcare team to be clear, concise, and noncontradictory in messages given. The nurse uses written instructions when possible, repeats verbal instructions when appropriate, and does not overwhelm the patient with too much information at one time. This goes a long way toward preventing misunderstanding or misinterpretation.

But for the truly noncompliant patient, this is not enough. The pressure to yield to or comply with negative factors is too great for them and they disrupt their healthcare regimens. This problem is most frequent in the adolescent population. So often, attention is concentrated on their physical recovery, letting their emotional adjustment suffer. As mentioned earlier, the cosmetic changes associated with long-term steroid and cyclosporine therapy are significant. For the adolescent in whom the "need to be normal" or "one of the crowd" is so important, the emotional magnitude of these changes cannot be underestimated. Their emotional stability is tenuous and can be further affected by factors that their adult support person may not recognize as important. Constant, but unobtrusive, monitoring of their feelings by the primary nurse is important if noncompliance is to be predicted and hopefully prevented.

There is not always a clear reason for noncompliance. Distress over appearance, power struggles with adults, boredom with routine, newfound religious beliefs that God will save them, or simply curiosity about their chances of beating the system can be enough to motivate adolescents to discontinue taking their medications.

Noncompliance with diet can result from frustration, anger, and a feeling of loss of control. Eating can provide short-term satisfaction, yet obesity only serves to increase feelings of isolation and being different.

Aggressive attention to modify troublesome side effects can be very effective in helping the adolescent cope with their transplant. Early dietary management and weight control can have long-term benefits. The nurse offers the patient choices between the dietician's menu planning and a more visible approach, such as a group weight-loss program, giving adolescents more control over the direction their lives are taking.

Regular dermatologic intervention to deal with superficial blemishes, encouragement to seek new hair styles, and a trip to the makeup counter at a large department store for ideas on how to conceal real or perceived faults can help these patients to deal with their stresses. Again, the nurse can suggest ways to provide them with a sense of control.

When there are multiple members of the transplant followup team, patients will often identify one of them as someone they feel comfortable talking with and to whom they would be more likely to verbalize anxieties and worries. Giving adolescents time and opportunity may increase their ability to share these concerns. But any member of the transplant team who notices unexplained weight loss, lessening of cushingoid features, or dissipation of previously existing drug-related conditions will recognize signs of noncompliance and investigate the possibility.

Noncompliance can result in a reduction of graft organ function or progress to a more serious loss of the organ graft. Clearly, this can be fatal in many transplant recipients.

The following case history is that of a 17-year-old male, 2 years following his cardiac transplant:

> On a routine surveillance biopsy, rejection was noted and treated according to protocol with an increase in oral steroids. Followup biopsy 14 days later showed resolution of the process. Two months later another routine surveillance biopsy again showed rejection and once again oral steroids were increased. During this two-month time period, 12-hour trough cyclosporine levels had been falling, so the daily dose of cyclosporine had been increased. Rebiopsy 14 days later showed continued rejection and a 3-day course of intravenous Solu-Medrol was given. While hospitalized for the Solu-Medrol, he admitted that he had not taken all doses of prednisone and cyclosporine the past few months because he was "mad at his dad." Because he did not report the cyclosporine noncompliance, the interim increase in the dose of the drug significantly impaired his renal function. A few weeks after his rejection cleared, he was readmitted with acute renal failure. This required placement of a Scribner shunt and dialysis. Biventricular congestive heart failure, ascites, and moderate pedal edema were also present. A cardiac catheterization revealed a restrictive cardiomyopathy with normal coronary arteries. The left ventricle displayed greatly decreased contractility with a cardiac output of 2.1 liters per minute and a cardiac index of 1.2. Endomyocardial biopsy showed no evidence of rejection, making the prospects for improvement with medical management limited. The situation was discussed with him and his parents and he agreed to proceed with elective retransplantation when and if a donor became available.

When the reality of noncompliance became apparent, his medical team arranged for him and his parents to meet with counselors in an effort to identify areas of disagreement and mechanisms to use in order to avoid such disagreements in the future.

Noncompliance in younger children is rarely a medical problem since parents maintain control over the child's medical regimen, assuring safety. However, their cooperation can be altered by changes in routine that adults may not notice or may take for granted. The following excerpt is from a letter written by the mother of a 3-year-old shortly following their return home:

. . . anyway, Amy's behavior needs to be worked on. It was so horrendous the first few days back, I felt like "Mommie Dearest." The first week home it was really a struggle to get her to take her meds. We had that problem with her when she was discharged from ICU too.

Unlike the older children in whom noncompliance can often be triggered by power struggles with adults, the sudden disruption of routine, transfer from hospital to home, or from one home to another was stressful enough to this 3-year-old that she rebelled by refusing to take her medications, testing her parents to see just how much of her life was changing.

EXERCISE/DIET

Following transplantation, much emphasis is placed on obtaining and maintaining an ideal body weight and developing regular exercise patterns. Dietary counseling is instituted while the patient is still in the hospital and continued throughout the patient's lifetime. Many of the drugs included in the management of patients will alter their response to calories, fluid balance, and lipids. While their post-transplant diet may be more liberal than pre-transplant, there still remain significant guidelines to follow.

Maintaining ideal body weight. Once patients have achieved their desirable body weight, it should be maintained. Excess weight can increase blood cholesterol and triglyceride and glucose levels. All of these factors increase the risk of arteriosclerosis, high blood pressure, and coronary artery disease. Long-term use of prednisone can also elevate triglyceride levels.

The nurse assists the patient in maintaining a weight graph to visualize sudden changes or subtle patterns of weight gain, and is available to help the patient identify and correct the problem.

Limiting sugar and concentrated sweets. High blood sugar levels can indirectly increase triglyceride levels. Patients are instructed by the nurse and dietician to keep the total amount of carbohydrates in their diet within a moderate range.

Modifying fat intake. High cholesterol levels are related to coronary artery disease. These patients may be at increased risk and are encouraged to restrict cholesterol intake, decrease total saturated fats, and substitute polyunsaturated fats. The nurse teaches the patient that these goals can be more easily achieved by limiting their intake of egg yolks and high-fat dairy food and meats, and by selecting in their place nonfat milk, poultry, fish, and lean cuts of red meat.

Restricting sodium intake. Although sodium levels vary, patients are instructed to follow a no-added-salt diet. While patients frequently take diuretics to control fluid balance, the diuretics are less effective if the body is taxed with excessive sodium.

Dietary principles are presented to patients as guidelines rather than as a specific dietary prescription. The goal of patient teaching is to assist the patient in selecting foods that promote sound nutritional health without aggravating the metabolic consequences of immunosuppressive therapy. The nurse includes the primary food preparer, if other than the patient, in all dietary teaching sessions (Stanford University Hospital, 1986).

Exercise is a major component of any wellness plan. As patients maintain their nutritional balance, the nurse will encourage enrollment in a complementary exercise program to maximize their potential for full rehabilitation. Prednisone (a catabolic steroid) is well known for its muscle wasting effects. Regular exercise is the only effective way to combat the loss of muscle mass and tone.

Programs and levels of exercise will change postoperatively as a reflection of continued recovery and strength. Some basics, however, are included in every program. Patients are taught to warm up with limbering and stretching activities. Following this is the time of peak activity, such as cycling, rapid walking, or swimming. Jogging is a less desirable form of peak activity due to the jarring effect on joints and bones. This is followed by a cool-down period with repetition of the stretching exercises.

Transplant patients (with hearts the exception) should be aware of their optimal target heart rates and check their rate frequently during exercise. Heart transplant patients will not have the normal rate responses to exercise and cool-down due to denervation of the graft and must rely on therapist guidelines (i.e., muscle fatigue and shortness of breath) to determine maximal exercise tolerance.

RENAL DYSFUNCTION/HYPERTENSION

Cyclosporine was introduced to the field of organ transplantation in the mid-1970s. It was one of the first drugs to qualify as an immunopharmacologic agent. These are compounds or methods that modulate specifically defined subpopulations of immunocompetent cells. Cyclosporine was quickly incorporated into the drug regimen of most organ transplant centers.

Gradually, the evidence began to grow, implicating cyclosporine in the induction of chronic renal injury. Most of the early experience was obtained from recipients of renal transplants, and the effects of the drug were difficult to distinguish from graft rejection in such patients. As the numbers of cardiac recipients receiving cyclosporine increased, there was an opportunity to study its effect on patients with previously normal renal function. The results of these studies clarified the effects of cyclosporine on the kidney, resulting in depressed glomerular filtration rates (GFRs) and reduced renal plasma flow. Examination of tissue obtained at renal biopsy showed "a variable degree of tubulointerstitial injury accompanied by focal glomerular sclerosis" (Myers, et al., 1984).

As the magnitude of the problem was recognized, centers began modifying protocols to ameliorate the deleterious effects of cyclosporine while maintaining adequate immunosuppression. Slowly, the dosages of cyclosporine were reduced while renal function and graft viability were closely monitored. Many centers currently obtain trough blood levels of the drug and use this information to adjust the dosage to a range thought to be consistent with maximum graft protection and minimum renal toxicity. The nurse emphasizes to the patient the importance of accurate timing for the drawing of blood.

It is therefore important for the nurse and physician to collaboratively evaluate the patient's renal status at regular intervals. Serum blood urea nitrogen (BUN) and creatinine levels can be monitored easily during routine blood sampling, but cannot be relied upon to adequately reflect the presence or absence of renal damage. Regular urine creatinine clearances are followed to track subtle changes in renal filtration rates, which are reflected by a gradual fall in creatinine clearance. The nurse teaches the patient how to collect an accurate 24-hour urine sample.

Should renal function deteriorate, suboptimal doses of cyclosporine may be necessary. If the patient's renal function continues to deteriorate, a decision to discontinue the drug would need to be evaluated.

Severe arterial hypertension, which is seen in 64% of patients within the first postoperative year (Myers, et al., 1984), is another important side effect associated with the use of cyclosporine. It is assumed to be associated with the same long-term sequelae as other forms of hypertension, and every effort is made for control. It is a very difficult form of hypertension to manage. Its mechanism of arterial hypertension is not well known, and no particular drug or class of drugs has been found to be especially effective. As with all hypertensive patients, transplant recipients must learn to monitor their blood pressure at home and be given parameters to follow. The nurse teaches the importance of correctly measuring blood pressure and of following recommended parameters carefully; identifies the symptoms of hypotension to be aware of; and stresses the vital importance of never discontinuing antihypertensive medications without medical supervision.

SUMMARY

There are a myriad of conditions and complications that can affect the morbidity and mortality of immunocompromised hosts. Steroid use can lead to transient or long-term glucose intolerance, visual disturbances, increased incidence of malignancy, and mood swings.

Cyclosporine is a powerful drug with a growing list of side effects and complications. The recognized number of drugs that affect the metabolism or potentiate the nephrotoxic effects of cyclosporine is growing also. Those currently identified are summarized in Table 10–2.

The addition or removal of any drug from a transplant patient's regimen should not be done lightly. The possible effect such a decision could have on the action of other drugs the patient is taking can be significant. Additionally, any change in wellness or well-being on the part of the patient is thoroughly and aggressively investigated, in order to rule out any pathology.

The role of the nurse is pivotal to the successful management of these patients. Often the first to learn of the symptoms of a presenting complication, the nurse will be relied upon by the medical staff to arrange consultations, schedule diagnostic procedures, obtain test results, and maintain communication between patient and doctor. With every change in treatment, the patient and physician will rely on the nurse to follow through on instructions, to verify comprehension, to be available to answer questions, and to offer encouragement and support.

Teaching is not static, but ongoing. For the patient, each new development is potentially stressful and the nurse must always be certain to first cover the basic information, and then incorporate any idiosyncrasy specific to organ transplantation.

The nurse serves a critical role in maintaining a successful transplant program.

Bibliography

Bradford, DS, et al: Osteonecrosis in the transplant recipient. Surg Gynecol Obstet 159:328–334, 1984.

Fine, RN, et al: Cadaver renal transplantation in children. Transplant Proc 9:133, 1977.

Fisher, DW and Bickel, WH: Corticosteroid-induced avascular necrosis. J Bone Joint Surg 53A:859–873, 1971.

Gao, SZ, et al: Accelerated coronary vascular disease in the heart transplant patient. J Am Coll Cardiol (August, 1988):334–340.

Ibels, LS, et al: Aseptic necrosis of bone following renal transplantation experience in 194 transplant recipients and review of the literature. Medicine 57:25–45, 1978.

Jowsey, J and Riggs, BL: Bone formation in hypercortisolins. Acta Endocrinol 63:21–28, 1970.

Kosek, JC, Hurley, EJ, and Lower, RR: Histopathology of orthotopic canine cardiac homografts. Lab Invest 19:97, 1968.

Kosek, JC, et al: Histopathology of orthotopic canine cardiac allografts and its clinical correlation. Transplant Proc 1:311, 1969.

Myers, BD, et al: Cyclosporine associated chronic nephropathy. N Engl J Med 311(11):699–705, 1984.

O'Connell, BM, et al: Dermatologic complications following heart transplantation. The Journal of Heart Transplantation 5:430–436, 1986.

Pietrogrande, V, and Mastomarino, R: Osteopatia da prolongato trattamento cortisonico. Ortop Traumatol 25:791–810, 1957.

Reznik, VM, et al: Changes in facial appearance during cyclosporine treatment. Lancet 20, (June, 1987)8547:1405–1406.

Stanford University Hospital: A Manual for Transplant Patients, pp 17–19, Stanford University, Stanford, CA, 1986.

Stinson, EB, et al: Infectious complications after cardiac transplantation in man. Ann Intern Med 74:22, 1971.

Urbach, F: Ultraviolet radiation carcinogenesis. J Dermatol Surg Oncol 9:597–599, 1983.

Patient Education: A Recipient Perspective

Tina Haberer-Weiss

PATIENT INVOLVEMENT

Transplantation comes with a lesson about life — about what is important in life. If they are willing to try, transplant recipients can learn a wonderful lesson. Their involvement can make the crucial difference between the success or failure of transplantation. The recipient's perception of the situation dictates whether or not he or she *will* try: to get out of that bed; to be a part of the transplant team; to take responsibility for recuperation. It is only when the recipient *does* try that he or she begins to realize the opportunities offered by transplantation.

The importance of involving patients in their own health care cannot be overemphasized. Patient involvement has a multifaceted effect on the success of any healthcare program, from weight loss to post-transplant maintenance care. The better patients understand the therapy and their personal responsibilities within that therapy, the better the therapy will work.

Transplantation may be considered a temporary solution to a permanent problem. Although it comes with its share of discomforts and challenges, it is well worth these obstacles. The potential transplant recipient is living a life of change — change so dramatic that it is seemingly beyond his or her control. It is vital that patients understand that they *can* control

241

their response to this change. The bottom line is that transplantation affords the recipient a quality of life that no other therapy has come close to matching. Granted, roles may have to change at home: breadwinner may become domestic engineer; mother may become child; child may have to contribute to family support. But this is all part of the change, and it is not necessarily bad. It is up to the recipient and the family to perceive this change positively, and to go on with life.

Nurses, as healthcare providers, infuse the patient with the energy to cope with the disease, and with the side effects of immunosuppressive therapy. This energy is delivered at every visit, often in subtle ways: a reassuring touch, a subtle acknowledgment of the patient's situation — each conveys the firm belief that the situation will ultimately improve. Healthcare providers must provide the role models that patients are looking for to help them see the way out of their tunnel.

PATIENT EDUCATION AND NONCOMPLIANCE

Transplant recipients make daily decisions that will ultimately affect the success of their therapy. These decisions are vast in scope, encompassing everything from choosing a diet and exercise regimen to recognizing and reporting signs and symptoms of rejection.

The most widely documented aspect of patient responsibility is the willingness to comply with medication regimens and clinic visits. Several studies have identified the patient as a major factor in any therapeutic regimen. The Merck Manual (1987) begins the section on Patient Compliance with the following statement:

> Even the most thorough and well-designed therapeutic regimen will fail without patient compliance. Depending on the variable studied and the strictness of definition, from 15% to 95% of patients studied have been found to be noncompliant. Overall, probably a third to a half of patients make some error with their medications — incorrect dose, errors in timing, adding unprescribed medications, or not taking medication.

Didlake and his associates at the University of Texas Transplant Division recently published a retrospective study of 500 renal transplant recipients over a five-year period (Didlake, et al., 1987). The study illustrates the effect that noncompliance with immunosuppressive therapy has on the success of transplantation. Overall, noncompliance was the third leading cause of graft loss, following rejection and infection.

The timing of noncompliance observed in this study presents an interesting implication for patient education. After 6 months of transplantation, noncompliance was equal to infection and rejection as a cause of graft loss. After the 36th month, noncompliance was responsible for all graft losses. For nurses and their transplant recipient patients, this means that patient education must be an ongoing process. The further along a transplant recipient is with post-transplant maintenance, the more likely he or she is to discontinue immunosuppression.

Didlake (1987) concluded that noncompliance was a major cause of *late* graft loss in cyclosporine-treated renal transplants. Demographic factors such as age, race, and level of education were *not* predictive of noncompliance. In addition, drug cost, taste, and side effects were not found to be statistically significant reasons for noncompliance.

Why *do* noncompliant patients stop taking their medication? In Didlake's study (1987), the patients had been out of the hospital for at least 6 months. One would assume that they must have been feeling good. All they had to do was spend 5 minutes out of the day to increase their odds of keeping the transplanted organ. Why didn't they?

A Personal Perspective

My personal experience with medication noncompliance involved antihypertensives. Twelve years ago I was placed on antihypertensives. I was given no reason, just a command . . . "Take your pills!" I went home and took my pills. But very quickly I grew tired of taking them. I decided "if I can't live naturally, without the aid of drugs, I do not want to live at all." When you are a young adolescent, that is a very rational thought. What is life anyway? I was willing to throw mine away. I flushed the pills down the toilet. I lied when asked if I had taken my pills.

Soon, however, it all caught up with me: intense headache, disorientation, and nausea. At the next clinic visit, my blood pressure was soaring. My doctor handed me a blood pressure cuff and told me to put it on. He *taught* me how to take my blood pressure. Then he *explained* why I should be taking those pills. It then became *my* responsibility to take my own blood pressure and my pills every day. No one was going to remind me. It was my job. I responded very well to this approach. I continued to take the medication.

Just as there were many reasons for the noncompliance described above, there are numerous reasons why any patient decides to discontinue medication. However, once the healthcare provider explains the rationale and gives the patient the responsibility for maintaining the regimen, there is often a positive response. Although there may appear to be little or no excuse for noncompliance, patients may have what they consider to be quite valid reasons, but because they may not be able to effectively communicate their reasons, the nurse may have difficulty understanding at first. Once the nurse has elicited and understands the reason, however, this knowledge can well become the key to assuring patient compliance with drug regimens.

It is also important to note that sometimes patients commit what could be termed intelligent noncompliance (Merck Manual, 1987). This refers to the circumstance in which the patient discontinues or decreases the dose of medication based on a correct interpretation of the clinical situation. While this may decrease adverse effects and improve therapeutic outcome, the healthcare provider is often not told of the manipulation. It is, therefore, important for the nurse to encourage an open and honest communication process with the patient.

THE ASSESSMENT

Transplant patient education begins the moment the patient is considered as a viable candidate for transplantation. The nurse initiates an assessment of the patient's ability to learn. Is there an impairment of vision, hearing, or learning ability? Can he or she read (Smith, et al., 1987)? These findings will dictate in what form informational materials should be supplied to a particular patient. For the visually impaired, an audio tape version of a lecture may be preferred. For the illiterate, there are scores of video programs available that will communicate at least the foundation of knowledge necessary for the patient to begin to ask questions and understand the available options. "Good communication involves using language appropriate for the audience, conscious awareness of nonverbal cues the patient gives, and careful listening to the questions asked, issues raised, or concerns expressed" (Smith, et al., 1987).

A Personal Perspective

I remember when I was first told that I had kidney failure, over a decade ago. The conversation went something like this: "You have had RENAL FAILURE due to GLOMERULAR NEPHRITIS; in a few days you will begin DIALYSIS, and later we will consider TRANSPLANTATION; do you have any questions?" At the time, I was sedated, my head was spinning with all these new words, and I had no idea what any of them meant. I didn't have any questions. All I had was fear and resentment. This is not patient education.

Patients must be spoken to in language that they can understand and act upon. Current literature reveals many alternative techniques that may be useful for effectively communicating with the transplant recipient; however, the fact remains that every patient is different, with an individual scope of ability and willingness to learn. It is the challenge of the healthcare provider to establish what, when, and how each patient will learn. While this challenge may seem insurmountable at times, assessing the patient's educational needs and abilities is a crucial step in the patient education process. Only with successful patient education can the healthcare provider assure patient involvement, which has a lasting effect on the success of transplantation.

THE WAITING PERIOD

Patients are made a part of the transplant team from the moment transplantation is considered as an option. At this time, potential recipients are given the challenge of proving to the transplant team that they will take part in their own recuperation. It may be helpful to give the potential recipient an active role in preparing for transplantation. This approach can be useful because when patients receive successful transplants, they have made a personal investment, and may then view the post-transplant regimen as a way of protecting that investment.

For the renal disease population, this approach is fairly easy to accomplish. During each dialysis treatment, responsibilities can be assigned. The nurse may begin by having the patient read a booklet on transplantation, and then subtly testing the patient for comprehension and effort. Or the potential recipient may be guided to understand and repeat to the nurse that medications and clinic visits are a long-term commitment, one that must be followed faithfully in order to maintain the transplant.

As the beginning of a very long relationship between the nurse and the transplant recipient, this is an ideal time to initiate habits that will enhance that relationship. It is important to remind patients that transplantation is only a temporary solution to a permanent problem, but that their active participation in the maintenance of the transplant can help to make that solution more permanent.

Frierson and his associates at the University of Louisville recommend strongly that the waiting period be used as an evaluation period for transplant candidacy. By doing so, they believed they were able to identify patients who were poor risks for long-term cardiac transplant success (Frierson, et al., 1987). The study examines criteria for proper patient selection. The criteria outlined included: compliance, history of alcohol or drug abuse, and personality disorders such as depression, paranoia, and antisocial behavior. The authors found that noncompliance was the major reason that patients were not considered for transplantation. Among other conclusions, they emphasize the appropriateness of using the waiting period to assess the suitability of the potential graft recipient in their statement, "As the number of heart transplants in this country increases, the competition for donor organs will intensify. Proper patient selection will be essential."

The importance of their own attitudes and behavior should be communicated to patients. The transplant team offers them the challenge of proving their compliance as potential transplant recipients, but it first provides them with the tools. The healthcare provider tells patients, in simple language that can be acted upon immediately, how they can best prepare for transplantation. Often, nurses feel that their patient education program is not effective enough, because it does not have all of the so-called bells and whistles that a similar program at another institution may include. The bells and whistles, however, are not what is important. An educational program may be ineffective simply because enough quality time has not been spent establishing a relationship with each patient, a relationship critical to effective two-way communication.

The most important factor in any patient education program is this relationship, which must be mutually open, honest, and respectful. The recipient must be willing to share needs, problems, and misunderstandings with the healthcare provider. Likewise, the healthcare provider must listen carefully for subtle hints that the recipient may be expressing (Smith, et al., 1987). For some patients, compliance may become much easier if they can shift the reason for adherence to a medication regimen away from doing it for their own well-being to reasons beyond themselves. For example, there was a television public service message developed by the American Heart Association that said, "If you can't take your medication for yourself, then take it for the ones you love." This concept could be expanded in urging the patient to take the immunosuppressive medication.

THE RELATIONSHIP BETWEEN HEALTHCARE PROVIDER AND PATIENT

In the late 1950s, Szasz identified three basic models of the physician-patient relationship (Szasz, et al., 1956). The models are correlated with different levels of illness, and the environmental settings that surround them. The first model is appropriate for the acute trauma patient. Such a patient is unable to respond, and therefore the healthcare provider makes all decisions and administers to the patient. This model is compared with the parent/infant prototype, and is labeled: Activity-Passivity.

The second model occurs in the acute infectious situation in which the patient is conscious and experiencing some sort of discomfort. The patient is dependent upon the healthcare provider for help. The healthcare provider tells the patient what to do, and the patient responds as instructed. The prototype model is the parent/adolescent relationship, and this model is labeled: Guidance-Cooperation.

Dorothea Orem (1985) identified similar phases of the nurse-patient interaction. The wholly compensatory nursing system, like the activity-passivity model, is for patients who are unable to care for themselves. The partially-compensatory system describes the interaction for those patients and families who need assistance, but can meet some of the patient's needs.

For the chronically ill patient, the relationship becomes two-way. The patient needs the healthcare provider, and the healthcare provider needs the patient's participation. This relationship is far more complex than those involved in the previous two models because it requires full participation on the part of both parties. A balance must be achieved that allows for the unique individuality of the both the observer and the observed. Both have approximately equal power, and their activity must be in some way satisfying to both. The prototype relationship for this model is the adult/adult interaction, and it is labeled: Mutual-Participation. This model is favored by patients who want to take care of themselves. It is not appropriate for the mentally deficient, very poorly educated, or profoundly immature.

Orem's Supportive-Educative System describes the nurse-patient/family relationship in similar terms to that of the mutual-participation model. Teaching, guiding, supporting, and providing a positive developmental environment are nursing role functions (Orem, 1985).

Once mutual-participation is achieved, everyone becomes a winner. Patients get what they need from the therapy and healthcare providers maintain a sense of accomplishment. To achieve mutual participation, it is necessary to understand the patient's environment: the setting in which he or she will be coping with the disease. The nurse assesses the obstacles that the patient will be facing. Help is given to assist the patient in diagnosing ways to overcome the obstacles. The more the patient participates in the early phases, the better prepared he or she will be for lifetime management of the disease.

Another approach that is particularly appealing for establishing a relationship of mutual-participation is called a contingency contract. Cameron and associates (1987) published their findings on this approach with chronically ill patients. The idea is to begin by determining where, in level of importance, patients place their medical regimen. From the healthcare provider's perspective, the medical regimen is obviously number one; however, to the patient, the regimen may be very low on the priority list.

The patient is treated as an equal. The nurse stresses that the patient's concerns are a vital part of the therapy. Assessing what the patient does during the day, the nurse evaluates the patient's life-style, including daily activities, diet, sleep, and exercise.

In return, patients share with the nurse what they want to do, and when. This allows the patient's unique individuality to be expressed. The healthcare regimen is adapted to fit the patient's life-style patterns, and often linked to a specific activity such as taking medication right after toothbrushing.

The next step is to set goals mutually agreed upon by the patient and the healthcare provider. In some cases, the patient chooses to work toward a tangible reward. The reward does not have to be exotic. Often, for example, all that is desired is some extra time with the healthcare provider in the hospital cafeteria. When the approach is shifted from "You *must* do this" to "*What* will you do?" the patient becomes a decision-maker. The healthcare provider is aware of the obstacles that successful therapy and the patient face, and can make suggestions to alter inappropriate behavior before it becomes a problem.

This type of interaction provides insight into the patient's motives, needs, and priorities so that an appropriate healthcare regimen can be worked out. Contingency contracting also informs the healthcare provider about the patient's understanding of the disease process. This will help to identify the need for more patient teaching information if necessary. Contingency contracting can be something that is implemented when the patient is immediately post transplant. Speeding up the process of discharge from the hospital is a wonderful incentive to motivate recipients. The sooner patients learn the names of their medications and the correct doses, the sooner they get to go home. Patients should be able to explain to the nurse why they are taking those medicines and why they have to return for clinic visits. Responsibility is usually given to the patient to arrange the first clinic visit, including assuring transportation arrangements and directions to the clinic.

THE FIRST STEPS OUT

Once the recipient does go home and is presumably taking the prescribed medication, a new obstacle — medication side effects — rears its head. The long-term use of corticosteroids, for example, presents a plethora of complications (Rimza, 1978). The complications are ophthalmologic, hematologic, gastrointestinal, metabolic, and cosmetic. Although each of these complications presents an unwanted challenge to the recipient, the cosmetic side effects of corticosteroids, especially for adolescent girls, can be devastating and have been implicated as contributing to noncompliance with immunosuppressive therapy (Korsch, et al., 1978). This is a sensitive subject to cover.

A Personal Perspective
I will never forget looking in the mirror and seeing myself as a stranger with a very fat face. I immediately resented the transplant, and accused the transplant team of not saving my life, but creating a monster! I was sure that I would never get a date to the prom. My reaction was anger and depression. I did not think of discontinuing my medication; however, many adolescent girls do consider it, and this cannot be ignored.

Korsch and associates (1978) at The Children's Hospital of Los Angeles evaluated 14 cases of noncompliant adolescents. In 12 of the cases, the patients were female. The cosmetic side effect of steroid therapy was a common reason given for interruption of therapy. "Several of the girls told us that their appearance was so repugnant to them and caused such problems in their social relationships that 'it was not worth it.'" Korsch and associates (1978) concluded in their study of noncompliance in children with renal transplants that "the experiences related to the treatment of end-stage renal disease are particularly stressful to the adolescent patients, especially adolescent girls, and that it is the combination of vulnerable personality and renal failure occurring during the critical period of adolescence that leads to severe maladaptation and noncompliance."

A Personal Perspective

The thing that I found very irritating was the hesitancy of people to acknowledge that I had changed physically. This included healthcare providers, family members, and friends. In retrospect, I understand and appreciate what they tried to do, but at the time I needed for someone to say it: "Wow, you look terrible." I also needed some tips on how to improve what I had. As for me, I used the time to work on my personality. I realized that if someone did not want to be my friend because of appearance, then he or she was never going to be a true friend anyway.

Given adequate encouragement, recipients can cope with side effects. There are post-transplant diets that help to decrease steroid side effects. There are cosmetologists who are ready and willing to counsel recipients back to a more pleasing appearance. Sharing these options with recipients will help to bring self-confidence back into their lives. It will let them enjoy their transplant a little more.

It is also important at this time to remind recipients that life is precious, and that there is no gain from being upset by what other people may think of one's appearance. Those other people have no idea what recipients have gone through in an effort to lead a so-called normal life. Perhaps this is one of the important lessons that recipients learn by going through transplantation.

This is a difficult time for recipients. New priorities are being set in their lives, new roles are being forced upon them, and healthcare regimens are now a vital part of their existence. The combination of these factors may affect patients' willingness to comply.

For the cardiac recipient population, these factors are especially significant. Unlike the renal population, cardiac recipients have no alternative therapy such as dialysis to rely on, and thus are forced to comply stringently with a specific medical regimen in order to stay alive. Rogers (1987), at The Tampa General Hospital, evaluated the nature of spousal support that influenced cardiac recipient compliance. In this study, it was concluded that the support given by the spouse was informational in nature. The spouse plays a significant role at home by reminding the recipient about specific medical regimens. Thus, Rogers recommends that the spouse be included in all teaching sessions regarding medical regimens, and further recommends that "it may be helpful for the coordinators to evaluate patients and spouses together and separately to determine what types of spousal behaviors are used preoperatively to promote patient compliance post-transplant" (Rogers, 1987). This research identifies a useful avenue that should be assessed and evaluated by the health-care provider.

THE PATIENT'S PERSPECTIVE

Transplant recipients receive a lot of new information. At first, all of it may seem to be of equal importance, and it can be difficult to set learning priorities. In addition, timing of patient education is difficult due to the unpredictability of donor organ availability.

A study by Berron (1986) at the Methodist Hospital of Indiana evaluated the transplant patient's perceptions about effective preoperative teaching. The purpose of this study was to identify what information cardiac recipients found to be most helpful as they started taking charge of their own recovery post transplant. Careful consideration was given to actual patient needs in order to incorporate them into future preoperative teaching plans. A two-part questionnaire was developed to assess perceived helpfulness. The first part of the questionnaire allowed recipients to rank (on a five-point Likert scale) information that they had received. The highest ranked categories included information relating to immuno-suppression, rejection, biopsy, and infection. The investigator goes further to conclude that it appears that patients perceive information about long-term survival to be more helpful than information about the actual surgical procedure and immediate post-transplant recovery.

The second part of the study identified an area that recipients felt should be added to preoperative teaching — they repeatedly mentioned the area of belief. Recipient comments (Berron, 1986) included:

- Develop and maintain utmost confidence in medical professionals on whom we depend.
- Be optimistic.
- Attitude is of number one importance.
- Mind over matter is a big healer.

A Personal Perspective

I couldn't agree with these recipients more. I learned first hand the effect that my attitude had over transplantation. Just a few days post transplant, I was recuperating rather smoothly; at least I felt good. A laboratory technician came by to record my daily test results. Being the inquisitive recipient that I was, I asked how the results were. The response: "You are in rejection!" And zip, she was gone. With her went all of my confidence. I understood rejection to be the end of the transplant. Why hadn't it worked for me? What did I do to deserve this? I shut the curtains in my room. I cried. I got in bed and stayed there. I withdrew from the staff. This went on for about 4 days. My test results were declining more quickly each day.

The thing I found very odd was that no one else would tell me that I was rejecting. Finally one of the nephrology residents got tired of my "bad attitude." He forced me to tell him my problem. When I told him that I had rejected, his response was total relief. He informed me that mild rejection was normal, and that I was still safe. I was going to keep this kidney!

What a difference that made. I got out of bed. I opened the curtains. I believed that I would beat this "mild" rejection. Within days, the test results improved. It has been 11 years since the transplant and I'm still going strong.

THE POSITIVE APPROACH

While it is vitally important to supply recipients with technical and instructional data, it is equally important to provide spiritual support. The mind and the body are related through reaction; what the mind believes, the body acts out.

> The Will to Live
> Is not a theoretical abstraction
> but a physiologic reality
> with therapeutic characteristics.
> — Norman Cousins

In his book *Anatomy of an Illness*, Cousins (1979) demonstrates what the mind can do to overcome illness. Cousins was diagnosed with a chronically debilitating disease. Instead of despairing, he decided to fight back. He took a holistic approach to his recuperation. This does not mean that he discontinued traditional medical intervention. Rather, he enhanced his therapy. The idea is to treat the whole patient instead of the disease — to include the *whole* environment in the treatment. Starting with an improvement in attitude and progressing onward, he used his will to live. He tapped into the power of optimism, and of positive thinking. Cousins used humor to overcome his disease. He prescribed for himself at least 4 hours of real laughter each day. He watched funny films, read funny books, and listened to jokes. Essentially, he induced his own mood change and reinforced his immune system's ability to fight his disease. This finding was published over a decade ago (Cousins, 1979).

Subsequent research has suggested that laughter elicits discernible physiological effects as well as subtle effects that are difficult to verify (Friedman, 1988). Cousins (1979) believes that patients must take responsibility for, and actively participate in, their recuperation. When the power of the mind is behind the therapy instead of fighting against it, recuperation is much more likely. *Anatomy of an Illness* delivered this message; it is up to the nurse to deliver the message to the patient.

Siegel, in his book *Love, Medicine and Miracles* (1986), reports case after case of the effect such a message can have on the patient. He found that if told a cancer patient that he had 3 months to live, he lived for 3 months to the day. Doubting that his powers of diagnosis could be that precise, he stopped telling patients how long they would live, and his patients started living longer! He found that patients could control the therapy and the disease by either wanting to live — or not wanting to live. Siegel subscribes strongly to Cousins's will-to-live premise. This approach allows patients to believe in their own strength. It gives the patient the license to try, along with a sense of power over his or her own destiny.

Siegel further found that patients were able to control the side effects of medication. His patients were on high doses of chemotherapy, during which hair loss and nausea can become a way of life. Through creative visualization and meditation, these patients were able to minimize unwanted side effects (Siegel, 1986).

Siegel's work relates to a basic experiment taught in introductory psychology: a patient is given a placebo and told he will have absolutely terrible side effects — and he responds accordingly. Siegel and his patients are using the same theory, but in reverse: real medicine, minimal side effects (Siegel, 1986).

These theories work, however, only if the patient wants them to work. Once the patient is involved, he or she can begin to perceive the situation positively. The effect a positive frame of mind has on the immune system has prompted the development of laughter therapy as an alternative for patients (Friedman, 1988). Again, this therapy in no way replaces conventional therapy; rather, it enhances any therapy that patients undergo.

Above all, give your patients hope. If you can give them nothing else, give them hope! Hope provides the will to live. The *zeitgeist* — today's general intellectual, moral, and cultural climate — has brought a new understanding of the interrelationship between the mind and the immune system. Today's magazines are filled with exercises for the mind, and so the mainstream of the population has become aware of this interrelationship. This general level of awareness makes it easier for transplant recipients to accept positive thinking as a recuperative modality.

Because end-stage organ failure brings emotional upheaval to a person's life, and it is common to get bogged down in the routine of daily existence during a chronic illness, it is easy for patients to feel self-pity and to allow their attitude to deteriorate. This is when it is most important to take a positive approach toward your patients. As important as it is to say the right thing, it is equally important to say it right — to be aware of the message being transmitted to patients. At the same time that the nurse is evaluating the patient for subtle hints of a message contrary to his or her spoken words, the patient is also reading the nurse's subtle hints. Instead of reminding patients that they are sick, the nurse communicates to them a feeling of continued progress.

TAKING CHARGE

After the recipient returns to the usual routine — job, family, and/or school — it is still vitally important for the nurse to reinforce the patient responsibilities in transplantation. It is time for recipients to begin to take charge of their own lives. This applies both to healthcare regimen and to social responsibilities.

As mentioned earlier, in Didlake's (1978) study, at 36 months post transplant, the only reason for graft failure in this group of recipients was noncompliance. These recipients simply stopped taking their medication 3 years after transplantation! What happened? Was the need for medication spontaneously forgotten? Did the recipient get tired of being a recipient? Was the recipient just burnt out?

To prevent recipients from spontaneously withdrawing their own medication, the nurse routinely reviews the relationship between immuno-suppression and graft survival. This is a clear message that can be communicated in language that the patient understands. It may be helpful for the nurse to return to the same materials used in the initial patient education process. Nurses who suspect that recipients are losing interest in their protocol should introduce them to other patients. By meeting with patients waiting for transplantation, recipients are reminded of how fortunate they are to have received their transplants. By meeting with patients who are experiencing graft rejection due to noncompliance, recipients get a graphic reminder of the reality of their situation.

What about the patient who is just tired of it all? Hoover (1983) reviewed patient burnout and other reasons for noncompliance in the diabetic population. Her findings are also applicable to the long-term transplant recipient. The patient most likely to burn out is the perfectionist — the patient who starts out wanting to do everything to just the right degree. After a while, patients may begin to question why they are still dependent on a healthcare regimen. Month after month the diabetic patient endures insulin injections and hospital visits (this is comparable with the transplant recipient who endures daily pills and repeated clinic visits). In the long term, diabetics are plagued with the chronic effects of the disease (likewise, transplant recipients face an unknown future of possible graft failure and the long-term effects of immunosuppression). When will they be "cured"? In order to effectively help a patient like this, the nurse must attempt to "truly understand his feelings and emotionally stand in his shoes" (Hoover, 1983). This patient is grappling with the reality of chronic illness; it is forever, but it doesn't have to be debilitating. And so patient education moves into a new phase: getting on with life.

Some recipients may require extra encouragement to get out and live their lives to the fullest. Post-transplant recipients are able to return to work. They are able to do just about anything they put their minds to. It is important that recipients view themselves as useful members of society. If they receive the right encouragement, they can return the energy that society has given to them. They do not have to be treated as if they are fragile — if they are treated as fragile, they will behave that way. They should not be given excuses for lack of achievement. It is up to each recipient to make the best of the situation. The recipient may respond very well to options offered by a vocational rehabilitation counselor — the opportunity to return to school, for example — or to start a garden. What is important is that there *is* something to live for, some reason for tomorrow.

SUMMARY

The transplant recipient has a lot of lessons to learn as well as to teach; these are not easy lessons, but they are long-lasting. The nurse's involvement in the education of the recipient will necessarily change with each encounter. Nurses are the crucial link in deciding what the patient needs to know, and when. Choose wisely and choose with compassion.

Bibliography

Berron, K: Transplant patient's perceptions about effective preoperative teaching. J Heart Transplant 5:162–165, 1986.

Cameron, K, et al: Chronic illness and compliance. Journal of Advanced Nursing 12:671–676, 1987.

Cousins, N: Anatomy of an Illness as Perceived by the Patient. WW Norton, New York, 1979.

Didlake, R, et al: Non-compliance: A major cause of late graft loss in cyclosporine-treated renal transplants. Transplantation 43:924, 1987.

Friedman, M: A Laugh a Day. New Realities 1:39–42, 1988.

Frierson, RL, et al: Heart transplant candidates rejected on psychiatric indications. Psychosomatics 7:347–355, 1987.

Hoover, J: Patient burnout and other reasons for noncompliance. The Diabetes Educator 3:41–43, 1983.

Korsch, BM, et al: Noncompliance in children with renal transplants. Pediatrics 6:872–876, 1978.

The Merck Manual, ed 15, ch 278. Merck Sharp & Dohme, Rahway, NJ, 1987, p 2467.

Orem, D: Nursing Concepts of Practice, ed 3. McGraw-Hill, New York, 1985.

Rimza, ME: Complications of corticosteroid therapy. Am J Dis Child 132:806–810, 1978.

Rogers, KR: Nature of spousal supportive behaviors that influence heart transplant patient compliance. J Heart Transplant 2:90–95, 1987.

Siegel, B: Love, Medicine and Miracles. Harper & Row, New York, 1986.

Smith, CE, et al (eds): Patient Education; Nurses in Partnership with Other Health Professionals. Grune & Stratton, NY, 1987.

Szasz, T, et al: A Contribution to the philosophy of medicine. AMA Archives of Internal Medicine 57:585–592, 1956.

CHAPTER

13

Tissue Transplantation

M. K. Gaedeke Norris, RN, MSN
Robert M. Duckworth, BS,
CPTC (ARTC)

For hundreds of years, tissue transplantation has been performed in attempts to benefit humankind. Perhaps the earliest bone transplantation was performed in the late 1600s by using a piece of dog skull bone to close an open area in a Russian soldier's cranium (Burchardt and Enneking, 1978). Skin is used to save the lives of burn victims, corneas to restore sight, while middle ear ossicles restore hearing. Heart valves can return a patient to the normal activities of daily living. New uses for donated human tissue are constantly being found. Table 13-1 lists many of the currently transplantable tissues, and the list is growing.

A large variety of tissue is presently being transplanted, and many of these procedures are being performed in community hospitals as well as in university transplant centers. Unlike solid vital organs for which transplantation can only be performed in approved centers, tissue transplants can be done almost anywhere. Bone transplants, in particular, are frequently done during orthopedic surgery to replace cancerous tumors, and fill defects caused by trauma, cystic growths, and congenital defects.

255

Table 13-1. Tissues Used for Transplantation

- Cornea
- Dura mater
- Fascia lata
- Skin
- Ilium
- Ulna
- Radius
- Humerus
- Femur
- Tibia
- Fibula

- Cartilage
- Mandible
- Heart valves
- Stapes
- Tympanic membrane
- Incus
- Malleus
- Tendons
- Ribs

CRITERIA FOR DONATION AND TRANSPLANTATION

The greatest obstacle to more successful transplantation of tissues is the same as that of organs — there is not enough supply. But unlike solid organs, the criteria for tissue transplantation are much broader, with far fewer restrictions.

The criteria for donating tissue, as with receiving tissue, are also much less restrictive than they are solid organs (Table 13-2). After circulation ceases, tissues have a much longer viability than highly metabolic vital organs. This allows tissues to be retrieved following cardiac death. Heart-beating cadavers are not necessary. Actually, tissues can be retrieved for a number of hours following cardiac death.

For eye donation, the only absolute contraindications recognized by most eye banks are acquired immune deficiency syndrome (AIDS), active

Table 13-2. Donor Criteria

Criterion	Heart Valves	Bone	Skin	Eye	Ear
Age (years)	0-55	16-55	15-75	100+	8-80
Active Infection	No	No	No	No	No
No Previous Disease of Organ	Yes	Yes	Yes	N/A	Yes
Blood Type	N/A	N/A	N/A	N/A	N/A
Tissue May Be Retrieved after Cardiac Death	Yes, up to 12 hr	Yes, up to 24 hr	Yes, up to 36 hr	Yes, up to 6 hr	Yes, up to 48 hr

N/A = not applicable.

hepatitis, rabies, and Cruetzfeld-Jakob disease. It is worth noting that even patients blind from noncorneal causes make excellent donors. In these cases, the donor family is often particularly receptive to eye research and treatment. The family receives great comfort in knowing their consent to donation may help to improve the quality of someone else's life. There are no age limitations for eye donation. This means that potential corneal donors can be identified in a majority of deaths.

The donation of most other tissues (such as skin, bone, middle ear, heart valves, and so forth) require that the donor must, in addition to other criteria, be free of malignancy (other than nonmetastasized, primary brain tumors), and have no unresolved infection at the time of death. A history of autoimmune or tissue-specific diseases, chronic intravenous drug abuse, homosexuality, or prolonged steroid use are also usually contraindications to donation. Generally, donors are under 60 years of age, but each organ and tissue procurement agency evaluates potential donors individually. Even with these additional restrictions, many of those who die in hospitals can still be multitissue donors.

NURSING CARE OF THE TISSUE DONOR

It is important for the nurse to assure that when family members give consent for tissue donation, they understand which tissues can be procured, specifically giving permission for each one. Occasionally a family gives blanket approval for "any needed tissue," and is unaware of the large numbers that can be procured. The nurse approaches the family's donation consent as an informed consent, assuring that the family's knowledge is complete. (See Appendix F for a general consent form.)

Once death has occurred and donation permission has been received from the family, the care of the tissue donor is minimal. However, as in the case of the cornea, nursing interventions can be crucial to the viability of the future graft.

For such eye donation, the nurse intervenes by simply closing the lids and applying light ice packs. This greatly assists in slowing deterioration that might hamper optimal vision for the recipient. Also, instilling sterile normal saline eye drops before closing the lids and elevating the head of the bed 30° add to the quality and viability of the tissue. The most successful procurements for transplantation occur within 4 to 6 hours after death. By assuring these simple interventions, the nurse greatly enhances the viability of the procured tissue.

At the opposite end of the spectrum, middle ear donors require virtually no specific nursing interventions. The tympanic membrane and ossicles can be retrieved up to 48 hours following death, even after embalming. Most other tissues need to be retrieved within 6 to 24 hours, depending on whether or not the body was refrigerated. Whenever possible, refrigeration or cooling is arranged.

All procedures are performed so as to assure that the appearance of the donor is not different, and will therefore not effect any open-casket funeral arrangements. In skin donation, a layer of skin only 12 to 15 thousandths of an inch is removed. This is similar to a mildly peeling sunburn. Skin is removed from areas such as the chest, back, buttocks, and thighs, which will be covered by clothing during the funeral. When the eyes are removed for corneal donation, they are replaced with a prosthesis to maintain an unaltered appearance. Surgically removed bones are replaced with dowels before incisions are sutured closed to maintain appearance.

Tissue donation does not need to affect the family's decision for funeral arrangements. Tissue donor care is minimal for the nurse, and the results of potentially dozens of people benefiting from a single donor make any such nursing effort worthwhile.

PROCURING AND PRESERVING TISSUES

Corneas

The preferred method for procuring corneas for transplantation is to remove each eye globe in its entirety from the donor. This procedure may be performed in the morgue, in the donor's private hospital room, or in the operating room following organ retrieval. The enucleation is performed under aseptic conditions. The area surrounding the eyes is prepared using an antimicrobial agent and sterile drapes are applied. After using a speculum to separate the lids, one cuts various tissues, including the optic nerve, rectus, and oblique muscles, to remove the left and right globe. Each eye is then placed in a special sterile container, and irrigated with either normal saline or an antibiotic solution. Cotton or gauze is placed under the eyelid by the procuring specialist, and a prosthesis is inserted before the lids are closed. The tissue containers are then transported on ice. Once the eye has arrived at the eye bank, the cornea is removed for microscopic evaluation and processing. The back, or poles, of the eye are used for research unless the family consented to "transplantation only."

A variant method of cornea procurement can also be utilized. Rather than performing an enucleation (removal of the whole eye), only the cornea and a small portion of the sclera (*in situ* excision) are removed. The eye bank specialist still places cotton or gauze under the lid, and typically inserts a prosthesis to ensure an unaltered appearance of the donor.

Corneas can be preserved in a variety of ways. Short-term preservation is accomplished by storing the entire eye in cool, moist jars at 4°C. By using a modified culture medium in cold storage, the preservation time can be extended. Cryopreservation also offers an option for longer-term preservation. However, because there are thousands of people in need of corneas each year, those corneas which are suitable are transplanted as soon as possible, minimizing storage times.

Skin

Skin procured from cadaveric donors must be preserved until quality control programs (cultures, etc.) are completed and the donor skin is needed for patient use. Immediate short-term preservation may be accomplished by immersion of the skin in a physiologic salt solution and cooling to the temperature of "wet" ice (approximately 4°C). Long-term storage resorts to more secure procedures at lower temperatures (−70° to −196°C, the temperatures of "dry" ice and liquid nitrogen, respectively) and using chemical cryoprotectants such as glycerol.

Following recovery, testing, and sizing, skin is packaged in a variety of sizes and formats. Typically it is sealed in plastic (Mylar) bags and frozen for long-term storage. Freezing methodologies vary with the skin bank responsible, and may involve rather complex rate-controlled freezing methods coupled with pretreatment of the skin with cryoprotectants. Other tissue banks will simply test, package, and freeze the donor skin in an ultra-low (−70°C) refrigerator. Expiration limits for cryopreserved skin are not well established. However, most agree that five-year preservation is possible.

The donor skin is rapidly thawed and washed in the operating room just prior to use. Portions of the donor skin that are not immediately utilized for the current procedure may be retained and utilized on the same patient within approximately 7 days after the initial thawing if properly cared for and refrigerated.

Bone

The recovery, processing, and preservation of cadaveric bone may be accomplished by two different methods. One method requires that all bone be recovered and processed under completely aseptic conditions. The other allows for recovery and processing under clean conditions with the allograft material subjected to terminal sterilization prior to preservation. At present, there is no clear indication as to which of these two methods is most appropriate.

Sterile recovery provides material that is free of damage caused by sterilization while clean recovery provides for greater applicability and thus larger amounts of recovered bone. Many tissue banks also operate surgical bone recovery programs in which patients who are undergoing elective orthopedic procedures (involving removal of autogenous bone) may donate this excised bone to the tissue bank.

Aseptic recovery takes place in the operating room, as would any sterile surgical procedure. All efforts are made by the procurement specialists to remove, process, and package the recovered bone without contamination. Each skeletal component is cultured immediately after removal, packaged in sterile materials, labeled, logged, and placed in crushed ice for transportation.

At the bone bank, the materials are processed into the desired bone components. These components are usually preserved by lyophilization (or freeze drying). This process renders the materials nonviable but stable for a number of years. Some components are preserved for short periods (less than 5 years) by freezing at $-70°C$. This maintains the viability of the cells. In many cases these fresh-frozen components are pretreated with cryoprotectant agents in order to improve recoverability of viable tissue cells.

The second methodology, clean recovery, is very similar to sterile procurement, with the exception that the recovery does not take place in the operating room. Clean recoveries may be performed in the morgue or funeral home. Otherwise, the recovery procedure differs little from that of aseptic and sterile recovery. A sterile environment is maintained during the recovery procedure. All instruments, drapes, gowns, gloves, and components are prepared as they would be in the operating room.

The processing of clean-recovered bone is identical to that of sterile bone except that clean conditions rather than sterility are maintained. After processing is complete, the components are subjected to a terminal sterilization procedure utilizing ethylene oxide gas. Other components are subjected to radiation sterilization. Clean recovery does not allow for the recovery and processing of fresh-frozen tissue. Therefore the cells are not viable.

Other Tissues

Other tissues such as middle ear and heart valves are processed at only a few centers around the country. The same principles of preservation which assure that there is no transmission of communicable diseases, and that the tissues are sterile, are part of the unique processing of these tissues.

TRANSPLANTING TISSUES

Evaluating the Recipient

Qualifying to receive a tissue transplant is a much less complex process than qualifying as a solid organ recipient. The restrictions are minimal, with none except perhaps a negative human immunodeficiency virus (HIV) status presently being recognized by most programs as a criterion for candidacy. The presence of a malignancy is frequently a contraindication for receiving a solid organ transplant, yet bone transplants are often done especially for patients with bone cancer. Transplantation of other tissues such as skin, cornea, middle ear, heart valves, and so forth is more dependent upon available supply than on the health or condition of the recipient. Corneal transplants have even been performed on patients over 100 years of age. Unlike the requirement for solid organ recipients, psychosocial evaluations are not considered necessary because postoperative recovery and long-term management are much less complex.

Cornea

As the transparent covering the eye, the cornea is critical to the quality of vision. Often damaged from trauma, chemical accidents, infection, and congenital defects, the dysfunctional cornea is responsible for most cases of blindness. In the United States it is a cause of blindness second only to diabetic retinopathy (Eye Bank Association, 1986). When damage to the cornea occurs, light rays are not properly transmitted through to the other structures of the eye, resulting in a loss of vision.

Corneal allografts, obtained from eye donors, can be used to replace a patient's own cornea and restore vision. Corneas are considered to be relatively immunoprivileged, that is not highly susceptible to rejection. This is because the cornea is without blood supply, making rejection much more unlikely than in the case of solid organs or vascularized tissues. Usually only local steroid drops are used to manage potential rejection. Most often performed as an outpatient procedure, the patient's own cornea is cut to remove a round disc of tissue. This same size "button" is then used to cut a replacement from the donor cornea, which is sutured into place. Common causes of failure of the transplant are infection, poor healing, and occasionally rejection. Figure 13–1 illustrates the corneal transplant process.

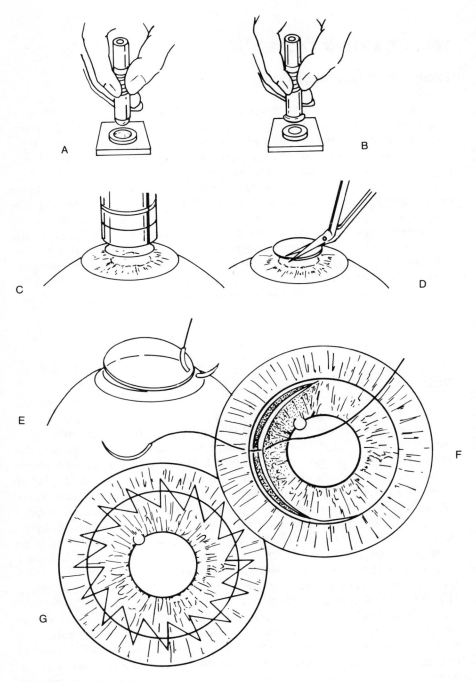

Figure 13-1

Penetrating keratoplasty. (*A*) The donor cornea with a scleral rim on the Teflon plate. (*B*) Donor tissue is punched with a trephine. (*C*) Incision of recipient cornea with a trephine. (*D*) Incision is completed with corneal scissors. (*E*) Corneal buttons are exchanged; the first cardinal suture is placed. (*F*) The fourth cardinal suture is placed. (*G*) Completed running sutures; the cardinal sutures have been removed.

Skin

Most recipients of skin allografts are burn victims. While generally only solid organs are spoken of as vital organs or lifesaving transplants, for many of the 2 million burn patients each year, these transplants *are* lifesaving. Without therapeutic replacement of their skin patients face both life-threatening fluid and electrolyte imbalances and infection.

Anatomically, the skin is composed of two major layers, the epidermis and the dermis. The epidermis is a thin layer performing such functions as the manufacture of keratin and melanin The dermis, lying under the epidermis, contains nerves and blood vessels. While both these layers are relevant to autograft transplantation, cadaveric allografts typically utilize a layer only 12 to 15 thousandths of an inch thick.

The skin serves several biological functions. The patient with large body-surface-area burns loses the protection from infection that an intact skin barrier provides. In addition, the burn patient also has alterations in temperature regulation as well as fluid and electrolyte balances.

To increase the potential surface area that it can cover, donated skin may undergo a procedure to mesh it to many times its original size in order to serve as a temporary biological dressing over the patient's burned areas. Allografts such as these are used to cover superficial to moderate second-degree burns. They are also used as a temporary dressing while the burn site is awaiting an autograft (Epstein and Epstein, 1987). Unlike most transplants, allograft skin is not usually expected to remain with the patient permanently. It serves only as a dressing. Typically the allograft skin is placed over the patient's own autograft. That is, skin is obtained from unburned areas of the patient and also meshed and stretched to cover the maximal area possible. This autograft is expected to be incorporated and heal fully by filling in the spaces of the meshed areas. The allograft of donated skin lies above the patient's own autograft to help minimize fluid losses and the potential for infection. These allografts also speed healing and reduce pain. This is called an overlay technique (Fig. 13–2). This technique helps assure that the patient's own skin can be maximally used to cover the largest areas. The donor skin only survives a few weeks before sloughing off. Depending upon each burn center's protocol, the skin may actually be changed every few days. It is often necessary to replace donor skin many times before an area has satisfactorily healed. Skin allografts are an excellent means to maximize the use of any autograft skin the patient may have. In burn patients, they play a particularly critical role in reducing sepsis, which is the most common cause of death.

In order for grafts to "take," the nurse must assure that they are kept undisturbed and stabilized by preventing movement of the tissue. This is frequently accomplished by having dressings or Steri-Strips applied at the time of grafting and left in place 2 to 3 days.

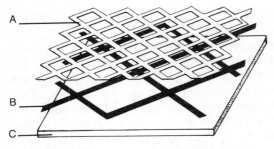

Figure 13-2

The overlay technique combines expanded donor skin (*A*) and expanded patient skin (*B*) in a single grafting procedure to the burn wound (*C*). The patient skin is expanded nine times the original size and the donor skin three times the original size.

Overlay technique of skin allograft transplantation

Bone

Bone is made of both living tissues and nonliving materials. The living portions include four cell types, blood vessels, nerves, the periosteum, endosteum, and marrow. Nonliving materials include calcium salts, collagen, and mucopolysaccharides that constitute the bone matrix, or "cement." The four bone cell types are important in understanding bone growth, healing, and the physiology of transplanted bone. All have different functions. Osteogenic cells are immature or early cells that must undergo differentiation to become osteoblasts. Located in growth plates, the periosteum and endosteum play critical role in growth and healing of fractures. Osteoblasts, also located in the periosteum, are cells designed to build bone on the outer aspects. In addition, they are instrumental in the formation of the bone matrix, which is the nonliving component, by forming collagen and helping with calcium and phosphorus activity. Osteocytes, the third cell type, help maintain the matrix between the living cells. When these cells die, resorption of the matrix occurs and greatly weakens the bone. The last bone cell type, osteoclasts, are the cells responsible for resorption. They may function normally in growth and development of bone, or in resorption of transplanted bone that is nonviable and/or rejected.

When bone is used for transplantation, it can take many forms. Entire bones may be used such as the tibia, femur, and ileum to replace cancerous, defective, or traumatized bones. Bone can also be treated and processed to form plugs, strips, particles, and other suitable shapes to fulfill a need or fit smaller spaces. When bone is processed, it has often been treated by freezing or freeze-drying. This helps decrease factors that would promote the recipient to reject it, and helps preserve the bone tissue for storage. When the selected preservation method does not promote the viability of the tissue, the transplanted bone is referred to as an implant. It is important that whatever the preservation method of the graft may be, it is a method that maximizes the graft's inductive capacity — the ability of the implant to encourage the recipient's native tissues to form new bone tissue in and around the graft. Both freeze-drying and freezing have been shown to maintain bone induction properties. (Cruess and Rennie, 1984). Infrequently, vascularized bone grafts may also be performed, wherein both the bone and the blood vessels that supply it are transplanted. This helps to maintain the viability of the graft and causes less resorption of the transplanted tissue. Generally, resorption of transplanted bone occurs more quickly than new bone can be formed to replace it. This resorption can be a long process, extending over months or even years. As this occurs, particularly in bones subjected to a weight-bearing load, stress fractures can occur. This is not an infrequent complication. The nurse assesses for pain, tenderness, and muscle spasms and instructs the patient to report these symptoms immediately. Short-term immunosuppression is sometimes utilized in bone transplantation to assist in reducing rejection and resorption.

Instead of utilizing a bone allograft for transplantation, autografts are often considered. These use bone from other areas of the patients themselves for the graft. While rejection is not a major issue in this type of graft, increased discomfort and risk of infection to the patient related to an additional surgical site are important considerations when selecting the type of graft.

Bone allograft is an excellent treatment option for most patients and may be utilized for dental procedures, spinal fusions, and joint replacements in addition to other uses previously mentioned. Bone transplantation can serve a wide variety of patient needs from speeding recovery from trauma to preventing amputation of a cancerous limb.

Middle Ear

Patients are thoroughly evaluated for the type of hearing loss they have experienced. Individuals who can benefit from receiving a middle ear transplant are only those patients with bone conduction hearing loss or damaged tympanic membranes. Those patients with nerve conduction hearing loss are not considered for this transplantation procedure. There are no additional evaluation processes unique to the middle ear transplant recipient. Additional criteria depend primarily upon surgeon and center preference.

Heart Valves

Patients who are considered for heart valve transplantation are those with symptomatic cardiac failure or cardiac compromise that has not effectively been treated by any other means. Evaluation of the patient is that typical to any cardiac patient. The final decision to use human heart valves versus porcine or mechanical valves depends upon availability and the preference of the physician. Tissue typing and compatibility are not necessary for heart valve transplantation because it is a relatively immunoprivileged tissue.

POSTOPERATIVE CARE OF RECIPIENTS

Preventing Infection

Most tissue transplant recipients do not require major immunosuppression as do organ donors. For instance, in corneal transplantation only locally applied steroid drops are used. Occasionally with other tissue transplants, such as bone, short-term immunosuppression may be used. Still, immediately postoperatively, the largest threats of infection are related to the surgical wound sites themselves. For burn patients undergoing skin allografts, the burn site is the area of most concern for infection. Secondary opportunistic infections are seen much less often in tissue than in organ recipients due to the lack of or minimal use of immunosuppression. The nursing interventions aimed at minimizing the potential for infection are standard ones. Impeccable hand washing and strict aseptic technique in caring for all wounds are critical. Including the patient, family, and visitors in teaching precautions against infection is also a nursing priority.

Corneal recipients are assessed for any signs of redness or pain in the eye. Because the procedure is often done on an outpatient basis, these patients are taught how to recognize and report these symptoms promptly. While these can be signs of rejection, they can also be signs of infection (Tooke, 1986). Teaching patients how to maintain aseptic technique while instilling eye drops is another important nursing intervention in reducing the long-term risk for infection

Reducing Anxiety and Fear

Tissue transplantation for many patients can be an exciting and hopeful experience. But with that anticipation can come reservations about undergoing the surgical procedure; fear of failure of the graft, resulting in disappointment; fear of recurrence of the underlying disease process such as musculoskeletal or cardiac disease; and so forth. Each patient has a unique set of experiences that has brought him or her to the point of needing a tissue transplant. It is vital that the patient be allowed to vent feelings even if they are not optimistic or positive in order to help deal with anxiety and increase coping skills. Frequently the patient's support persons cannot cope with this type of negativism. Nursing interventions and support aimed at allowing the patient to freely explore his or her anxieties and to express them openly are priorities of care. This is a necessary step in assisting the patient to make a positive adjustment and develops a foundation for patient compliance with future care.

Promoting Positive Self-Concept

For burn patients, disturbances in body image begin as soon as the patients are aware of their appearance. While autografts and allografts are certainly employed to achieve optimal cosmetic outcomes, these seldom reach the pre-injury condition. These patients need a great deal of support from nursing staff and family or significant others. The nurse refers the patient to additional counseling sources to minimize negative self-concepts.

Corneal transplant recipients will generally experience improvement in their body image resulting from successful transplantation. Effects are dramatic and rapid.

Bone transplant recipients' disturbances will vary greatly depending upon the underlying condition. For an individual who has undergone cosmetic maxillofacial reconstruction, the positive outcomes will usually far outweigh pre-existing negative self-concepts. For a young, athletic, trauma patient undergoing extensive reconstruction, the disturbances will be considerably different. The pre-existing condition that necessitated the tissue transplant will most often be the major factor in self-concept alterations. Nursing interventions are specifically individualized for each patient.

Monitoring for Rejection

Rejection, even in relatively immunoprivileged tissues, is always a threat. Patients are taught by their nurse to recognize the signs and symptoms of rejection for their graft and to seek medical attention immediately.

For all tissues, fever and pain are critical indicators and are reported to the physician immediately. In many of these tissues (such as tendons and fascia), rejection is difficult to detect by signs and symptoms alone. Vague, general responses such as an elevated temperature and pain may be the major indicators. Nurses stress with tissue transplant patients that the symptoms may often be subtle and to report any changes or symptoms immediately.

SUMMARY

Tissue donation and transplantation include both the oldest and some of the newest transplantable grafts. Almost every hospital death offers the nurse an opportunity to be involved in some type of tissue donation, and many of the patients we care for every day are receiving transplanted tissues. This makes *all* nurses, regardless of where they may work, in an acute care hospital a potential member of the transplant team. Unlike potential organ donors and recipients, tissue donors and recipients are everywhere. All nurses, not only those in critical care, have the opportunity to play an important role in increasing the availability of tissue for transplantation and in caring for transplant recipients.

Bibliography

Burchardt, H and Enneking, W: Transplantation of Bone. Surg Clin North Am 58(2):403–423, April, 1978.

Cruess, RJ, and Rennie, W: Adult Orthopaedics. Churchill Livingstone, New York, 1984.

Epstein, E and Epstein, E Jr: Skin Surgery. WB Saunders, Philadelphia, 1987.

Eye Bank Association of America: Fact Sheet. Washington, DC, May 1, 1986.

Illinois Transplant Society, Inc. ITS News 3(2), Summer, 1986

Technical Manual for Tissue Banking. The American Association of Tissue Banks, McLean, VA, 1987.

Tooke, MC, Elders, J, and Johnson, DE: Corneal Transplantation. American Journal of Nursing (June, 1986):685–687.

Issues in Organ Procurement and Transplantation

Mary L. Stoeckle, RN, MSN, CCRN
M.K. Gaedeke Norris, RN, MSN

LEGISLATIVE AND LEGAL ISSUES

Legislative and legal issues in transplantation are complex, as is often true in areas of health care. This subject is relatively new and it has evoked powerful emotional response. Through media attention, a demand for immediate response has caused transplantation regulations to come about rapidly and from numerous sources. State legislation and regulations, federal legislation and regulations, and Joint Commission on Accreditation on Healthcare Organizations (JCAHO) requirements are the major sources of the regulatory response to the need for organ and tissue donations for transplantation. A list and summary of legal milestones and current legal issues in the transplant continuum follows.

Public Law 92-603

This federal legislation passed in 1972 was to provide Medicare insurance coverage for victims of end-stage renal disease. This amendment to the Social Security Act made dialysis and renal transplantation available to all end-stage renal disease (ESRD) patients. It had taken

269

nearly two decades of progress in the fields of dialysis and transplantation, as well as the efforts of patients and the National Kidney Foundation,
among others, to bring this monumental legislation to fruition.

Successes in the technology of dialysis and progress in transplantation coupled with the enormous costs of treatment drove the federal
government to approve funding for this select population of ESRD patients. Providing coverage for the medical expenses of those with renal
disease, with no regard to age or ability to pay, was unique in this
country's history with regard to healthcare insurance coverage.

One problem associated with this legislation included a decrease in
home dialysis due to the lack of incentives for this less expensive alternative to in-center treatment. Another problem was that while nurses no
longer had to see patients dying because they couldn't afford treatment,
the legislation by no means took care of all the financial burdens. The time
commitment of dialysis treatments made employment difficult for patients. However, followup clinic visits for transplant patients often made
employment as difficult for them as when they required dialysis. Even
when schedules and health permitted, employment could be difficult because of an inability to return to their previous occupation, or difficulty in
being hired due to medical history. Nurses were no longer facing the
challenge of keeping patients with ESRD alive, but were now facing new
challenges of rehabilitation and restoration of role functions. This problem
was not a direct result of PL 92–603, but was a problem nonetheless that
is still an issue today for all transplant patients.

Public Law 95-292

This federal law, passed in 1978, helped address two of the problems
associated with PL 92–603: specifically, that the previous legislation had
unintentionally been structured not to favor home dialysis and transplantation, which are both cost-effective alternatives to in-center dialysis.

Some progressive insurance companies such as Blue Cross of Roches-
ter, New York, reimbursed nurses directly for dialysis treatments provided
in the home. A direct fee-for-service payment proved cost-effective for
the insurance companies; provided more flexibility for patients, especially
in rural settings; and provided alternative autonomous settings for nursing
practice.

Uniform Determination of Death Act

In 1980 this act was introduced to serve as a model for the declaration of death to be adopted by all states. Simply, it recognizes either
cardiopulmonary cessation or whole brain function cessation as death.

Specific criteria for determination were not specified, but were left open by referring to accepted medical standards as the basis. All but six states have adopted a form of this act (Flye, 1989).

While the determination of death is not new legislation, confusion remains today concerning both the knowledge and concepts of brain death among physicians and nurses (Youngner, et al., 1989). Youngner has suggested that healthcare professionals who are neither knowledgeable about legal criteria nor accurate in their concepts of brain death are ill prepared to discuss this issue with potential donor families. Furthermore, it may be a major factor in the stress nurses feel when maintaining donors, their resentment of required request laws, and their reluctance to approach donor families (Youngner, et al., 1989).

Uniform Anatomical Gift Act

Adopted in all 50 states, the purpose of this legislation was to have a consistent, simple approach in all states to obtaining cadaver organs and tissues (Flye, 1989). Signed by the holder and witnessed by two individuals, the donor card is a legal document consenting to donation. In practice, however, organ and tissue procurement agencies still approach families for consent and do not rely on this document as anything more than an expression of desire by the holder. Nurses may find a similarity between this and the living will. Both find that healthcare systems, fearing legal retribution from the remaining family members, do not honor the wishes of the deceased if the family does not also consent. Nurses, whose role functions include acting as a patient advocate, may find great frustration in knowing the wishes of their patients can be overturned by their families. The patient's wishes are more likely to be honored when the nurse focuses the request to the family around the wishes of the patient, not the feelings of the individual family members.

Public Law 98-507

The National Organ Transplant Act was passed in 1984. Even 6 years later this important legislation still is a major director of procurement and transplant activities in the United States. PL 98-507 called for the establishment of a task force on both organ procurement and transplantation to tackle the spectrum of associated medical, legal, ethical, financial, and social issues (Flye, 1989). The task force was specifically charged with establishing a national organ procurement and transplantation network (OPTN), a registry of recipients, and a registry of bone marrow donors. This legislation was also the first to explicitly prohibit the sale of organs and tissues for profit. This was later amended to include fetal tissues. In

1986 the contract for the OPTN was given to the United Network for Organ Sharing (UNOS). Chapter 1 discusses UNOS in more detail.

Public Law 99-272

The Consolidated Omnibus Budget Reconciliation Act (COBRA) of April 1986 was the first time that the federal government recognized liver transplantation as the accepted therapy for adults with end-stage liver disease. It did not, however, provide financial coverage for this treatment.

Public Law 99-509

The Omnibus Budget Reconciliation Act (OBRA) passed in October of 1986 was the beginning of federal required-request legislation. As a condition of Medicare and Medicaid reimbursement, hospitals are now required to have in place policies and procedures to identify potential donors and routinely inform their families of the option to donate organs and tissues. Failure to comply can result in the loss of Medicare reimbursement for the healthcare institution.

In this same act, coverage for immunosuppressive therapy was made available for 1 year following transplantation. Nurses will find that the enormous expense of immunosuppressive therapy is a major issue with transplant patients. With graft survivals extending often for 10 years and more, this legislation can be only a beginning for families faced with such a financial burden.

Joint Commission on Accreditation of Healthcare Organizations Regulations

Standards initiated in 1988 also require hospitals to have policies and procedures in effect to identify and refer potential donors to their designated organ procurement organization. Fry of the JCAHO has said that the intention of the regulations is to further facilitate the organ and tissue donation process and that there is presently no plan to specify methods or extend the regulations (Hospital Risk Management, 1987).

State Required-Request Legislation

Forty-three states and the District of Columbia have adopted their own required-request legislation. Common to all is the call to hospitals for establishing policies and procedures to identify potential donors and make requests to families. Most states have not included sanctions in their laws for noncompliance, but some have. Kentucky, for instance, has included penalties in their legislation that can result in loss of licensure for any hospital failing to comply.

MEDICARE REIMBURSEMENT

Although patients with end-stage renal disease were allocated Medicare funding for dialysis and transplantation in 1972 by PL 92-603 (Medicare reimbursement), no other types of transplantation have received such unlimited funding. The Health Care Financing Administration (HCFA), which administers Medicare, considered transplantation of other organs experimental and therefore ineligible for funding. However, in 1979 HCFA gave tentative authorization for payment to Medicare beneficiaries for cardiac transplants performed at Stanford University Medical Center. In 1980 the funding was withdrawn (Marsden, 1988).

The limited funding approval by Medicare helped change the status of cardiac transplantation from experimental to that of an accepted therapy. It also provided access to the procedure for those who did not have private insurance or personal funds (Marsden, 1988). Medicare funding, however, is for those over 65 years of age or individuals with a work history who have been disabled for two years. Medicare, primarily designed to provide health care to the elderly, is currently allocating a substantial amount of funding resources to procedures that benefit only a minority of its beneficiaries. Is it fair that a large amount of Medicare recipients do not benefit from these regulations?

The costs of transplantation are staggering, ranging from $30,000 for a kidney transplant to $338,000 for a liver. Appendix D summarizes the current costs for transplantation. Providing wider access to organ transplantation means that access to other kinds of health care will likely be limited. Despite the fact that most fatal illnesses are preventable, only 1% of health care dollars has been spent on prevention in the last decade (Marsden, 1988). If prevention is more effective than curative care, isn't society morally bound to change the allocation to resources?

The President's Commission for the Study of Ethical Problems in Medicine and Biomedical and Behavioral Research (1983) studied the ethical implications of differences in access to health care. The commission concluded that society has an ethical obligation to ensure all its members equal access to an adequate level of health care. However, society has been unable to reach a consensus on the meaning of an adequate level of health care and how it is to be allocated. Therefore, it is highly unlikely that our society will decide to change its current policy of providing funds for more advanced technologies utilized by so few to providing basic health care to all.

Nurses are affected by the ethical and economic questions related to transplantation. They participate in the allocation of resources through involvement with recipient selection and organ procurement activities. Through professional involvement, scientific research, and participation in public policy debates, nurses play an important role in determining the allocation of health care and government funding. Chapter 2 discusses more of the nurse's role in procurement of organs. In addition, Chapter 13 discusses the nurse's role in tissue transplantation.

FETAL TISSUE TRANSPLANTS

The use of fetal tissue for transplantation is a highly controversial practice. Doctors have transplanted fetal organs into infants and are using fetal cells as treatment for Parkinson's disease. Experimental evidence is also strong that fetal islet cell transplants will restore insulin function in diabetics. The essential fetal tissue controversy is between procuring tissue from miscarriages and procuring tissue from abortions. The latter generates further controversy between procuring tissue from abortions performed for family planning reasons and procuring tissue from abortions performed expressly to provide tissue for transplants.

Right-to-life advocates object strongly to fetal tissue transplants unless the tissue comes as the product of a miscarriage. However, tissue from elective abortions may be used without implying approval of abortions to produce tissue. With an ample supply of tissue available from elective abortions, the use of abortions for the purpose of producing fetal tissue may never occur.

Each year in the United States over 1.3 million elective abortions are performed. Nearly 80% of these abortions are performed between the 6th and 11th weeks of gestation, at which time neural and other tissue is sufficiently developed to be used for transplantation (Fine, 1988; Robertson, 1988). Therefore, tissue from approximately 90,000 appropriately aged fetuses could be available for transplantation. The annual incidence of Parkinson's disease in the United States is 60,000 new cases diagnosed per year. Thus it would appear that the potential supply of fetal neural tissue for transplantation from elective abortions would exceed the anticipated demand.

Another issue of the fetal tissue transplant controversy involves tissue procurement procedures. If fetal transplants occur, questions about the process of consent and the circumstances and procedures by which fetal tissue will be retrieved must be addressed.

Currently there are legal barriers to the therapeutic use or research of donated fetal tissue. The Uniform Anatomical Gift Act (UAGA) treats fetal remains like other cadaver remains and allows the next of kin to donate the tissue (Nolan, 1988; Robertson, 1988). Some ethicists claim that the decision to abort disqualifies the mother from playing any role in the disposition of fetal remains (Robertson, 1988). If the mother exercises her right to determine whether fetal tissue is used for therapy or research, the main concern is to assure that her choice for abortion and tissue donation is informed and free. Separation of these two decisions will assure that tissue donation is not a prerequisite for the abortion. Therefore, the request to donate fetal tissue must be made only after a woman has consented to abortion.

Prior to having the option to donate, women routinely furnished tissue from electively aborted fetuses without any thought of a gift. In 1985, most research institutions had, as part of their consent forms, statements authorizing the hospital to dispose or preserve fetal tissue for diagnostic, research, or teaching purposes (Nolan, 1988). Thus, women undergoing abortions were routinely requested to authorize any reasonable use of fetal tissue as permitted by the 1968 UAGA.

The increased interest in postmortem disposition of fetal tissue raises the issue of potential procedural changes. The possibility exists that pregnant woman considering an elective abortion could have an interest in pursuing transplantation to relieve guilt, or to receive payment. Some women have indicated a willingness to conceive and then abort a fetus for the purpose of donating tissue to a relative. The National Organ Transplant Act of 1984, which bans payment for donation of solid organs, was amended in 1988 to ban sales of fetal organs and "subparts thereof" (Robertson, 1988). Federal regulations governing fetal research also state that no procedural changes that may cause greater risk to the fetus or pregnant woman will be introduced into the procedure for terminating the pregnancy solely in the interest of research (Robertson, 1988). While this policy is intended to protect a fetus from later and more painful abortions, it also aims at protecting women from prolonging pregnancy and undergoing more difficult procedures to obtain tissue.

The use of fetal tissue inevitably invokes the strong feelings surrounding abortion. Research with fetal tissue transplants as a therapy for serious illness should not be barred by ethical concerns. The issues raised can be treated separately so that ethical and political concerns associated with abortion do not interrupt the progress of important research.

Nurses involved in ethics committees and in professional organizations can help society in making decisions about fetal tissue transplants. As educators, nurses can increase public awareness of the issue and help implement public policies.

ANENCEPHALIC INFANTS: A SOURCE OF TRANSPLANTABLE ORGANS

Transplantation of neonatal solid organs is now capable of saving thousands of fatally ill newborns. As transplantation techniques are advanced, the already acute shortage of small organs will likely grow worse unless new sources of organs are identified.

Missing both cerebral hemispheres and having little, if any, brain function above the brain stem, anencephalics are severely impaired. Although many anencephalic infants are stillborn, 25% to 45% are live births. Forty percent of these live births survive at least 24 hours. Of these survivors, 1 of 3 will be living at the end of 3 days and 1 of 20 will live at least 7 days (Walters and Ashwal, 1988). These live anencephalic infants perform circulatory and respiratory functions naturally. Thus, these infants are not dead according to currently accepted standards for the determination of death.

Historically, anencephalic infants were first used as organ donors in the 1960s. However, deviation from the usual standards were noted in two anencephalic heart transplant cases. Instead of using the criteria of a flat electroencephalogram and absence of all neurological functions, the timing of cardiac excision was based on the moment when the heart stopped beating spontaneously, not irreversibly (Shewmon, et al., 1989).

The usual mode of death of anencephalic infants is cardiopulmonary failure, which makes their organs unsuitable for transplantation. Thus proposals to remove the organs of anencephalic infants in ways that would be ethically and legally acceptable require changing the Uniform Determination of Death Act (UDDA) to make anencephalics exempt or devising a way of removing their organs that does not violate the current rules. The positions most frequently advocated include waiting for traditional death, maintaining cardiopulmonary support until brain death occurs, and redefining brain death.

Most anencephalic infants die within a few days of birth but little is known of the actual cause of death. The causes of death probably include infection, aspiration, adrenal insufficiency, and poor temperature regulation (Fost, 1988). The life-ending event is presumably cardiopulmonary failure rendering the solid organs unsuitable for transplantation. Skin and corneas may be retrieved, but the demand for these tissues from neonates is minimal. For medical reasons, then, brain death must occur prior to cardiopulmonary collapse if removal of organs for transplantation is to proceed under the current guidelines.

The clinical criteria to determine brain death include coma, absence of brain stem reflexes, and apnea testing with the $PaCO_2$ greater than 60 mmHg. In order to permit brain death to occur naturally and maintain proper oxygenation of organs, protocols for use of ventilatory assistance in anencephalic infants have been established in the United States and Canada. Currently, the protocol at Loma Linda University Medical Center limits ventilator assistance to 7 days. However, not all anencephalic infants meet the criteria for brain death within the 7-day period and ventilatory support is discontinued (Ashwal, et al., 1987; Walters and Ashwal, 1988; Fost, 1988; Pomerance, et al., 1989). In Canada, similar protocols are used with a maximum time limit of 14 days. The reasons for limiting ventilatory support include not prolonging the suffering of the potential donor's family and not permitting infants to receive ventilator assistance until cardiopulmonary arrest occurs.

Because of these difficulties some physicians and ethicists have suggested adding a special "brain absent" category to the UDDA for anencephalic infants. This special category would avoid redefining or reconsidering death. It would, in essence, constitute a special exemption from those parts of the criminal code dealing with battery and homicide and allow anencephalics to be considered as suitable sources of organs.

The main objection to the "special category" theory is that it takes the first step down the so-called slippery slope. The slippery-slope argument suggests that if anencephalics are considered to represent a special case for organ donation, then others, such as patients in chronic vegetative states, microcephalic, or hydroencephalics might also become special cases. Slippery-slope concerns are over real consequences. Erosion of present barriers against promoting death can lead to desensitization of society, and the inclusion of other vulnerable patients can widen rapidly (Fost, 1988). Slippery-slope questions are concerns that must be examined, but their role in shaping policies is unclear. The questions raised are fundamentally empirical questions that may not be answered for many years.

The role of the nurse is important in shaping the policies for the use of anencephalics as organ donors. Participation in ethics committees and policy and procedure committees will allow nurses to participate as an advocate for the rights of these infants. Nurses can also help to achieve a social consensus by participating in professional and legislative organizations, and informing the public of current trends in organ transplantation and the use of anencephalic infants as donors.

RELIGIOUS ISSUES

Organ and tissue donation is a personal and emotional decision for all those faced with the option. For those presenting the option of donation who wish to support the surviving family members, each family's beliefs and desires are major considerations. For the family members who are making the decision, the beliefs and desires of their deceased loved one are major considerations in the decision process, but these are not the only considerations. Religious beliefs, or perceptions of religious beliefs, are important in the decision for many. In a Gallup poll, 9% of the respondents who said they would not donate cited religious reasons (Gallup, 1987).

In contrast to the fact that a small percentage of individuals may cite religious reasons for not donating organs, *no* major religion in the United States opposes organ donation. In fact, many religions have taken a firm position encouraging organ donation as the highest charitable gift, a gift that is given to preserve the sanctity of life. Even churches that have not actively supported donation do not oppose it. Jehovah's Witnesses, commonly believed to be opposed to donation and transplantation, may find it acceptable provided all blood is removed from the organ prior to transplantation (NATCO Training Manual, 1987). Overwhelmingly, the common theme uniting all religious groups is the preservation of the sanctity of life. From Moslems to Jews to Christians of many denominations, the goal of preserving or saving human life is the basis of support for donation and transplantation. Some geographic or ethnic groups such as Appalachians, native Americans, and blacks believe that their bodies must be whole for the afterlife. In actuality, their churches seldom, if ever, intend this literally to prevent donation.

When presenting the option for donation to family members, religious issues are seldom truly an obstacle. However, it is important for the nurse to recognize that families may sincerely believe that their religion prohibits donation. Validating the family's belief about their church's position and offering to contact someone from the pastoral care department or the family's own church can help address any misconceptions. The nurse assures that the family's decision is based on accurate information to prevent feelings of guilt later should the family discover that their church actually encourages donation. Table 14–1 summarizes the position of major religions and denominations. The nurse also recognizes that patients and families frequently make decisions that may not necessarily be in agreement with the position of their church. Many Catholics practice birth control; some Jehovah's Witnesses accept blood transfusions. Unless state laws prohibit approaching a family whose religion clearly opposes donation, or unless the family has stated they are opposed to donation, the nurse should assure that family members have the option to consider donation.

NEWS MEDIA INVOLVEMENT IN THE SEARCH FOR ORGANS

Families of patients with end-stage organ failure often find it difficult to wait for the lifesaving organ. This is especially true when the patient is a child. The feelings of helplessness and desperation have turned families to

Table 14–1. Opinions Held on Organ and Tissue Donation and Transplantation by Religious Groups		
Religion	**Acceptable**	**Opposed**
Amish	X	
Baptist	X	
Buddhist	X	
Catholic	X	
Christian Science	X	
Disciples of Christ	X	
Episcopal	X	
Greek Orthodox	X	
Gypsies		X (generally)
Hindu	X	
Islamic	X	
Jehovah's Witness	X	
Judaism	X	
Lutheran	X	
Mennonite	X	
Methodist	X	
Mormon	X	
Presbyterian	X	
Unitarian Universalist	X	

the news media for help in finding the much-needed organ. Frequently, those families able to involve the media are well-educated, upper-middle-class professionals who understand their child's prognosis but do not accept it. Media attention is gained when time is short and the needed organ is not available.

Once the media are involved, the story of the dying child is repeated many times on the radio, television, and in the newspaper. Every time the story is told, the parents are informing the public about medical advances in transplantation and the need for organ donation. In this way media attention increases the supply of organs. With national coverage, almost everyone is informed of the need for organ donation, including the families of other patients on the waiting list.

The National Organ Transplant Act of 1984 made it illegal to use financial status as a criterion for obtaining organs. In 1986 the United Network for Organ Sharing became the official registry for those on the waiting list for an organ. This waiting list is based on the severity of need combined with the likelihood of benefit regardless of race, religion, ethnic, educational, or economic status (Erikson and Mitchell, 1988). Although this registry is in effect and the use of financial status to obtain organs is illegal, acts of desperation will continue to involve the media until the supply meets the demand.

Nurses caring for patients with end-stage organ failure are often confronted by angry, distraught families when another family's plea for organs is highlighted by the media. These families frequently feel that everything is not being done for their loved one because of their economic status, education, or race. It can be difficult for a nurse to handle charges of discrimination, especially when he or she thinks that the accusation is false.

Nurses can help ease this type of situation by taking the complaint seriously. The similarities and differences between the media case and the patient's case are explained using facts. If the family is still not convinced, involve the hospital's Public Affairs department, which handles media contacts. Once the family has met with the local media, whether or not their story is used, the family is usually reassured that everything is indeed being done for their loved one.

BUYING AND SELLING KIDNEYS

Humans were made with two kidneys, while only one is necessary for life. This simple fact has opened the door to the buying and selling of kidneys between living, unrelated individuals. Turkey, Brazil, Japan, and India are a few of the countries where living donors are actively sought for cash payments. For the poor in these countries, the few thousand dollars they receive may be used to pay for housing, food, or medical care for families. For the wealthy who buy the kidneys, the return to better health is well worth the price, and often is their only hope for a transplant.

Few people feel that the selling of organs is right. It was outlawed by the National Organ Transplant Act of 1984 as well as many state statutes. But it is difficult to argue why it is morally correct (even admirable) to donate a kidney, yet reprehensible to sell one. Clearly, in either case, the kidney is received by someone who will be freed from dialysis and restored to improved function of activities of daily living — the objective of all nursing and health care. When money benefits the living donor by providing opportunities that would otherwise be unavailable, and benefits the recipient as well, the ethical issues of buying and selling kidneys become clouded.

Nurses throughout the world can help prevent the need for the marketing of organs or tissues from living donors — right or wrong — by identifying and referring potential cadaveric donors. Nurses, by assuring that all families of potential cadaveric donors are given the option to donate, can make the difference in eliminating the need for a black market in kidneys.

Another perspective on the selling of organs is the current discussion that families of cadaveric donors should be financially compensated for their gifts. Suggestions have been made that it would be morally and ethically correct to compensate families when they donate any organs because of the overall positive effect that is achieved by the outcome of a transplantation. These are issues in which nurses will find themselves involved in the future. Becoming involved by serving on ethics committees, review boards, and acting as a patient advocate for all those in the transplant spectrum will assure that nurses play a critical role in grappling with difficult ethical issues.

MINORITY ISSUES

Overwhelmingly, Americans have a high awareness of and support for organ and tissue donation. Over 94% of Americans surveyed stated they had heard of organ and tissue transplantation. Individuals have strongly expressed their willingness to donate their own organs, and the organs of their loved ones, including the organs of their children. The American public has clearly stood behind the transplant system with a support that is committed enough to have been responsible for the passage of major transplant legislation (see "Legislative and Legal Issues").

But for some groups, a reluctance to donate is strong. African Americans, perhaps more than any other minority group, have been especially hesitant to consent to donate organs and tissues. In a recent survey (Manninen and Evans, 1985), only 35% of blacks said they would be willing to donate their kidneys at their death. This is well below the national level of 52.3% in that same survey. (Table 14-2 shows differences in attitudes related to demographic characteristics.

What are the causes that account for these differences? A variety of explanations have been offered (Callender, et al., 1982). First, far fewer blacks than whites are aware of donation and transplantation. Lack of knowledge is clearly an issue in lower donation rates (Callender, et al., 1982). Studies of blacks have concluded that there is a need for more education about organ transplantation as well as donation (Callender, 1987a, 1987b).

Another factor identified was religious myth and superstition. Many blacks and other minority groups believe in the concept of the afterlife and that they must leave this world whole, with an intact body. Yet, it bears repetition that no major religious groups oppose donation. Clarence Page, a black syndicated columnist, made a convincing point when he said, "After a couple of years in the ground, there is little left of the body anyway. Why not use one's body in death to help someone else save life?" (Chicago Tribune, 1988).

A general distrust among blacks of the healthcare community was another identified block cited in the pilot study by Callender and asso-

Table 14-2. Differences in Attitudes Toward Organ Donation by Sociodemographic Characteristics of Individuals

Sociodemographic Characteristic	Currently Carry Organ Donor Card, %	Willingness to Donate, %				
		Relative's Organs	Own Kidneys	Own Corneas	Own Heart	Own Liver
Age*						
18–24	14.5	50.2	56.7	44.7	49.5	50.4
25–34	20.9	56.7	54.7	51.8	51.5	52.1
35–44	25.4	63.0	57.0	56.3	54.7	56.0
45–54	18.1	52.9	49.9	48.7	46.5	48.7
55+	17.5	46.4	38.7	37.2	35.3	35.6
Sex						
Male	20.3	52.6	49.8	47.8	47.0	47.5
Female	18.3	53.0	49.5	44.9	44.9	46.0
Race*						
White	29.8	54.6	52.3	49.4	48.9	49.4
Other	12.9	41.6	35.0	27.8	28.3	31.1
Education*						
Less than high school graduate	10.7	41.0	36.1	32.7	32.8	32.6
High school graduate	15.3	51.0	50.4	46.5	45.8	47.2
More than high school graduate	26.4	62.4	57.7	54.6	54.4	55.2
Income, $*						
<10,000	17.9	41.6	36.6	32.2	32.8	32.4
10,000–14,999	15.8	48.2	50.9	42.7	48.4	48.8
15,000–19,999	15.2	57.4	47.2	41.6	41.9	44.9
20,000–24,999	16.1	56.6	58.6	53.4	54.8	53.5
25,000–29,999	21.0	60.9	52.6	50.7	49.3	51.3
30,000–34,999	23.4	63.9	61.5	60.1	61.7	60.2
35,000–39,999	28.6	73.6	65.2	66.2	62.7	64.8
40,000+	30.1	70.5	62.4	64.3	59.4	60.9
Don't know	12.7	39.6	43.3	39.7	38.5	41.2

* Difference between groups was significant at the .05 confidence level using one-way analysis of variance.
From Manninen and Evans (1985), with permission.

ciates (1982). Fears were stated that organs might be taken before death, though this is not a concern unique to minority groups. Overall, a lack of communication and trust between blacks and the predominantly white healthcare system appears to be one reason blacks are reluctant to give consent. Significantly, though, there is another reason for this apparent reluctance that may fall clearly into the laps of white healthcare professionals: it appears that blacks and other minorities may not ever be approached for donation; that such requests are often not even made. White healthcare workers may be hesitant to approach minority groups because of large family sizes common to some minorities, or a discomfort and lack of knowledge about other cultures. Simply, minority groups are often just not given the *opportunity* to donate.

Whenever potential donors are lost, it is a loss everyone shares. Those waiting for organs and tissues, their families, and those of us sharing healthcare costs through group insurance and government healthcare programs are all affected. Sadly low donor rates among blacks are hurting blacks in other ways. The need for kidney transplants among this group is high. Renal failure is at least three times more common among blacks with hypertension than among hypertensive whites (De Palma, 1989). Most dialysis centers have large numbers of black patients. These numbers are far in excess of black demographic representation within the respective community. Lack of cadaveric kidneys from any source hits this ethnic group hard. But there is another issue. Many feel that if blacks were to donate more, there would be better tissue matches for blacks receiving organs (Callender, 1987b). Graft viability in blacks is often found to be less than in whites. One reason is believed to be differences seen in tissue matching among this population. Increasing organ donations by blacks will benefit society as a whole by making a larger number of organs available. However it may turn out to benefit the black community even more by making better tissue matches available to black transplant candidates.

Nurses can do a great deal to address this issue. As educators, nurses can increase awareness of organ and tissue donation and the need for transplantation. Improving communication and relationships among all ethnic groups in the healthcare system can help increase the donor pool and make available better matches for those awaiting transplantation. Assuring that all families have the opportunity to give the gift of life benefits both the donor families and the transplant recipients.

The Future

The Cooperative Organ Transplantation Contributions Act of 1989 is considering establishing a national trust fund for end-stage organ disease patients who could not otherwise afford the cost of transplantation. At the time of this writing it has not yet passed Congress.

While federal legislation has recognized transplantation as the therapy for adults with end-stage liver disease, as of 1989, it does not cover liver transplantation under Medicare for adults. Adults receiving coverage have had to resort to litigation based on age discrimination because children *are* currently covered. Congressman Walgren of Pennsylvania pointed out in a letter to the Secretary of the Department of Health and Human Services that insurance companies and state Medicaid programs depend upon the position Medicare takes when they formulate their own coverage (Transplant Action, 1989). Without this lead from Medicare, nurses are likely to continue to see adult patients with end-stage liver disease struggling to raise money for transplantation to save their own lives.

Federal regulations will most likely soon extend from organ procurement organizations to tissue banks. Standards of care that would both provide quality of care and offer legal protection are also likely to come soon. It is difficult to predict just how far the federal government will go in providing coverage for all those with end-stage organ disease. Will the current coverage for all those with ESRD be extended to those with liver and pancreatic failure? Or will current coverage of ESRD be revoked so that basic health care needs may be provided to all? Oregon has recently taken steps in this direction. Will immunosuppressive costs post transplantation be covered for more than 1 year? Will families of potential donors bring suits against hospitals who fail to inform them of their option to donate? Will fetal tissue transplants become acceptable therapeutic treatment for seriously debilitating illnesses? Will the federal government monitor required-request policies in hospitals and actually deny reimbursement for those who fail to comply? Will JCAHO enforce their regulations during surveys or even deny accreditation? The questions are endless and all impact on nursing practice. Nurses can play a major role in deciding these issues by becoming involved in appropriate hospital committees and by making the needs of their patients and their practice known to their representatives at local, state, and federal government levels.

Bibliography

American Council on Transplantation: US Transplant Stat Sheet. Lifesource, Summer, 1989.
Ashwal, S, et al: Considerations of Anencephalic Infants as Organ Donors. Loma Linda University Medical Center: A Working Document, 1987.
Benjamin, M (Chair): Anencephalic infants as sources of transplantable organs. Hastings Center Report (October/November, 1988); 28–30.
Callender, CO, et al: Attitudes among blacks toward donating kidneys for transplantation: A pilot study. Journal of the American National Medical Association. 74(8):807–809, 1982.
Callender, CO: Organ donation in blacks: A community approach. Transplant Proc 19(1):1551–1554, 1987a.
Callender, CO: Organ donation in the black population: Where do we go from here? Transplant Proc 19(2) (Suppl 2):36–40, 1987b.
De Palma, JR: Black Americans and the ESRD program. Contemporary Dialysis and Nephrology 10(4):33–37, 1989.
Erikson, I and Mitchell, C: Which child gets the transplant? American Journal of Nursing (March, 1988):287–288.

Flye, MW: Principles of Organ Transplantation. WB Saunders, Philadelphia, 1989.

Fine, A: The ethics of fetal tissue transplants. Hastings Center Report (June/July, 1988):5–8.

Fost, N: Organs from anencephalic infants: An idea whose time has not yet come. Hastings Center Report (November, 1988):5–10.

Gallup: The U.S. Public's Attitudes Toward Organ Transplantation and Organ Donation. April, 1987.

Hospital Risk Management. Following organ donor laws carefully to avoid negligence suits. 9:5, 1987.

Langone, J: One womb to another. Time (April 3, 1989):71.

Manninen, DL and Evans, RW: Public attitudes and behavior regarding organ donation. JAMA 253(21):3111–3115, 1985.

Marsden, C: Ethical issues in cardiac transplantation. Journal of Cardiovascular Nursing 2:23–30, 1988.

NATCO Training Manual, North American Transplant Coordinators Organization, Lenexa, KS, 1987.

Nolan, K: Genug ist Genug: A fetus is not a kidney. Hastings Center Report (December, 1988):13–19.

Page, Clarence: Blacks reluctant to donate organs. The Chicago Tribune, February 15, 1988.

Pomerance, JJ, et al: Anencephalic infants: Life expectancy and organ donation. Journal of Perinatology 9:33–37, 1989.

President's Commission for the Study of Ethical Problems in Medicine and Behavioral Research: Securing Access to Health Care, Vol 1. US Government Printing Office, Washington, DC, 1983.

Robertson, J: Rights, symbolism, and public policy on fetal tissue transplants. Hastings Center Report (December, 1988):5–12.

Shewmon, DA: Anencephaly: Selected medical aspects. Hastings Center Report (November, 1988):11–18.

Shewmon, DA, et al: The use of anencephalic infants as organ sources. JAMA 261(12):1773–1781, 1989.

Transplant Action. Legislative Update. The American Council on Transplantation, March–April, 1989, pp 1,3.

Youngner, SJ, et al: "Brain death" and organ retrieval: A cross-sectional survey of knowledge and concepts among health professionals. JAMA 261(15):2205–2210, 1989.

Walters, JW and Ashwal, S: Organ prolongation in anencephalic infants: Ethical and medical issues. Hastings Center Report (November, 1988):19–27.

Nursing Care Plan for the Organ Donor

Marguerite E. Brown

NURSING DIAGNOSIS:	BODY TEMPERATURE, ALTERED POTENTIAL
Possibly related to:	Injury to the hypothalamus resulting in hypo/hyperthermia Infection resulting in hyperthermia
Possibly manifested by:	Increased body temperature; decreased body temperature
Desired donor outcomes:	The donor will not exhibit alteration of body temperature and will have normal skin color and temperature.

ACTIONS/INTERVENTIONS

Independent

- Monitor for and report signs and symptoms of hypothermia (temperature <36.6°C, cool skin, bradycardia).
- Monitor for and report signs and symptoms of hyperthermia (temperature >38°C, hot, dry trunk, cold extremities).
- Monitor for possible sources of infection.

287

- Use strict aseptic technique at all times.
- Perform aggressive pulmonary care to prevent pulmonary infections:
  - aseptic technique in suctioning
  - suction frequently
  - turn, sigh, and percuss as indicated
- Assess for dehydration with hyperthermia.
- Protect the skin from thermal injury when using warming devices.
- Explain to family need for regulating body temperature with brain death.

Collaborative

- If hypothermia occurs, implement measures to gradually increase donor's body temperature:
  - warming blanket
  - warming light
  - warm infused fluids
  - warm infused blood
  - warm inspired gases
  - increased room temperature
- If hyperthermia occurs, implement measures to gradually decrease donor's temperature:
  - cooling blanket
  - decreased room temperature
  - ice bags to groin and axilla
  - administer antipyretics
- Monitor laboratory results for signs of infection.

NURSING DIAGNOSIS:	FLUID VOLUME DEFICIT, ACTUAL
Possibly related to:	Loss of hormonal regulatory function of fluid conservation resulting in diabetes insipidus Fluid restrictions secondary to management of intracranial pressure Loss of blood volume secondary to injury Loss of circulating volume secondary to diaphoresis
Possibly manifested by:	Dilute urine; weight loss; increased urine output; altered serum and urine sodium levels; increased serum osmolarity; increased urine specific gravity; poor skin turgor; decreased venous filling time; dry

mucous membranes; hypotension; tachy-cardia; decreased pulse volume and pressure; hemoconcentration

Desired donor outcome: Donor will exhibit adequate fluid volume as evidenced by moist mucous membranes, adequate skin turgor, stable weight, and laboratory values reflecting fluid status within normal limits.

ACTIONS/INTERVENTIONS

Independent

• Record and evaluate intake and output hourly or more often as needed.
• Monitor for and report signs of fluid volume deficit.
• Monitor all laboratory values for signs of fluid volume deficit.
• Evaluate effectiveness of fluid volume replacements.
• Provide eye care to prevent corneal drying if a potential eye donor.

Collaborative

• Administer fluids and/or blood to achieve normal central venous pressure and pulmonary capillary wedge pressure.
• If polyuria develops, maintain fluid intake to equal output plus about 50 cc or as ordered.
• Transfuse blood to maintain a packed cell volume (hematocrit) of approximately 30 mg% or as ordered.
• Administer antidiuretic hormone medications as ordered: (vasopressin; 1-desamino-8-d-arginine-vasopressin [DDAVP]).

NURSING DIAGNOSIS: CARDIAC OUTPUT, ALTERED: DECREASED

Possibly related to: Fluid volume deficit
Blood volume deficit
Decreased preload secondary to impaired vasomotor tone

Possibly manifested by: Hypotension (decrease in systolic pressure of 20 mmHg or systolic <80 mmHg); decreased hemodynamic parameters; decreased or absent peripheral pulses; dysrhythmias; tachycardia; brad-

ycardia; cold, clammy skin; poor capillary refill; cyanosis; decreased urine output (<30 cc)

Desired donor outcomes: Donor will have adequate cardiac output
as evidenced by signs of adequate organ
and peripheral perfusion.

ACTIONS/INTERVENTIONS

Independent

- Record and evaluate intake and output hourly or more often as needed.
- Monitor for signs and symptoms of decreased cardiac output.
- Raise legs 20°–30° temporarily to increase venous return.
- Weigh daily.

Collaborative

- Restore volume deficit by administering fluids/blood products to maintain central venous pressure (CVP) at 5–10 mmHg or as ordered.
- Administer pressor agents, inotropic agents, and antidysrhythmics as
ordered. Monitor effectiveness.
- Administer oxygen as ordered to maximize tissue and myocardial
oxygenation.

NURSING DIAGNOSIS:	BREATHING PATTERN, INEFFECTIVE
Possibly related to:	Loss of respiratory mechanics secondary brain stem death
Possibly manifested by:	Apnea; absent cough reflex; loss of gag reflex; decreased PaO_2 and increased $PaCO_2$; respiratory acidosis; metabolic acidosis secondary to anaerobic metabolism
Desired donor outcome:	Donor will maintain effective breathing patterns with mechanical assistance as evidenced by blood gas values within normal limits.

ACTIONS/INTERVENTIONS

Independent

- Evaluate for bilateral breath sounds to validate proper endotracheal placement.
- Evaluate breath sounds at least every 4 hours or as indicated.
- Review blood gas results for PaO_2 and $PaCO_2$, saturation, pH, HCO_3^-, and base excess.
- Reposition to promote lung expansion and mobilize secretions if donor is stable enough to tolerate.
- Suction as needed.

Collaborative

- Decompress abdomen with nasogastric tube to decrease abdominal distension.
- Implement the use of a volume-cycled respirator with tidal volume at 10–15 cc/kg with approximately 5 cm positive end-expiratory pressure (PEEP) or as ordered.
- Evaluate chest x-rays for endotracheal tube placement and infiltrates.
- Assist with insertion of chest tubes when needed.

NURSING DIAGNOSIS:	GAS EXCHANGE, IMPAIRED
Possibly related to:	Alveolar-capillary changes secondary to neurogenic pulmonary edema Altered blood flow to peripheral tissues Pulmonary secretions
Possibly manifested by:	Adventitious breath sounds; poor capillary refill; cold, clammy extremities; absent or weak peripheral pulses; hypoxia; tachycardia; abnormal blood gas values
Desired donor outcome:	The donor will exhibit adequate oxygen/carbon dioxide exchange as evidenced by blood gas values within normal limits, absence of significant adventitious breath sounds, and warm, dry skin.

ACTIONS/INTERVENTIONS

Independent

• Maintain airway through frequent suctioning and verification of tube placement.
• Monitor effectiveness of oxygen and mechanical ventilatory therapy.

See also interventions for breathing pattern, ineffective (above)

Collaborative

• If neurogenic pulmonary edema is present, use PEEP as ordered.
• Monitor and adjust ventilator settings as indicated.
• Administer medications as indicated: antibiotics, bronchodilators, expectorants, diuretics, etc.

NURSING DIAGNOSIS:	**TISSUE PERFUSION, ALTERED: PERIPHERAL, RENAL, CARDIAC, PANCREATIC, HEPATIC**
Possibly related to:	Hypovolemia Hypotension secondary to loss of vasomotor tone Vasoconstriction secondary to hypothermia
Possibly manifested by:	Cold extremities; impaired renal function (decreased urinary output, edema, hypertension); impaired hepatic function (alteration in hepatic enzymes); impaired cardiac function (dysrhythmias); impaired pancreatic function
Desired donor outcome:	The donor will maintain adequate perfusion of peripheral tissues and vital organs as evidenced by blood pressure and pulse rate within normal range, palpable peripheral pulses, warm and dry skin, and vital organ function within normal limits.

ACTIONS/INTERVENTIONS

Independent

- Monitor vital signs and hemodynamic parameters to assist in monitoring perfusion of peripheral tissues and vital organs.
- Evaluate peripheral pulses, skin temperature.
- Continuous cardiac monitoring.
- Auscultate heart sounds every 4 hours or as needed.
- Monitor hourly urine output.
- Avoid use of knee gatch.
- Apply antithromboembolic hose or elastic wraps to lower extremities.

Collaborative

- Monitor effectiveness of fluid and/or blood replacements.
- Administer medications such as pressor agents to improve vasomotor tone.
- Evaluate laboratory and diagnostic tests for vital organ function.

COLLABORATIVE PROBLEM:	ELECTROLYTE IMBALANCE

ACTIONS/INTERVENTIONS

- Monitor and report signs of metabolic acidosis:
  - decreased pH <7.35
  - decreased $Paco_2$
  - negative base excess
  - anion gap >15 mEq/liter
- Improve cardiac output to promote adequate tissue oxygenation and minimize anaerobic metabolism, which results in lactic acid production. See nursing diagnosis for Cardiac Output, altered: decreased, page 289.
- Assess for hyperkalemia:
  - K^+ >5.0 mEq/L
  - dysrhythmias
  - tented T waves
  - prolonged P – R interval
  - widened QRS complex
- Assess for hypokalemia:
  - K^+ <3.5 mEq/L
  - dysrhythmias

- ○ ST segment depression
- ○ T wave inversion
- ○ U waves present
- Treat hyperkalemia as ordered:
  - ○ remove K^+ from IV solutions
  - ○ administer ion exchange resins
  - ○ administer insulin and glucose
  - ○ administer sodium bicarbonate
- Treat hypokalemia as ordered:
  - ○ add K^+ to IV solutions
- Assess for other electrolyte imbalances that may occur with diabetes insipidus and treat as ordered.

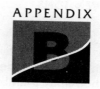

Nursing Care Plan for the Organ Donor Family

Rachel I. Rhude

NURSING DIAGNOSIS:	POWERLESSNESS
Possibly related to:	Suddenness of death Circumstances surrounding cause of death Perception of lack of control
Possibly manifested by:	Nonparticipation in organ donation decision; verbalizations of lack of control; expressions by family member(s) that they are unsure of their role(s) in donation process.
Desired family outcome:	The family is involved in the decision to donate organs and will make choices related to the process. They will express some sense of control over the donation process.

ACTIONS/INTERVENTIONS

Independent

- Assess for other contributing factors to the perception of powerlessness other than the nature of the death.
- Assess where the family members' sense of control comes from: externally ("We always have bad luck") or internally ("I should have been able to see this coming").
- Determine if there have been any recent changes in the relationships between the donor and other family members.
- Assess for poor eye contact, lack of verbal responses, lack of emotional displays.
- Allot time to the family and show concern for them as individuals and as a family unit.
- Assist families in identifying feelings toward organ donation.
- Allow family to express anger and hopelessness.
- Acknowledge/reinforce statements regarding the reality of the situation.
- Encourage the family to make as many decisions as possible. Support the decisions they make, regardless of whether they are for or against donation.
- Allow the family to be with the donor as much as possible before going to the operating room.
- Provide accurate verbal and written material concerning brain death and donation. Assure the family is getting consistent information.

Collaborative

- In cooperation with the organ procurement coordinator, provide information to the family to assure an informed consent.
- Assure the organ donor coordinator follows up with the family regarding the transplantation of the organs if they have asked to have this information.
- Refer to counseling or support services as needed.

NURSING DIAGNOSIS:	FAMILY PROCESS, ALTERED
Possibly related to:	Sudden death of donor Changes in roles secondary to death of donor
Possibly manifested by:	Inability to seek or accept assistance from the healthcare team; destructive management of crisis; inability to ex-

press or accept each other's feelings regarding brain death or donation; inability
to make a decision regarding organ
donation.

Desired family outcomes: Family is able to express openly feelings
regarding brain death and/or organ do-
nation. They are able to reach an agreed-
upon decision that is sensitive to and respectful of family members' input.

ACTIONS/INTERVENTIONS

Independent

- Determine if there were pre-existing problems with family process or if the present situation has precipitated an acute problem.
- Determine who the principal decision-makers are and any significant others who may not be direct family members.
- Assess for any significant religious or cultural factors that might influence their decision regarding donation or acceptance of brain death.
- Encourage all family members to participate in decision except the very young child.
- If a family member or significant other is being particularly destructive and not allowing the legal next-of-kin to make his or her own decision, consider moving the legal decision-maker to another area to be able to make his or her own decision more easily.

Collaborative

- Refer to clergy if appropriate.
- Utilize expertise of organ procurement coordinator whenever possible.
- Seek the assistance of other counseling services as needed.

NURSING DIAGNOSIS: **COPING, INEFFECTIVE FAMILY: COMPROMISED**

Possibly related to: Sudden change of roles
Feelings of anger or guilt
Conflicting coping styles of family members
Inability to utilize problem-solving pro-
cesses

Possibly manifested by:	Failure to visit donor; hostility of family members toward the healthcare team and/or each other; denial of death of donor; failure to care for other family members
Desired family outcomes:	Family members visit donor at least until declaration of death and typically make a final visit before the donor goes to the operating room. They are able to interact constructively with family members and healthcare team and meet basic needs of each other.

ACTIONS/INTERVENTIONS

- Assess for pre-existing ineffective coping behaviors.
- Assist the family in identifying previous successful coping mechanisms.
- Determine if there are contributing factors that are blocking the use of effective coping mechanisms.
- Assist the family through the problem-solving process:
  - identifying the problem
  - identifying alternative actions
  - determining the perceived benefits and drawbacks of each action
  - selecting the action to take
- Be with family members as they enter the unit to visit the donor to be available to answer any questions.

Collaborative

- Act as a liaison between the family and various members of the health-care team, especially the transplant coordinator.
- Seek assistance from counseling services as needed.
- Assure all information given to the family is consistent and in terms the family can understand.

NURSING DIAGNOSIS:	**COMMUNICATION, IMPAIRED: VERBAL**
Possibly related to:	Cultural differences Difficulty understanding complex medical terminology Difficulty understanding complex medical concepts such as brain death

Possibly manifested by:	Inability to understand communication from healthcare personnel; failure to ask questions as needed; misinterpretation of information given; failure to accept that death has occurred.
Desired family outcomes:	Family will understand information given them by clarifying and asking questions as needed. This will result in an acceptance of death and the ability to make an informed decision regarding organ donation.

ACTIONS/INTERVENTIONS

Independent

- Assess cultural orientation and education levels of family members.
- Determine knowledge level of complex medical terminology and concepts.
- Use metaphors to explain complex concepts.
- Minimize the use of medical terminology and explain all that must be used.
- Give the family every opportunity to ask questions by asking: "What questions do you have?" This is a very open statement that gives permission for questions to be asked in a way that indicates questions are *expected.*
- Validate that the healthcare personnel's perception of what the family is saying is accurate by restating.
- Discuss brain death, organ donation, and other critical matters only in private areas allowing for adequate time with the family.
- Repeat information given both often and consistently.

Collaborative

- Be present whenever possible when other healthcare personnel discuss information with the family.
- Assure information is consistent.
- Assure family has the opportunity to clarify and ask questions.
- Seek a "bridge" for the family if necessary, such as family member who has lived both within the family's culture and outside it, or clergy who might be better able to communicate complex information that could be totally foreign to the family.

NURSING DIAGNOSIS:	GRIEVING, DYSFUNCTIONAL
Possibly related to:	Lack of opportunity for anticipatory grieving secondary to sudden death Circumstances surrounding sudden death
Possibly manifested by:	Failure to meet basic physiological needs; inappropriate affect; failure to accept death; inability to discuss or become involved in issues related to the death such as organ donation, selection of funeral home, and notifying other relatives and friends of the death
Desired family outcomes:	The family will accept and verbalize the death of the donor and begin proceeding through the grieving process.

ACTIONS/INTERVENTIONS

Independent

- Assess the family's knowledge regarding death. Do they know death has occurred? Or do they see the donor as in a coma from which he or she may awaken?
- Assure that explanations are consistent, and that a minimal number of healthcare personnel are involved in discussions with the family to decrease the chances of confusion.
- Identify influential cultural factors.
- Encourage the family to express their understanding of the donor's condition without being confrontational about the reality of death.
- Determine previous coping mechanisms and assist the family in employing them.
- Identify stage of grieving: denial, anger, bargaining, depression, or acceptance.
- Allow the family to express anger.
- Involve significant family members in decision making.
- Do NOT approach topic of organ donation unless the family has accepted that death has occurred.
- Avoid using the term *brain death* frequently. This can sound to families as though it's different from being dead and sends mixed messages. Use the term *death*.
- Do not refer to ventilators and other devices as *life support*. This sends the family a message that there is life to support and that perhaps death has not occurred.

- Use the term *ventilator* rather than *respirator*. A dead person does not have respirations, but can be artificially ventilated.

Collaborative

- Seek the assistance of a grief counselor, social services, clergy, the transplant coordinator, or other experienced individual who can offer the family guidance in dealing with the death.
- Notify the physician to speak with the family again if they do not express understanding that death has occurred. Be present when the physician explains brain death to the family again.
- Refer to support groups and/or counseling as indicated.

NURSING DIAGNOSIS:	**HOPELESSNESS**
Possibly related to:	Death of the donor
Possibly manifested by:	Verbalizations; lack of involvement in decision making; withdrawal; inability to reflect on life achievements of donor
Desired family outcomes:	Family verbalizes feelings and begins to use effective coping mechanisms to process feelings. Family will express that organ donation was a positive experience giving them a sense of hope for the potential recipients.

ACTIONS/INTERVENTIONS

Independent

- Assess family's previous coping mechanisms and sense of hope.
- Determine if there are coexisting factors.
- Assist the family in employing previously successful methods to deal with difficult situations.

Collaborative

- Refer the family to counseling and other support services as needed.
- Assure that transplant coordinator gives the family feedback on recipients if they have expressed a desire to do so.

NURSING DIAGNOSIS:	SPIRITUAL DISTRESS
Possibly related to:	Sense of abandonment by God Decision to terminate ventilatory support if brain death is not understood
Possibly manifested by:	Verbalizations about the meaning of life; verbalizations about the senselessness of death; verbalizations about conflict with spiritual beliefs; belief that the death was a punishment
Desired family outcomes:	The family will discuss beliefs or values as appropriate, not differing significantly from those that they held before the donor's death.

ACTIONS/INTERVENTIONS

Independent

- Determine the family's religious beliefs.
- Determine if family members hold the same beliefs/values.
- Allow the family to verbalize all feelings, projecting acceptance of these feelings.
- Assess present and past support systems.

Collaborative

- Refer to appropriate clergy as family wishes.
- Assist in locating support groups relevant to the family's needs.

APPENDIX

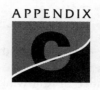

Nursing Care Plan for the Post-Transplant Patient

Joyce A. Slusher
M.K. Gaedeke Norris

NURSING DIAGNOSIS:	KNOWLEDGE DEFICIT
Possibly related to:	Lack of information about immunosuppressive therapy
Possibly manifested by:	Inability to describe purpose of medications; inability to take medications without guidance; inability to identify side effects
Desired patient outcomes:	Patient and family will verbalize and demonstrate understanding by identifying medications prescribed and the schedule for administering them. Patient and family will recognize side effects of drugs and demonstrate appropriate techniques of self-care.

ACTIONS/INTERVENTIONS

Independent

- Provide list of medications with dosages and schedule.
- List side effects of each drug.
- Explain importance of following prescribed dosage and schedule. Have patient and family repeat information.
- Explain that dosage of immunosuppression may change depending upon blood level.
- Warn the patient and family that **severe** rejection/death may occur if immunosuppressant is stopped suddenly.
- Suggest emollient lotions for dry, irritated skin.
- Allow patient adequate opportunity to express concerns/fears about changes in skin/hair that effect appearance.

Collaborative

- Wash face twice a day with pHisoHex for acne.
- Administer prescribed oral and/or topical medications.
- If Accutane is used, instruct patient in decreased triglyceride diet.
- Instruct patient on need to consider birth control measures; individualize to type of transplant and sex of patient.

NURSING DIAGNOSIS:	**KNOWLEDGE DEFICIT**
Possibly related to:	Signs and symptoms of infection
Possibly manifested by:	Inability to verbalize symptoms; inability to identify when to notify physician or clinical nurse specialist; inability to verbalize or demonstrate how to monitor for infection
Desired patient outcome:	Patient and family will verbalize sign and symptoms of infection and demonstrate behaviors needed to monitor for infection.

ACTIONS/INTERVENTIONS

Independent

- Teach patient and family to take and record temperature daily. Take temperature in mid-afternoon to monitor for low-grade infections
- Instruct patient/family to report immediately a cold, cough, fever, de-

creased urine output, pain with urination, hematuria, tenderness over implant, jaundice, anorexia, weight changes, severe headache associated with emesis, rash, and any other patient-specific information.
• Provide the patient with phone numbers to report any symptoms 24 hours a day.
• Keep accurate medication, weight, and vital sign records.

NURSING DIAGNOSIS:	NUTRITION, ALTERED: POTENTIAL FOR MORE THAN BODY REQUIREMENTS
Possibly related to:	Alterations in metabolism secondary to immunosuppressant therapy
Possibly manifested by:	Weight gain
Desired patient outcomes:	Patient will maintain weight within 10% of ideal body weight for age and height.

ACTIONS/INTERVENTIONS

Independent

• Stress importance of regular exercise program including warm-up phase, peak activity, and cool down.
• Monitor weight daily.
• Instruct patient and family in importance of monitoring weight in the home setting.

Collaborative

• Instruct the patient/family in dietary guidelines to follow a low-cholesterol, no-added-salt diet with a moderate amount of carbohydrates.
• Present the patient with a diet that is structured to allow choices, which enhances feelings of control.

NURSING DIAGNOSIS:	ACTIVITY INTOLERANCE
Possibly related to:	Generalized weakness secondary to prolonged organ failure Effects of pharmacological therapy Postoperative recovery period Chronic rejection

Possibly manifested by:	Verbalizations of fatigue; weakness; alteration in vital signs; decreased or poor participation in activities
Desired patient outcomes:	Patient can identify factors, both positive and negative, that affect activity tolerance, and can make beneficial adaptations.

ACTIONS/INTERVENTIONS

Independent

- Assess response to activity by subjective and objective (vital signs, dyspnea) findings.
- Assist patient to evaluate his or her individual activity tolerance with minimal guidance.
- Evaluate current activity tolerance in relation to previous activity tolerance.
- Assess patient's desired activity level.
- Assist patient to plan activities with rest periods as needed.
- Involve patient and family in planning activities.

Collaborative

- Involve exercise physiologist, occupational therapist, physical therapist, and physician when evaluating maximal activity levels.
- Refer to appropriate sources to assist the patient in finding possibly assistive devices to maximize activity levels.

NURSING DIAGNOSIS:	ANXIETY
Possibly related to:	Threat of graft rejection Threat to health status, secondary to graft rejection
Possibly manifested by:	Verbalizations of tension; complaints of feeling scared; shaking; sleeplessness; somatic complaints
Desired patient outcomes:	Patient will verbalize decrease in anxiety. Manifestations will be resolved.

ACTIONS/INTERVENTIONS

Independent

- Review past history and family history for contributing problems.
- Assist the patient in identifying source of anxiety
- Observe for physical signs of anxiety such as restlessness, irritability, quivering voice, increase in vital signs, preoccupation with self, withdrawal, use of drugs or alcohol, defense mechanisms.
- Establish a therapeutic relationship with patient/family.
- Acknowledge anxiety with patient/family.
- Assist the patient in identifying what may exacerbate anxiety and what may lessen it.
- Identify previous effective coping mechanisms.

Collaborative

- Refer to other healthcare team members as needed.

NURSING DIAGNOSIS:	COPING, INEFFECTIVE INDIVIDUAL/FAMILY
Possibly related to:	Vulnerability of health status Inadequate coping methods Uncertainty regarding graft survival
Possibly manifested by:	Tension; worry; conflict; verbalizations; depression; use of alcohol or drugs to cope; abandonment; neglect
Desired patient outcomes:	Patient and family will successfully identify and use previous coping mechanisms and/or develop new coping techniques.

ACTIONS/INTERVENTIONS

Independent

- Assess for compounding factors that may be preventing effective use of coping mechanisms.
- Clarify role functions. Assist in transition to new functions as needed.
- Assess level of knowledge regarding areas that cause worry. Supply information as indicated.
- Encourage and support open communication with staff.

Collaborative

• Refer to other healthcare team members as needed.

NURSING DIAGNOSIS:	DIVERSIONAL ACTIVITY DEFICIT
Possibly related to:	Lack of opportunities in the environment Failure to reestablish previous activities
Possibly manifested by:	Verbalizations of boredom; failure to resume previous hobbies or interests; withdrawal; disinterest; flat affect
Desired patient outcomes:	Patient will identify fulfilling activities and participate in them appropriately.

ACTIONS/INTERVENTIONS

Independent

• Assess previous diversional activities.
• Encourage patient to develop a variety of activities.
• Involve patient in schedule of activities in hospital.
• Take the patient outside or off the unit whenever possible.
• Assess for mobility needs.
• Assess for fine motor function and special needs.
• Accept patient's feelings and perceptions regarding boredom.

Collaborative

• Refer to occupational therapy, physical therapy, and other healthcare team members as needed.
• Refer to community agencies to address diversional activity in the home environment.

NURSING DIAGNOSIS:	FAMILY PROCESS, ALTERED
Possibly related to:	Change from sick role functions Development of other family roles for the transplant patient following improved health status
Possibly manifested by:	Inability of family to accept new roles; failure of family unit to meet basic emo-

tional/physical needs; failure to accomplish developmental tasks; failure to communicate effectively

Desired family outcomes: Family is communicating needs effectively and able to meet basic physical as well as emotional needs.

ACTIONS/INTERVENTIONS

Independent

• Assess for factors that are causing the family to be unable to communicate or meet needs.
• Identify family's developmental stage.
• Evaluate communication patterns in family.
• Assess role functions of various members.
• Evaluate cultural or religious factors.
• Assist the family to communicate openly and accept varying opinions and needs.

Collaborative

• Refer patients and families to community support groups as needed.
• Refer patients and families to counseling services as needed.

NURSING DIAGNOSIS:	**HEALTH MAINTENANCE, ALTERED**
Possibly related to:	Lack of support community/family resources to access the healthcare system
	Perceptual/cognitive impairment secondary to steroid therapy
	Financial restraints preventing proper utilization of healthcare resources or treatments
Possibly manifested by:	Lack of ability to demonstrate critical behaviors such as immunosuppressive therapy; lack of transportation or communication resources; unsupportive family system; difficulty adapting to new information or change

Desired patient outcome:	Patient/family can verbalize and demonstrate critical behaviors essential to maintaining graft function or recognize dangerous symptoms. Patient and family will have the resources to contact the transplant team and utilize prescribed treatments.

ACTIONS/INTERVENTIONS

Independent

- Assess level of knowledge, ability to perform necessary skills, and individual behaviors regarding immunosuppressive therapy.
- Assess level of patient independence in accessing transplant team.
- Assess ability of patient/family to communicate with the transplant team.
- Evaluate how the patient uses professional services.
- Develop individualized plan to assist the patient to manage usual health practices such as monitoring for rejection, recognizing signs and symptoms of infection, and taking immunosuppressive medications.
- Assist the patient/family in establishing effective communication with the transplant team.

Collaborative

- Assist in coordinating home health services as needed.
- Refer patient to community resources as needed.
- Refer to support groups as appropriate.

NURSING DIAGNOSIS:	HOME MAINTENANCE MANAGEMENT, IMPAIRED
Possibly related to:	Impaired cognitive or emotional functioning secondary to steroid therapy Inadequate support systems
Possibly manifested by:	Verbal expressions by the patient/family of difficulty managing home; requests for assistance in managing home; stressed family members; failure to meet basic hygienic and environmental needs

| **Desired   patient/family outcomes:** | The patient/family will identify factors that prevent effective home management as well as those that help promote it. Family is able to meet basic hygiene needs and provide safe and nurturing environment. |

ACTIONS/INTERVENTIONS

Independent

• Evaluate home environment.
• Evaluate patient/family's perception of home environment and how it meets their needs.
• Identify support systems in home and community.
• Assist the patient/family with plan of care in managing home environment.

Collaborative

• Identify community resources and support systems.
• Coordinate planning with appropriate community agencies at the time of discharge.
• Refer patient/family in order to identify financial assistance options.

NURSING DIAGNOSIS:	**INFECTION, POTENTIAL FOR**
Possibly related to:	Compromised immune function secondary to immunosuppressive therapy Insufficient knowledge to avoid exposure
Possibly manifested by:	Leukopenia; inability to identify risk factors
Desired patient outcomes:	Patient will be able to identify potential risk factors and signs and symptoms of developing infections.

ACTIONS/INTERVENTIONS

Independent

- Monitor for signs and symptoms of infection. Teach patient/family these.
- Teach importance of hand washing.
- Monitor visitors and staff that come in contact with patient.

Collaborative

- Collect specimens to assess for infection as needed.
- Establish isolation if ordered (center preference).
- Monitor white blood cell counts.

NURSING DIAGNOSIS:	MOBILITY, IMPAIRED PHYSICAL
Possibly related to:	Musculoskeletal impairment secondary to osteonecrosis from long-term steroid therapy Intolerance to activity secondary to post-operative status
Possibly manifested by:	Verbal complaints regarding movement; pain with range of motion; impairment of range of motion; inability to meet basic physical and social needs
Desired patient outcomes:	Patient will be able to meet basic physical needs, participate in at least some activities to meet social needs.

ACTIONS/INTERVENTIONS

Independent

- Assess motor function, including range of joint motion.
- Assess pain with activity.
- Assess activity level before transplantation.
- Evaluate activities that cause the most difficulty to the patient as well as those most easily performed.
- Determine patient's desire for activity.
- Involve patient/family in decision making regarding activity.
- Evaluate and provide for safety needs in the acute care and home settings.
- Evaluate emotional and behavioral responses to limited activity.

- Encourage patient to perform activities of daily living independently when possible.
- Encourage careful ambulation.

Collaborative

- Refer to occupational and physical therapy as needed.
- Administer analgesics and anti-inflammatory medications. Alert to possible drug interactions.
- Plan and maintain exercise program in conjunction with physician and physical therapy.
- Assist patient in use of adjunctive mobility devices.
- Encourage patient to achieve ideal weight through weight loss if needed.
- Instruct patient to avoid sitting when experiencing back pain.

NURSING DIAGNOSIS:	NONCOMPLIANCE: IMMUNOSUPPRESSIVE THERAPY
Possibly related to:	Side effects of immunosuppressant therapy Cost of immunosuppressant therapy Failure to comprehend that graft loss results from failure to adhere to prescribed immunosuppressive therapy
Possibly manifested by:	Patient's failure to follow prescribed immunosuppressant therapy; failing graft function; failure to keep scheduled appointments
Desired patient outcomes:	Patient participates in planning goals and treatments and adheres to prescribed treatment designs.

ACTIONS/INTERVENTIONS

Independent

- Determine patient/family's perceptions of treatment plans.
- Determine patient/family's perceptions of relationship between treatment plans and graft survival.
- Assess value system that may be interfering (religious, cultural, folk values).

- Encourage patient/family to verbalize feelings and complaints.
- Determine length of pretransplant illness (patients often become non-compliant the longer they have suffered a chronic illness).
- Evaluate support systems of patient.
- Determine economic resources.
- Provide for continuity in caregivers.
- Assure that information given to patient/family is consistent.
- Have patient/family repeat back and demonstrate any information (including rationale) that is critical to graft survival and overall health of patient.
- Assist patient in self-monitoring behaviors of health status.

Collaborative

- Refer patient/family to counseling services as necessary.
- Refer patient/family for financial evaluation and assistance as needed.
- Use contracting with patient.

NURSING DIAGNOSIS:	POWERLESSNESS
Possibly related to:	Perceived inability to control graft survival Perceived inability to control health status
Possibly manifested by:	Verbal complaints of lack of control; failure to participate in planning goals; poor eye contact; withdrawal; passivity
Desired patient outcome:	Patient will express sense of control regarding graft survival by acknowledging link between patient's compliance with immunosuppressant therapy and graft survival.

ACTIONS/INTERVENTIONS

Independent

- Assess individual factors affecting patient's perception of lack of control.
- Assure that healthcare team does not take control from patient by making all decisions and not consulting patient, often done to "protect" the patient.
- Encourage patient to verbalize feelings, especially those that identify

major lack of control versus those that provide the patient with more feelings of control.
- Insure that patient is given reasons for treatment plans and how they relate to graft survival and overall health status.
- Avoid using logic or arguing with patient. Accept feelings and reiterate facts. Use patient teaching aids to reinforce material.
- Involve patient in all decision making possible.

Collaborative

- Refer to counseling and support groups as needed.
- Expose the transplant patient to other patients who can share their experiences.

NURSING DIAGNOSIS:	SELF-CONCEPT, DISTURBANCE IN: BODY IMAGE
Possibly related to:	Change in facial appearance secondary to steroid therapy Change in body appearance secondary to steroid therapy
Possibly manifested by:	Verbal complaints regarding appearance; failure to look in a mirror; new lack of interest in clothing or grooming; refusal to discuss or acknowledge changes; anger; withdrawal; reduced social contact; discontinuance of immunosuppressive therapy
Desired patient outcome:	The patient will acknowledge changes in facial and body appearance and seek information to cope with or modify appearance to meet the patient's needs.

ACTIONS/INTERVENTIONS

Independent

- Assess patient's feelings regarding present appearance.
- Emphasize positive aspects of the patient's physical and emotional being.
- Encourage activities to increase self-esteem (new hairstyle, makeup, bleaching of body hair).

- Encourage and assist in maintaining ideal body weight.
- Accept patient's negative feelings and allow expression.
- Set limits on maladaptive behavior, such as negative verbalizations.

Collaborative

- Refer to counseling and support groups as needed.
- Refer to cosmetologist, weight loss program, and so forth as needed.

NURSING DIAGNOSIS:	SKIN INTEGRITY, IMPAIRED: POTENTIAL
Possibly related to:	Immunological deficit
Possibly manifested by:	Skin infections; tumors of the skin
Desired patient outcomes:	Patient will have intact skin and will recognize potential abnormal skin conditions.

ACTIONS/INTERVENTIONS

Independent

- Assess skin surfaces each day.
- Teach patient/family to recognize breaks in skin and abnormal growths and to seek medical attention for these.
- Monitor for complications in wound healing.
- Identify any individual risk factors.
- Instruct patient in importance of using sun blocks.
- Advise in the use of emollient lotions to help prevent dryness.
- Allow the patient to express concerns or fears about changes in skin appearance.
- Maintain good skin hygiene, assisting patient to perform independently.

Collaborative

- Apply/administer prescribed medications.
- Refer to registered dietician for contributing nutritional problems.

NURSING DIAGNOSIS:	SLEEP PATTERN DISTURBANCE
Possibly related to:	Pharmacological side effects Anxiety

Possibly manifested by:	Complaints of difficulty sleeping; changes in sleep patterns
Desired patient outcome:	Patient will report improvement in sleep pattern and identify factors that promote or inhibit satisfactory cycles.

ACTIONS/INTERVENTIONS

Independent

- Determine previous sleep patterns.
- Determine patient's perception of satisfactory sleep/rest.
- Assist the patient in determining factors that promote or inhibit the patient's normal sleep pattern.
- Arrange care to provide for uninterrupted periods of rest/sleep.
- Instruct the patient in relaxation techniques.
- Evaluate diet for contributing causes of difficulty with sleep such as caffeine intake.
- Assess for pain as contributing cause.

Collaborative

- Encourage regular exercise program as permitted.
- Refer to sleep disorder center as needed.
- Administer sleeping medications as ordered. Observe for dependency and discourage prolonged use.
- Refer for counseling to decrease anxiety as needed.

NURSING DIAGNOSIS:	SOCIAL INTERACTION, IMPAIRED
Possibly related to:	Perceived changes in appearance
Possibly manifested by:	Refusal to participate in social activities; inability to interact when in a social situation; withdrawal; avoidance of interaction
Desired patient outcome:	Patient is involved in social activities at the same or improved level compared with pre-transplant.

ACTIONS/INTERVENTIONS

Independent

- Encourage patient to verbalize reluctance to socialize.
- Assist the patient to specify factors that most inhibit desire to interact.
- Assess if there has been a concomitant change in socioeconomic levels, geographic location, etc., that could make it difficult for the patient to interact in the same social system as before the transplant.
- Provide positive reinforcement for gains in social interactions.
- Involve the family in plans for increasing social interactions.

Collaborative

- Refer for counseling as needed.
- Seek community resources and support groups to assist the patient.

NURSING DIAGNOSIS:	**THOUGHT PROCESSES, ALTERED**
Possibly related to:	Pharmacological side effects secondary to steroid therapy Altered sleep patterns Stress
Possibly manifested by:	Memory deficit; confusion; change in attention span; disorientation; difficulty in decision making; difficulty in learning; inappropriate thought processes
Desired patient outcome:	Patient will remain oriented and have normal thought processes. When abnormal thought processes occur, the patient/family will recognize these and seek assistance from the healthcare system.

ACTIONS/INTERVENTIONS

Independent

- Identify factors responsible for physiological causes.
- Assist the patient in identifying stress-related causes.
- Assist the patient in identifying ways to promote effective sleep patterns.

See also nursing diagnoses for Sleep Pattern Disturbance, p. 316, and Anxiety, p. 306.

Collaborative

- Assure psychiatric referral as needed
- Arrange referral to sleep disorder center as needed.

American Council on Transplantation U.S. Transplant Stat Sheet

The following chart provides approximate numbers for certain organs and tissue transplants together with patient survival rates at one year, approximate numbers for those medically approved and actually awaiting transplant, and numbers of centers.

| Organ or Tissue | Transplants Performed In The U.S. | | | | | | | Aggregate Number of Transplants | Numbers Waiting Transplants | Number of Centers | Graft Survival | Cost ® Range |
	Before 1982	1982	1983	1984	1985	1986	1987					
Kidneys	33,799 e	5,358 c	6,112 c	6,968 c	7,695 e	8,976 e	8,967 e	77,872	13,100 g	201 e	**LR 89 % i CD 80 %	$30-40,000
Hearts	403	103 c	172 c	346 c	731 d	1,368 d	1,512 d	4,635	900 g	131 g	82 % h	$80-140,000
Heart/Lung	5	7 c	20 d	22 d	30 c	45 d	43 d	172	180 g	45 g	68-70 % h	$130-200,000
Liver	119	62 c	164 c	308 c	605 d	924 d	1,182 d	3,364 d	450 g	66 g	77 % i	$135-338,000
Pancreas	113 f	38 f	51 f	52 f	120 f	173 f	129 f	*676 f	150 g	51 g	44 % i	$30-40,000
Cornea	78,924 b	18,500 c	21,250 c	24,000 c	26,326 c	31,000 b	35,000 b	235,000 b	5,000 b	400 b	90-95 % b	$3,500-7,000
Bone Marrow	675 a	800 a	990 a	1,000 a	1,297 a	1,578 a	1,659 a	7,999 a		72 a		$80-110,000
Skin						2,000 j	5,000 j					
Bone Deposits					200,000 j	250,000 j						
Lung	14 h						9 h	23 h		32 g	35 % h	

Sources:
(a) International Bone Marrow Transplant Registry
(b) Eye Bank Association of America
(c) Division of Organ Transplantation, DHHS
(d) Office of Health Technology Assessment, DHHS
(e) Health Care Financing Administration, DHHS
(f) International Pancreas Registry
(g) United Network for Organ Sharing (OPTN)
(h) International Heart Transplant Registry
(i) Clinical Transplants, 1987
(j) American Association of Tissue Banks

Medicare coverage for ESRD began July 1, 1973
FDA approval of cyclosporine began November 14, 1983
* Includes Canadian and Mexico Data
** Patient survival for living related and cadaveric kidney transplantation is 96 % and 93 % respectively.
® The cost ranges for transplantation listed on this chart includes items such as laboratory fees, acquisition, hospitalization and other charges These figures should be used only as estimates for related transplantation cost.

APPENDIX

LifeSource Organ Donor Review Chart

APPENDIX E
LifeSource Organ Donor Review Chart

	KIDNEY	HEART	LIVER	PANCREAS	HEART FOR VALVES	BONE	SKIN	EYE	EAR
Age	0 – 55	2 – 45	1 mo. – 50	1 – 55	0 – 55	16 – 55	14 – 75	0 – 100 +	8 – 100 +
Cardiac arrest resuscitated	Prob. OK	Prob. OK	Prob. OK	Prob. OK	OK	Heart beating cadaver not mandatory	Heart beating cadaver not mandatory	Heart beating cadaver not mandatory	Heart beating cadaver not mandatory
Importance of Chest / Abd. trauma to suitability	Important	EXTREMELY IMPORTANT	EXTREMELY IMPORTANT	Important	Little Importance	Little Importance	Little Importance	Not Important	Not Important
No active infections	MANDATORY	MANDATORY	MANDATORY	MANDATORY	MANDATORY	MANDATORY	MANDATORY	N/A	MANDATORY
No previous disease of organs	MANDATORY	MANDATORY	MANDATORY	MANDATORY	MANDATORY	MANDATORY	MANDATORY	N/A	MANDATORY
No presence of communicable disease	MANDATORY	MANDATORY	MANDATORY	MANDATORY	MANDATORY	MANDATORY	MANDATORY	MANDATORY	MANDATORY
Episodes of Hypotension	Sensitive	VERY SENSITIVE	VERY SENSITIVE	Sensitive	N/A	N/A	N/A	N/A	N/A
Need to consider Vasopressor, i.e., Dopamine Sensitive	Yes	VERY	VERY	Yes	N/A	N/A	N/A	N/A	N/A
Weight important	No	Yes	Yes	No	No	No	>100 lbs.	No	No
Body build important	No	Yes	Yes	No	No	No	No	No	No
Blood type evaluation	MANDATORY	MANDATORY	MANDATORY	MANDATORY	N/A	N/A	N/A	N/A	N/A
Additional physician consults required	Usually Not	Yes	Possibly	Usually Not	No	No	No	No	No
Additional Lab needed	Yes Kidney specific	Yes Heart specific	Yes Liver specific	Yes Pancreas specific	No	No	No	No	No
Time needed to set up additional teams	No	Yes	Yes	Yes	No	No	Possible	No	No
Tissue may be retrieved after cardiac death	No	No	No	No	Yes, up to 12 hours after death. The whole heart is retrieved in the OR.	Yes, up to 24 hours in the OR under sterile conditions.	Yes, up to 36 hours if refrigerated.	Yes, up to 6 hours. Place ice packs on the eyes after closing them.	Yes, up to 48 hours. May be procured following embalming.

Adapted from the Ohio Valley Organ Procurement Center, Cincinnati, Ohio.

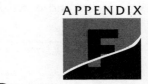

Organ and Tissue Donation Consent

I hereby make this anatomical donation as a gift from the body of
_____ who died on _____ at _____.
(name)   (date)   (name of institution)

The initials noted in the appropriate spaces and the words filling the blanks below indicate my relationship to the deceased and my desire to make an anatomical gift as noted.

I am the next of kin or other authorized person (this list is by priority according to the Uniform Anatomical Gift Act)

_____ spouse

_____ adult son or daughter

_____ parent

_____ adult brother or sister

_____ guardian

_____ _____
(name of other authorized person)

I give:

_____ any needed organs or tissues

_____ the following organs or tissues

_____

_____

_____

_____

to the following authorized organ or tissue center:

_____

for the following uses:

_____ transplantation, therapy, and research

_____ transplantation only

(continued)

After the donated organs and/or tissues are recovered, the body shall be referred to

_____

(name of funeral home or responsible party)

_____   _____

(date)   *(signature of responsible party)*

                           _____

                           _____

                                           (address)

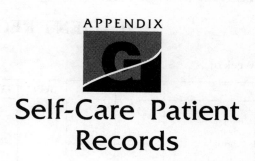

APPENDIX

Self-Care Patient Records

PATIENT RECORD

Week of _____

	MON	TUE	WED	THURS	FRI	SAT	SUN
Temperature before breakfast							
Before dinner							
Weight							
Blood Pressure							
24-hr urine volume							
Urine Clarity (blood or cloudiness)							

Things to mention to my Transplant Team _____

_____

_____

_____

_____

_____

MEDICINE SCHEDULE

MEDICATIONS

MEDICINE	Breakfast TIME: ___	Lunch TIME: ___	Dinner TIME: ___	Bedtime TIME: ___	Other TIME: ___
SANDIMMUNE® **(cyclosporine)** Oral Solution 100 mg per mL Take ___ mg, ___ mL, ___ time(s) per day					
PREDNISONE tablet size ___ Take ___ mg, ___ tablet(s), ___ time(s) per day					
IMURAN® (azathioprine) 50 mg tablets Take ___ mg, ___ tablet(s), ___ time(s) per day					
ANTACID Name: ___ Take ___ mL/tablet(s), one to two hours after each meal and before going to bed.					
DIURETIC/ ANTIHYPERTENSIVE Name: ___ Take ___ mg, ___ tablet(s), ___ time(s) per day					
ANTIFUNGAL Name: ___ Take ___ mL/tablet(s), ___ time(s) per day					

(From Sandoz Pharmaceuticals Corp., 1988, with permission.)

Index

A "t" indicates a table.

331